Yáng Jìzhōu's 楊繼洲

針 灸 大 成

The Great Compendium of Acupuncture and Moxibustion

Zhēn Jiǔ Dà Chéng

Volume V

Lorraine Wilcox, L.Ac., Ph.D.

The Chinese Medicine Database
www.cm-db.com
Portland, Oregon

The Great Compendium of Acupuncture and Moxibustion

針灸大成

Zhēn Jiǔ Dà Chéng

Volume V

Lorraine Wilcox

Copyright © 2010 The Chinese Medicine Database

1017 SW Morrison #306
Portland, OR 97205 USA

COMP designation original Chinese work and English translation

Cover Design by Jonathan Schell L.Ac.
Library of Congress Cataloging-in-Publication Data:

Yang, Jizhou, fl.
    [The Great Compendium of Acupuncture and Moxibustion. English]
    Zhen Jiu Da Cheng = The Great Compendium of Acupuncture and
Moxibustion/ translation Lorraine Wilcox
        p. cm.
Includes Index.
ISBN 978-0-9799552-4-2 (alk. paper)
Medicine, Chinese   I. Wilcox, Lorraine. II. Title: The
Great Compendium of Acupuncture and Moxibustion.
III. Title: Vol. 5

International Standard Book Number (ISBN): 978-0-9799552-4-2
Printed in the United States of America

Contents

Translation

Volume V

Contents

5

Contents

Contents

Illustrations

Contents

Tables & Diagrams

Appendix A: Stems and Branches

Introduction to Volume V

The main topic of Volume V of the *Great Compendium of Acupuncture-Moxibustion* is categories of acu-moxa points and how they are used (or how they were used during the *Míng* Dynasty). The point categories that are covered in this volume are the five transport points, yuán source points, luò network points, and the eight confluence points of the eight extraordinary vessels. The location, indications, and manipulation techniques for these points are described.

Yáng Jìzhōu 楊繼洲 also discussed point combinations. He explained the paired use of yuan source points and luo network points, calling this the host-guest relationship. Yáng also filled many pages with point combinations for the eight confluence points of the eight extraordinary vessels.

In addition, these are the points that are commonly used in chrono-acupuncture methods such as the midnight-noon flowing and pooling method (Zǐ Wǔ Liú Zhù 子午流注) and the eight methods of the mystical tortoise (Líng Guī Bā Fǎ 靈龜八法). These two methods of chrono-acupuncture are described in detail, although Yáng Jìzhōu let the reader know he prefered the former.

In this Volume, Yáng laid out the calculations for these points, but he also gave tables so that the practitioner could look them up quickly. He was concerned that a quick calculation might lead to an error and so provided the tables to make the practice more convenient.

I have also written extensive notes to help the motivated reader understand the calculations. However, the calculation is fairly complicated and if one is only interested in clinical practice, it is not necessary to understand the method of arriving at each point. The reader should feel free to skip over the discussion of calculation and simply use the tables if he or she only cares about its use in clinic.

Even if the reader is not interested in using chrono-acupuncture, Yáng Jìzhōu provides a great deal of information on the use of these point categories and the individual points within the categories. Most modern practitioners do not have a good understanding of how the ancients used points, before point functions were devised in the twentieth century. In earlier times, acupuncturists chose points based on indications and category, rather than by point function. Yáng Jìzhōu described the clinical use of these points from a *Míng* Dynasty perspective.

Chrono-Acupuncture

While the use of the ten heavenly stems and the twelve earthly branches may seem quite esoteric today, Chinese doctors of the past (and in fact, Chinese people in general) would be as familiar with them as we are with the days of the week. The stems and branches were an essential part of the every day calendar and were commonly used by all.

Time and timing has always been an essential part of Chinese medicine. The *Yellow Emperor's Inner Classic* constantly refers to the cycles of day and night, the four seasons, and the phases of the moon. The *Inner Classic* emphasizes that timing has a great bearing on the diseases we contract and in proper treatment. We are also advised to follow the appropriate lifestyle for the current season. In the *Inner Canon*, most of the emphasis is on the observable aspects of time (sun, moon, seasons, etc.). However, the stems and branches were also discussed in the *Inner Classic* in a number of chapters and were emphasized in the seven great treatises (Chapters 66 through 71 and Chapter 74) on the Five Transports and the Six Qì (Wǔ Yùn Liù Qì 五運六氣).

As time passed more and more emphasis was placed on the calculation arts and the use of the stems and branches. Medical day selection became more prominent from the *Táng* Dynasty onward. Most authors of acupuncture texts, from the time of Sūn Sīmiǎo onward, gave formulas for finding days when acupuncture and/or moxibustion was prohibited. There were other formulas for good days to treat patients.

The complexity also increased regarding the choice of treatment according to time. Early books might refer to the circadian clock and the daily tide of qì through the twelve channels. By the *Míng* Dynasty, this idea had fully given way to more complex calculations using the day stem and branch and the hour stem and branch. Instead of a whole channel being open, individual points were open during a time period. Instead of the sequence repeating every day, sequences repeated every five days, every ten days, or even every sixty days.

Some might say these doctors fell in love with the mysterious calculations and lost track of the natural observable rhythms. Others might say timing has little to do with medicine, that this is only superstition. Western medicine has gone through a long period of denying that timing and the cycles of nature have much effect on human illness and its treatment. Perhaps the decline of chrono-acupuncture during the *Qīng* Dynasty and into the 20th century is related to the influx of Western medicine. But in recent years, a new field of Western medicine called chrono-biology has emerged. It may also be a good time to re-investigate the time-related aspects of Chinese medicine.

In fact, there is some recent research in China regarding the efficacy of chrono-acupuncture.[1][2][3][4][5][6]

It is hard for an individual practitioner to gauge the effectiveness of chrono-acupuncture, but it is certainly something that can be tried experimentally in clinic with no harm to the patient. One can use the points that are open at the time of the patient's visit, or better yet, schedule the patient at a time when an indicated point will be open.

Characteristics of Volume V

Volume V is visually one of the more interesting parts of the *Great Compendium*. Yáng included a large number of diagrams and illustrations in this volume. He also drew up a couple of tables showing the points and the times in which they are open to make the information more quickly accessible in the clinic.

Many sections of the *Great Compendium* are written in verse. These poems or songs were designed to aid in memorization so clinicians could easily recall information. However, they are quite challenging to translate as they often leave out or include extra words to fit the meter. Sometimes they are just lists of point with a few extra words to glue them together. These poems were never meant for reading; they were simply used as memory devices. The data they contain would often be put into tables today, but tables were less commonly used in old Chinese medical books.

1. [Effects of Linggui Bafa on the therapeutic effect and quality of life in patients of post-stroke depression] Guo RY, Su L, Liu LA, Wang CX. Zhongguo Zhen Jiu. 2009 Oct;29(10):785-90.

2. Observation on therapeutic effect of acupuncture on stroke by "Najia method of Ziwu Liuzhu"] Liu DR, Hao SF, Liu ZY. Zhongguo Zhen Jiu. 2009 May;29(5):353-6.

3. [Effects of heavenly stem-prescription of point selection of needling methods of Ziwu Liuzhu on ischemic cerebrovascular diseases] Han ZX, Liu YG, Wei JL. Zhongguo Zhen Jiu. 2008 Dec;28(12):865-8.

4. [Effects of Ziwuliuzhu combined selection of the source point and the collateral point on athletic injuries and the state of channels] Deng BY, Zhang JF, Luo MR, Liang L. Zhongguo Zhen Jiu. 2006 Oct;26(10):707-9.

5. [Effect of opening point method of ziwu liuzhu on myocardial ischemia in the patient of stroke] Guan ZH, Yi R, Ye J, Ding LL, Zhu XY, Guo CP. Zhongguo Zhen Jiu. 2005 Nov;25(11):823-4.

6. [Clinical research and mechanical inquiry in the treatment of chronic superficial gastritis using ziwuliuzhu day-prescription of acupoint] Zhou ZL. Zhong Xi Yi Jie He Za Zhi. 1991 Feb;11(2):94-6, 69.

針灸大成・卷之五

Yáng's Sources

In general, if an earlier source gave an adequate description of a topic, Yáng quoted it verbatim. He wove together passages from various books, adding his own commentary or memorization poems as he saw fit. Yáng Jìzhōu used a number of sources for Volume V. Early works quoted by Yáng include:

*   *Líng Shū* 《 靈樞 》 (Magic Pivot)
*   *Sù Wèn* 《 素問 》 (Elementary Questions) as well as Wáng Bīng's 王冰 notes
*   *Nàn Jīng* 《 難經 》 (Classic of Difficulties)
*   *Zhēn Jiŭ Jiă Yĭ Jīng* 《 針灸甲已經 》 (the Systematic Classic of Acupuncture and Moxibustion) compiled by Huángfŭ Mì 皇甫謐 and published in 282 C.E.

Besides these classics, Yáng used earlier Míng Dynasty sources:
*   *Zhēn Jiŭ Dà Quán* 《 針灸大全 》 (Great Completion of Acupuncture and Moxibustion) by Xú Fèng 徐鳳 and published c. 1439.
*   *Zhēn Jiŭ Jù Yīng* 《 針灸聚英 》 (Gatherings from Eminent Acupuncturists) by Gāo Wŭ 高武 and published in 1529.
*   *Yī Xué Rù Mén* 《 醫學入門 》 (Entering the Gate of Medicine) by Lĭ Chān 李梴 and published in 1575.

The above are Yáng's most important sources, but he also occasionally cited other books and included commentaries from other authors on passages from the classics. Whenever possible, I give information about these minor sources.

Translation notes

In order to make a smoother translation I often made the following additions or subtractions of words:
*   I frequently added or removed the word 'point.' The Chinese text often simply said well, brook, stream, source, etc. without the word point or said "Sān Lĭ point" when in English, Sān Lĭ (ST 36) was adequate.
*   I add 'hour' after a branch name when the text is obviously discussing the twelve hours.
*   I add 'channel' after a six-channel name when it is obviously discussing the channel.
*   I added 'stem' or 'branch' after wu to clarify (wù 戊 stem or wŭ 午 branch). Sometimes I added 'branch' after yŏu 酉 or yín 寅 as these Pin Yin syllables are easily confused with other words.
*   (zhù) 注 may be translated as pool or pour, depending on the context.
*   The memorization poems have extra words, are missing words, or sometimes the words

15

in them make little sense and are only there to fill the meter or rhyme. They are not to be read in the same way as literary poetry and are more similar to our "Thirty days hath September..." than to the sonnets of Shakespeare.

•   I have followed the terminology of Nigel Wiseman and his associates. For explanation of unfamiliar terms, please see the *Practical Dictionary of Chinese Medicine.*

Acknowledgements

I am very grateful to Yue Lu and Jerome Jiang for the help with difficult passages. Jonathan Schell has done a wonderful job turning the manuscript into a beautiful book and making this project happen. Besides this, I want to thank Master Larry Sang of the American Feng Shui Institute for all he has taught me regarding Chinese calculation arts. He also has generously given us permission to use some pages from his *Ten Thousand Year Calendar.*

Publisher's Note

針灸大成・卷之五

In this series, the *Great Compendium of Acupuncture and Moxibustion,* the Chinese Medicine Database elected to use multiple translators to translate the different volumes. We did this so that our community would have access to the corpus of this text, sooner rather then later. There are many, many books that need to be translated, and if each translator did all of one large book, it would consume much of their life.

We have come to look at each volume as its own work, with each translator providing a slightly different, but similar voice to the translation. Everyone who has participated in this project has come to agreement that even though the same base translation dictionaries will be used, there is no way to produce a homogenous translation from one volume to the next. Expect to see small variations in reference to channel names like GV versus Du, as each translator uses the style that she feels the most comfortable with. I believe that the discrepancies are mostly superficial, and I hope that the reader who has waited for years to the read the *Great Compendium,* will feel the same way.

There have been a number of sacrifices on the part of the translators to certain individual standards as the Database works out the best way to present this material. For example, we believe that inclusion of point numbers help modern readers understand the content of the classics better. We have appreciated the "team spirit" that everyone has shared in the project, and the willingness to work through difficult issues together.

十二經井穴圖（楊氏）[1]

The Well Points of the Twelve Channels, Illustrated (Master Yáng)[1]

手太陰井

人病膨脹，喘咳，缺盆痛，心煩，掌熱，肩背疼，
咽痛喉腫。斯乃以脈循胃上膈入肺中，橫過腋關，
穿過尺澤，入少商。故邪客於手太陰之絡，而生是
病。
可刺手太陰肺經井穴，少商也，手大指側。刺同身
寸之一分，行六陰之數各一痏，左取右，右取左，
如食頃已。灸三壯。

**The Hand Tàiyīn Well Point
[Shào Shāng 少商, LU 11]**

The patient sickens with inflation[2], panting and cough,
pain at the supraclavicular fossa [Quē Pén 缺盆, also the
name of ST 12], heart vexation, hot palms, pain of the
shoulder and upper back, and throat pain or swelling.
This is because the vessel[3] follows the stomach, ascends
through the diaphragm to enter into the lungs. It passes

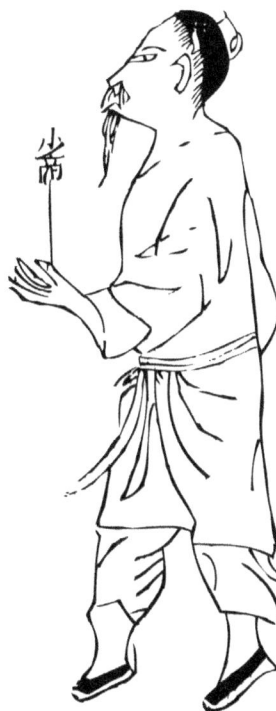

Fig. 5.1

---

1. This section is adapted from《黃帝內經・素問・繆刺論篇第六十三》*Elementary Questions*,
Chapter 63 and Wáng Bīng's notes. There is also some information taken from Zhēn Jiǔ Jiǎ Yǐ
Jīng《針灸甲乙經》the *Systematic Classic*. Yáng Jìzhōu edited and supplemented it as he saw
fit. This section uses an older style of writing and more archaic terminology than many other sections of this volume because it is based on *Elementary Questions*.

2. Wiseman glosses *péng zhàng* 膨脹 as inflation. Mathews defines it as fat, bloated, or swollen.

3. In the *Yellow Emperor's Inner Classic*, the terms 脈 vessel and 經 channel are often used as
synonyms. The term 經脈 channel-vessel is also used. In this section, the term 'vessel' refers to
what we would call 'channel' today.

horizontally through the axillary joint, penetrates through Chǐ Zé 尺澤 (LU 5), and enters Shào Shāng 少商 (LU 11). Thus when evil intrudes into the network[4] of the hand tàiyīn, it engenders these illnesses.

You can pierce[5] the well point of the hand tàiyīn lung channel, Shào Shāng 少商 (LU 11), located on the side of the thumb. Insert one *fēn* deep based on the same person's *cùn*. Move [the needle] six times, a yīn number,[6] on each site.[7] For problems of the left, treat the right; for problems of the right, treat the left. The patient should recover in the time it takes to eat a meal. Apply three cones of moxibustion.

---

4. This same sentence is used for all twelve channels. *Elementary Questions*, Chapter 63 uses the term *luò* 絡 or network, and yet the treatment given most often in this chapter is the jing well point. Yáng Jìzhōu 楊繼洲 follows Chapter 63 of *Elementary Questions* when he uses the term 'network.' Here it does not seem to refer specifically to the network vessels (絡脈), but probably means the sphere of influence of the channel as a whole. Wáng Bīng's notes explain that the evil intrudes into both the network branch divergence (*luò zhī bié* 絡支別) and the main channel.

5. *Cì* 刺 literally means 'to prick' or 'to pierce.' In terms of acupuncture, it can mean pricking to let blood or needling with a filiform needle. Wiseman glosses *cì* 刺 as 'needle' or 'insert' but that tends to exclude the technique of pricking to bleed. *Elementary Questions*, Chapter 63, the basis of this section, is not always clear on whether to bleed the point or needle it. To preserve either possibility, *cì* 刺 is translated in this section as 'pierce' or 'insert.' In other sections where the context makes it clear, *cì* 刺 may be translated as 'needle.'

6. Six is a yīn number. *Magic Pivot*, Chapter 5 states, "The dao of yīn is even. The dao of yáng is odd." In Yì Jīng 《易經》 numerology, six represents yīn and nine represents yáng. Yáng Jìzhōu tells us to move the needle six times for eleven of the twelve entries in this section. Six (the yīn number) drains. Nine (the yáng number) supplements. These numbers can be applied to rotation or to lift and thrust. Since Yáng discusses the well points in this passage, it is more likely that he had rotation in mind (assuming he intended needling with the filiform needle). This sentence "Move [the needle] six times, a yīn number" is not in *Elementary Questions*, nor in Wáng Bīng's notes, so it is likely that Yáng added it. It also implies that Yáng had in mind the use of the filiform needle, not bleeding.

7. The word 'site' is not really a translation of *wěi* 痏, which literally means 'a sore.' This refers to the sore left after the needle has been removed. *Wěi* 痏 is a common term in the *Inner Classic*, but was less frequently used during the Míng dynasty except when quoting the Classic. The use of the term *wěi* 痏 (a sore) may imply bleeding, as bleeding leaves more of a sore than does acupuncture with a filiform needle. Bleeding was more commonly used in the *Inner Classic* than it is today or during the Míng dynasty. Other chapters of *Elementary Questions* specify piercing a point two or three *wěi*. This probably means bleeding or needling the point two or three times in one session. This section of Volume 5 and Chapter 63 of *Elementary Questions* does not clearly state whether the treatment should be acupuncture with the filiform needle or bleeding. Only one *wěi* is prescribed for each point. Bleeding is specifically prescribed for a few of the points, but not all. Yáng does not specifically mention bleeding until we get to the seventh channel, the foot tàiyáng urinary bladder channel. However, the order is different in *Elementary Questions*, Chapter 63, where bleeding is mentioned for the first channel.

手陽明井

人病氣滿，胸中緊痛，煩熱，喘而不已息。斯乃以其脈自肩端入缺盆絡肺。其支別者，從缺盆中，直而上頸，故邪客於手陽明之絡，而有是病。可刺手陽明大腸井穴，商陽也，在手大指次指爪甲角，刺入一分，行六陰之數，左取右，右取左，如食頃已。灸三壯。

The Hand Yángmíng Well Point
[**Shāng Yáng** 商陽, LI 1]

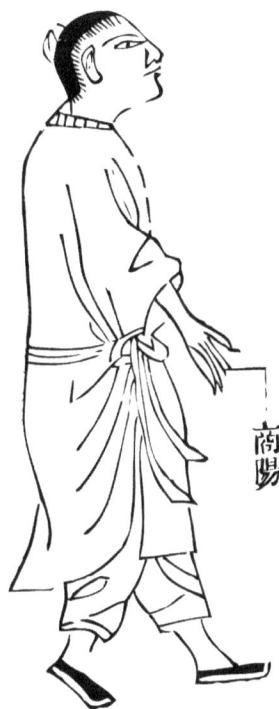

商陽

Fig. 5.2

The patient sickens with qì fullness, tight pain in the chest, vexing heat, and panting with inability to catch one's breath. This is because the vessel goes from the end of the shoulder, enters the supraclavicular fossa [**Quē Pén** 缺盆, also the name of ST 12], and networks to the lungs. Its branch diverges from within the supraclavicular fossa and goes straight up the neck. Thus when evil intrudes into the network of the hand yángmíng, there are these illnesses.

You can pierce the well point of the hand yángmíng large intestine channel, Shāng Yáng 商陽 (LI 1), located on the corner of the nail of the index finger. Insert one *fèn* deep. Move [the needle] six times, a yīn number. For problems of the left, treat the right; for problems of the right, treat the left. The patient should recover in the time it takes to eat a meal. Apply three cones of moxibustion.

足陽明井

人病腹心悶，惡人火，聞響心惕，鼻衄唇喎，瘧狂，足痛，氣蠱，瘡疥，齒寒。乃脈起於鼻交頞中，下循鼻外，入上齒中，還出俠口環唇，下交承漿。卻循頤後下廉，出大迎，循頰車，上耳前。故邪客於足陽明之絡，而有是病。

可刺足陽明胃經井厲兌，足次指爪甲上與肉交者韭許，刺一分，行六陰數，左取右，食頃已。

The Foot Yángmíng Well Point
[Lì Duì 厲兌, ST 45]

The patient sickens with oppression of the abdomen and heart, aversion to people and fire [or heat], apprehensive when hearing noises, nosebleeds, deviated lips, malaria, mania, foot pain, qì gǔ,[8] sores and scabs, and cold teeth. This vessel arises at the intersection of the nose and the brow, runs downward lateral to the nose, and enters into the upper teeth. It returns to emerge near the mouth, circles the lips, and descends to intersect with Chéng Jiāng 承漿 (Ren 24). Furthermore, it follows the posterior lower aspect of the jaw, emerges at Dà Yíng 大迎 (ST 5), follows through Jiá Chē 頰車 (ST 6) and ascends in front of the ears. Thus when evil intrudes into the network of the foot yángmíng, there are these illnesses.

You can pierce the well point of the foot yángmíng stomach channel, Lì Duì 厲兌 (ST 45), located above the nail on the second toe, about the distance of a leek leaf into the flesh. Insert one *fèn* deep. Move [the needle] six times, a yīn number. For problems of the left, treat the right. The patient should recover in the time it takes to eat a meal.

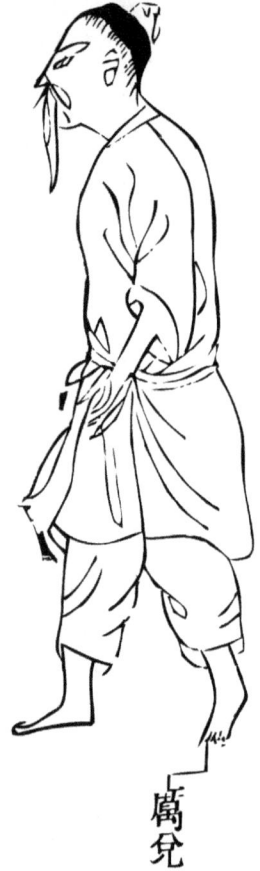

厲兌

足太陰井

Fig. 5.3

人病尸厥暴死，脈猶如常人而動。然陰盛於上，則邪氣重上，而邪氣逆，陽氣亂，五絡閉塞，結而不通。故狀若尸厥，身脈動，不知人事，邪客手足少陰、太陰、足陽明絡，此五絡，命所關。

可初刺足太陰脾隱白，二刺足少陰腎湧泉，三刺足陽明胃厲兌，四刺手太陰

---

8. *Gǔ* 蠱 is a type of poison from insects or reptiles, although it is sometimes associated with *gǔ zhàng* 鼓脹 (drum distention). In this passage, the *gǔ* condition is related to qì stagnation. This reference to gǔ is not from *Elementary Questions*, Chapter 63.

肺少商，五刺手少陰心少衝。五井穴各二分，左右皆六陰數。不愈，刺神門；不愈，以竹管吹兩耳，以指掩管口，勿泄氣，必須極吹甕，纏脈絡通，每極三度。甚者灸維會三壯。針前後各二分，瀉三度，後再灸。

The Foot Tàiyīn Well Point
[Yǐn Bái 隱白, SP 1]

The patient sickens with deathlike reversal or sudden death, [but] the pulse stirs like that of a normal person.[9] Like this, when yīn is exuberant in the upper body, evil qì repeatedly ascends, and evil qì counterflows. Yáng qì is chaotic. The five networks are blocked. They bind up and do not flow freely. Thus the condition is deathlike reversal: the patient's pulse stirs and there is loss of consciousness. Evil intrudes into the hand and foot shàoyīn and tàiyīn, and the foot yángmíng. These are the five networks that are related to life.

You can first pierce [the well point of] the foot tàiyīn spleen [channel], Yǐn Bái 隱白 (SP 1). Second, pierce [the well point of] the foot shàoyīn kidney [channel], Yǒng Quán 湧泉 (KI 1). Third, pierce [the well point of] the foot yángmíng stomach [channel], Lì Duì 厲兌 (ST 45). Fourth, pierce [the well point of] the hand tàiyīn lung [channel], Shào Shāng 少商 (LU 11). Fifth, pierce [the well point of] the hand shàoyīn heart [channel], Shào Chōng 少衝 (HT 9). [Pierce] each of these five well points two *fèn* deep, on both the left and right, [moving the needle] six times, a yīn number. If the patient does not recover, pierce Shén Mén 神門 (HT 7). If the patient [still] does not recover, blow in the two ears through a bamboo tube. Cover the mouth of the tube with a finger. Do not let the qì drain out. You must blow forcefully; then the vessels and networks will flow freely. [Blow into] each [ear] three times. If the condition is severe, apply three cones of moxibustion to Wéi Huì 維會.[10] Needle in front and in back [of Wéi Huì], each two *fèn* deep, drain it three times and afterwards reapply moxibustion.

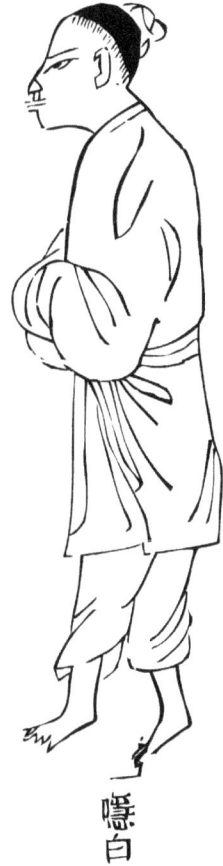

隱白

Fig. 5.4

---

9. This doesn't mean the patient's pulse is healthy. The person otherwise appears to be dead, but the pulse continues to beat.

10. In Volume 2, Yáng says Wéi Huì 維會 is on the gall bladder channel, located three cun above the lateral malleolus. This places it at or around Jué Gǔ 絕骨 (GB 39). Elsewhere Wéi Huì is an alternate name for Shén Què 神闕 (Ren 8) or Bǎi Huì 百會 (Du 20).

手少陰井

人病心痛煩渴，臂厥，脅肋疼，心中熱悶，呆癡忘事，顛狂。斯乃以其脈起於心，支從心系俠喉嚨，出向後腕骨之下；直從肺，行腋下臑內，循廉肘內通臂，循廉抵腕，直過神門脈，入少衝。

可刺手心經井少衝，手小指內側，交肉者如韭葉。刺一分，行六陰數，右取左。若灸三炷，如麥大，不已，復刺神門穴。

The Hand Shàoyīn Well Point
[Shào Chōng 少衝, HT 9]

The patient sickens with heart pain, vexing thirst, reversal cold in the arms, rib-side pain, heat oppression in the heart, feeble-mindedness, forgetfulness, and mania-withdrawal. This is because its vessel arises in the heart. A branch travels from the heart tie[11] on both sides of the throat, emerging toward the back below Wàn Gǔ 腕骨 (SI 4).[12] It travels straight from the lungs to the subaxillary region, to the medial upper arm, and follows the ridge of the medial elbow. It passes through the arm and follows the ridge. It arrives at the wrist, passes directly through the vessel at Shén Mén 神門 (HT 7), and enters Shào Chōng 少衝 (HT 9).

You can pierce the well point of the hand [shàoyīn] heart channel, Shào Chōng 少衝 (HT 9), located on the inner aspect of the little finger, the distance of a leek leaf into the flesh. Insert one *fèn* deep. Move [the needle] six times, a yīn number. For problems of the right, treat the left. If you apply three cones of moxibustion the size of a grain-of-wheat but the patient does not recover, also pierce Shén Mén 神門 (HT 7).

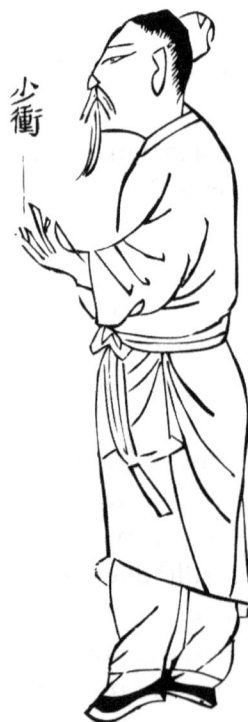

Fig. 5.5

11. According to Wiseman's *Practical Dictionary of Chinese Medicine*, the heart tie refers to the large blood vessels around the heart.

12. "A branch travels from the heart tie on both sides of the throat, emerging toward the back below Wàn Gǔ 腕骨 (SI 4)." This description seems to be based on the channel divergence of the pericardium described in *Zhēn Jiǔ Jiǎ Yǐ Jīng* 《針灸甲已經》 (the Systematic Classic). Yáng wrote 腕骨 wrist bone but the Systematic Classic had 完骨 which is also pronounced Wán Gǔ and is the mastoid process or GB 12.

手太陽井

人病頷腫，項強難顧，肩似拔，臑似折，肘臂疼，外廉痛。斯乃以其脈起小指，自少澤過前谷，上循臂內至肩，入缺盆，向腋，絡心間，循咽下膈，抵胃；支從缺盆上頸頰，至目銳眥入耳，復循頰入鼻頞，斜貫於顴。故邪客於太陽絡，生是病。

可刺手小腸井少澤，小指外側與肉相交如韭葉。刺一分，六陰數，各一痏，左病右取。若灸，如小麥炷，三壯止。

The Hand Tàiyáng Well Point
[Shào Zé 少澤, SI 1]

The patient sickens with submandibular swelling, stiff nape, and difficulty turning the neck. The shoulders feel like they are dislocated; the arms feel like they are broken. There is pain on the lateral aspect of the elbows and arms. This is because the vessel arises in the little finger, passes from Shào Zé 少澤 (SI 1) to Qián Gǔ 前谷 (SI 2), and runs up the medial arms to the shoulder. It enters the supraclavicular fossa [or Quē Pén 缺盆, ST 12], moves toward the axilla, and networks to the space of the heart. It follows the throat down through the diaphragm and arrives at the stomach. A branch ascends from the supraclavicular fossa to the neck and cheeks, arrives at the outer canthus, and enters into the ears. It also follows the cheeks to enter the nose and brow, and moves diagonally to pass into the cheekbones. Thus when evil intrudes into the network of the [hand] tàiyáng, it engenders these illnesses.

You can pierce the well point of the hand [tàiyáng] small intestine [channel], Shào Zé 少澤 (SI 1), located on the outside of the little finger, the distance of a leek leaf into the flesh. Insert one *fèn* deep. [Move the needle] six times, a yīn number, on each site. For disease of the left, treat the right. If you apply three cones of moxibustion the size of a small grain-of-wheat, the disease will stop.

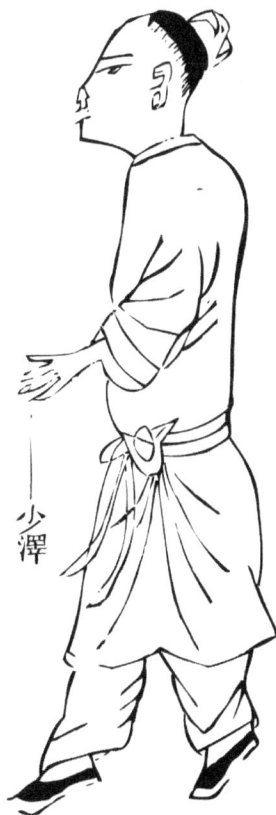

少澤

Fig. 5.6

足太陽井

人病頭項肩背腰目疼，脊痛，痔瘻，癲狂，目黃淚出，鼻流血。斯乃經之正者，從腦出別下項；支別者，從髆內左右別下；又其絡從上行，循眥上額。故邪客於足太陽絡，而有是病。

可刺足太陽膀胱井至陰，小指外側韭葉。行六陰數。不已，刺金門五分，灸三壯；不已，刺申脈一寸三分，如人行十里愈。

有所墜，瘀血留腹內，滿脹不得行，先以利藥，次刺然谷前脈，出血立已。

不已，刺衝陽三分，（胃之原）及大敦見血（肝之井）。

The Foot Tàiyáng Well Point
[Zhì Yīn 至陰, UB 67]

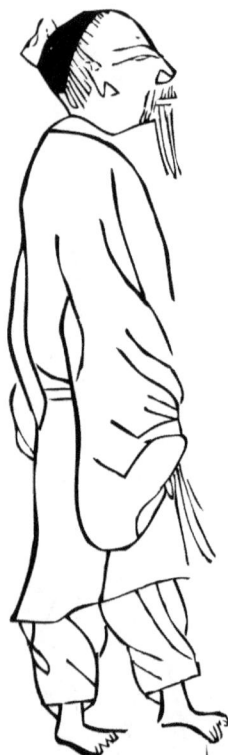

The patient sickens with pain of the head, nape, shoulder, back, and eyes, pain of the spine, hemorrhoids, malaria, mania-withdrawal, yellow eyes, tearing, runny nose or nose-bleeds. This is because the main channel emerges from the brain and diverges down the nape. A branch divergence travels bilaterally from the inner arms and diverges downward. In addition, its network travels upward and follows the [inner] canthus up the forehead. Thus when evil intrudes into the network of the foot tàiyáng, there are these illnesses.

You can pierce the well point of the foot tàiyáng urinary bladder [channel], Zhì Yīn 至陰 (UB 67), located on the outside of the little toe, [the distance of] a leek leaf. Move [the needle] six times, a yīn number. If the patient does not recover, pierce Jīn Mén 金門 (UB 63) five *fèn* deep and apply three cones of moxibustion. If the patient does not recover, pierce Shēn Mài 申脈 (UB 62) one *cùn* three *fèn* deep[13] for the length of time it takes to walk ten *lǐ* and the patient will recover.

When someone has fallen down, static blood remains inside the abdomen so fullness and distention cannot be moved. First take disinhibiting medicinals. Next, pierce the vessel in

---

13. The *Zhēn Jiǔ Jiǎ Yǐ Jīng* 《針灸甲已經》(Systematic Classic) specifies 3 *fèn* deep for Shēn Mài (UB 62).

front of Rán Gǔ 然谷 (KI 2). When you let out blood, there will be immediate recovery. If the patient doesn't recover, pierce Chōng Yáng 衝陽 (ST 42) three *fèn* deep (the source point of the stomach) and Dà Dūn 大敦 (LV 1) to make blood appear (the well point of the liver).

足少陰井

人病卒心痛，暴脹，胸脅支滿。斯逎脈上貫肝膈，走於心內。故邪客於足少陰之絡，而有是病。

可刺足少陰腎井湧泉，足心中。刺三分，行六陰數，見血出，令人立飢欲食。左取右，《素》有此病新發，刺五日愈，灸三壯。

The Foot Shàoyīn Well Point
[Yǒng Quán 湧泉, KI 1]

The patient sickens with sudden heart pain, abrupt onset of distention, and propping fullness of the chest and rib-sides. This is because the vessel ascends to pass through the liver and diaphragm, and runs into the heart. Thus when evil intrudes into the network of the foot shàoyīn, there are these illnesses.

You can pierce the well point of the foot shàoyīn kidney [channel], Yǒng Quán 湧泉 (KI 1), located in the heart of the foot. Insert three *fèn* deep. Move [the needle] six times, a yīn number. When you see blood, it makes the person immediately hungry and desire food. For diseases of the left, treat the right. *Elementary Questions* says that if this is a relapse of the disease, the patient will recover five days after you pierce it. Apply three cones of moxibustion.

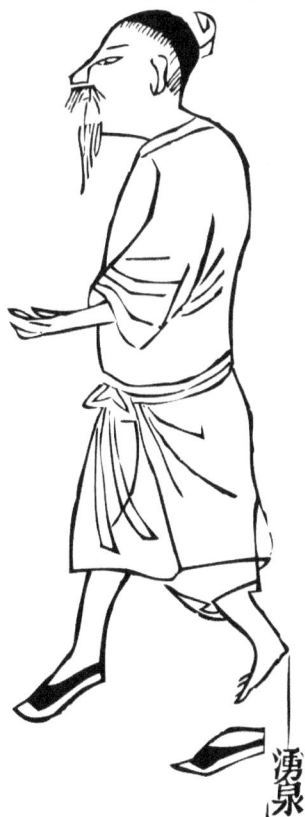

Fig. 5.8

湧泉

手厥陰井

人病卒然心痛，掌中熱，胸滿膨，手攣臂痛，不能伸屈，腋下腫平，面赤目黃，善笑，心胸熱，耳聾響。斯乃以其包絡之脈，循脅過腋下，通臑內，至間使人勞宮，循經直入中衝；支別從掌循小指，過次指關衝。故邪客於手厥陰絡，生是病。
可刺手厥陰心包井中衝，中指內端，去甲韭葉。刺一分，行六陰數，左取右，如食頃已。若灸，可三壯，如小麥炷。

The Hand Juéyīn Well Point
[Zhōng Chōng 中衝, PC 9]

The patient sickens with sudden heart pain, heat in the center of the palms, chest fullness and inflation, hypertonicity of the hands, arm pain, inability to bend and stretch, swelling below the axilla [making it] level, red face, yellow eyes, frequent laughter, heat in the heart and chest, and deafness. This is because the pericardium vessel follows the rib-sides, passes below the axilla, and flows through the medial upper arm. It reaches Jiān Shǐ 間使 (PC 5), enters Láo Gōng 勞宮 (PC 8), and follows the channel directly to enter Zhōng Chōng 中衝 (PC 9). A branch diverges from the palm, follows the ring finger, and passes through to Guān Chōng 關衝 (SJ 1). Thus when evil intrudes into the network of the hand juéyīn, it engenders these illnesses.

You can pierce the well point of the hand juéyīn pericardium [channel], Zhōng Chōng 中衝 (PC 9), located on the inner end of the middle finger, the distance of a leek leaf from the nail. Insert one *fèn* deep. Move [the needle] six times, a yīn number. For diseases of the left, treat the right. The patient should recover in the time it takes to eat a meal. If you apply moxibustion, you can use three grain-of-wheat size cones.

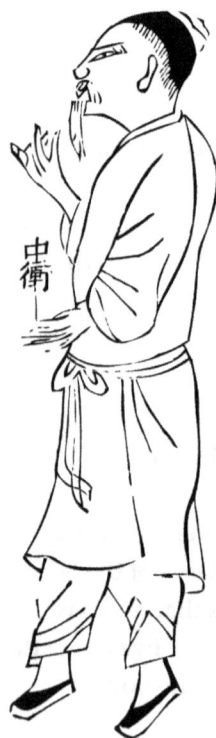

Fig. 5.9

28

手少陽井

人病耳聾痛，渾渾，目疼，肘痛，脊間心後痛甚。斯乃以其脈上臂，貫臑外，循肩上，交出少陽缺盆，膻中、膈內；支出頸頂耳後，直入耳中，循遍目內眥。故邪氣客於少陽絡，生是病。

可刺手少陽三焦井穴，關衝也，手小指次指，去爪甲與肉交者，如韭葉許。刺一分，各一痏，右取左，如食頃已，如灸三壯不已，復刺少陽俞中渚穴。

The Hand Shàoyáng Well Point
[Guān Chōng 關衝, SJ 1]

The patient sickens with deafness, ear pain, sounds are muffled and indistinct, eye pain, elbow pain, and severe pain between the spine and the back of the heart. This is because the vessel ascends the arm, passes through the lateral upper arm, and runs up the shoulder. It joins and emerges with the [foot] shàoyáng [channel] at the supraclavicular fossa (Quē Pén 缺盆 ST 12), and [continues on to] Dàn Zhōng 膻中 (Ren 17), inside the diaphragm. A branch emerges at the neck, [goes on to] the vertex, and behind the ear. It enters directly into the ear and follows to the inner canthus. Thus when evil intrudes into the network of the [hand] shàoyáng, it engenders these illnesses.

You can pierce the well point of the hand shàoyáng triple burner [channel], Guān Chōng 關衝 (SJ 1), located on the ring finger, the distance of a leek leaf from the nail into the flesh. Pierce each site one *fèn* deep. For diseases of the right, treat the left. The patient should recover in the time it takes to eat a meal. If you apply three cones of moxibustion but the patient does not recover, also pierce the shàoyáng transport point, Zhōng Zhǔ 中渚 (SJ 3).

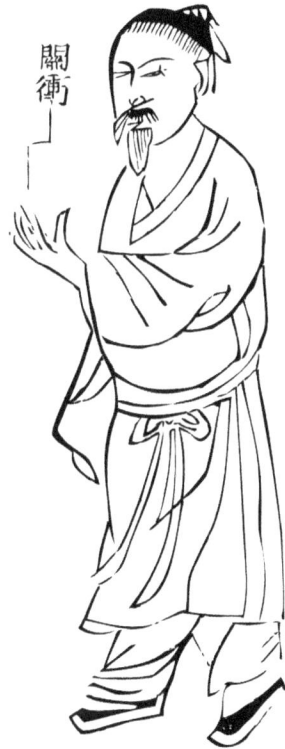

關衝

Fig. 5.10

29

足少陽井

人病胸脅足痛，面滯，頭目疼，缺盆腋腫汗多，頸項瘦瘤強硬，瘧生寒熱。乃脈支別者，從目銳下大迎，合手少陽抵項，下頰車，下頸合缺盆以下胸，交中貫膈，絡肝膽，循脅。故邪客於足少陽之絡，而有是病。

可刺足少陽膽井竅陰，在次指與肉交者，如韭葉許。刺一分，行六陰數，各一痏，左病右取，如食頃已。灸可三壯。

The Foot Shàoyáng Well Point
[Zú Qiào Yīn 足竅陰, GB 44]

The patient sickens with chest, rib-side,[14] and leg pain, the facial [complexion shows] stagnation, pain of the head and eyes, swelling in the supra-clavicular fossa or axilla, copious sweating, hard goiters and tumors on the neck, and malaria engendering sensations of cold and heat. A vessel branch diverges from the [outer] canthus down to Dà Yíng 大迎 (ST 5) and unites with the hand shàoyáng [channel]. It arrives at the nape, descends to Jiá Chē 頰車 (ST 6), descends the neck to unite with the supraclavicular fossa (Quē Pén 缺盆 - ST 12), and descends into the chest. It intersects the center [of the chest], passes through the diaphragm, networks with the liver and gall bladder, and follows the rib-sides. Thus when evil intrudes into the network of the foot shàoyáng, there are these illnesses.

You can pierce the well point of the foot shàoyáng gall bladder [channel], Qiào Yīn 竅陰 (GB 44), located on the fourth toe, the distance of a leek leaf into the flesh. Insert one *fēn* deep. Move [the needle] six times, a yīn number, on each site. For disease of the left, treat the right. The patient should recover in the time it takes to eat a meal. You can apply three cones of moxibustion.

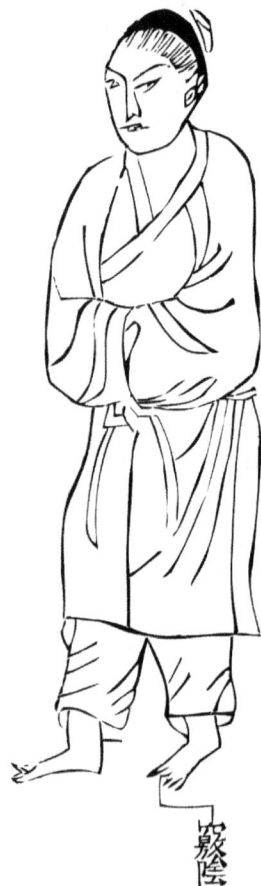

Fig. 5.11

---

14. Some editions have *gé* 膈 (diaphragm) instead of *xié* 脅 (rib-sides).

針灸大成 · 卷之五

足厥陰井

人病卒疝暴痛，及腹繞臍上下急痛。斯乃肝絡，去內踝上五寸，別走少陽；其支別者，循經上睪，結於莖。故邪客於足厥陰之絡，而有是病。
可刺足厥陰肝經井大敦，大指端，行六陰數，左取右。《素》有此病再發，刺之三日已。若灸者，可五壯止。

The Foot Juéyīn Well Point
[Dà Dūn 大敦, LV 1]

The patient sickens from sudden *shàn* 疝 (mounting) with abrupt onset of pain, and at the same time acute pain in the abdomen that winds around above and below the umbilicus. This is the liver network vessel which is five *cùn* above the medial malleolus. It diverges and runs into the shàoyáng [channel]. Its branch diverges to follow the channel up to the testicles and binds in the penis. Thus when evil intrudes into the network of the foot juéyīn, there are these illnesses.

You can pierce the well point of the foot juéyīn liver channel, Dà Dūn 大敦 (LV 1), located on the end of the big toe. Move [the needle] six times, a yīn number. For diseases of the left, treat the right. *Elementary Questions* says that if someone has had a relapse of this disease, pierce it and the patient will recover in three days. If you apply moxibustion, you can use five cones and the disease will stop.

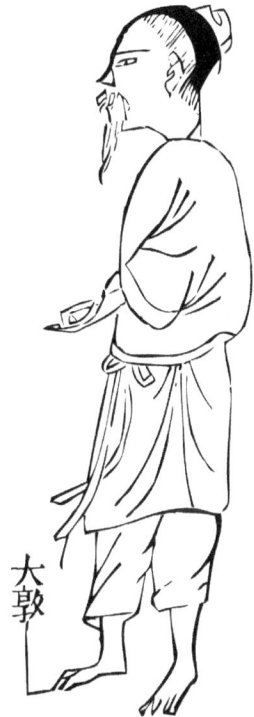

大敦

Fig. 5.12

井滎俞原經合歌（《醫經小學》）
Song of the Well, Brook, Stream, Source, River, and Uniting Points (from *Primary Studies of the Medical Classics - Yī Jīng Xiǎo Xué*[15])

少商魚際與太淵，經渠尺澤肺相連。

---

15. Published in 1388 (*Míng*), by Liú Chún 劉純. This poem simply lists the well, brook, stream, source, river, and uniting points in order for each channel. The name of the channel is mentioned in every line because the Chinese name of the point, unlike the English alpha-numeric system, does not specify the channel to which it belongs. Yáng summarizes these points in the table that follows.

商陽二三間合谷，陽谿曲池大腸牽 。
隱白大都太白脾，商邱陰陵泉要知，
厲兌內庭陷谷胃，衝陽解谿三里隨 。
少衝少府屬於心，神門靈道少海尋，
少澤前谷後谿腕，陽谷小海小腸經 。
湧泉然谷與太谿，復溜陰谷腎所宜，
至陰通谷束京骨，崑崙委中膀胱知 。
中衝勞宮心包絡，大陵間使傳曲澤，
關衝液門中渚焦，陽池支溝天井索 。
大敦行間太衝看，中封曲泉屬於肝，
竅陰俠谿臨泣膽，邱墟陽輔陽陵泉 。

Shào Shāng 少商 (LU 11), Yú Jì 魚際 (LU 10), Tài Yuān 太淵 (LU 9); Jīng Qú 經渠 (LU 8), and Chǐ Zé 尺澤 (LU 5) link up with the lungs.

Shāng Yáng 商陽 (LI 1), Èr 二 and Sān Jiān 三間 (LI 2 and LI 3), Hé Gǔ 合谷 (LI 4); Yáng Xī 陽谿 (LI 5), and Qū Chí 曲池 (LI 11) involve the large intestine.

Yīn Bái 隱白 (SP 1), Dà Dū 大都 (SP 2), and Tài Bái 太白 (SP 3) are spleen; Shāng Qiū 商邱 (SP 5) and Yīn Líng Quán 陰陵泉 (SP 9) are important to know.

Lì Duì 厲兌 (ST 45), Nèi Tíng 內庭 (ST 44), and Xiàn Gǔ 陷谷 (ST 43) are stomach; Chōng Yáng 衝陽 (ST 42), Jiě Xī 解谿 (ST 41), and Sān Lǐ 三里 (ST 36) follow.

Shào Chōng 少衝 (HT 9) and Shào Fǔ 少府 (HT 8) belong to the heart; seek Shén Mén 神門 (HT 7), Líng Dào 靈道 (HT 4), and Shào Hǎi 少海 (HT 3).

Shào Zé 少澤 (SI 1), Qián Gǔ 前谷 (SI 2), Hòu Xī 後谿 (SI 3), Wàn 腕 and Yáng Gǔ 陽谷 (SI 4 and SI 5) and Xiǎo Hǎi 小海 (SI 8) are small intestine channel.

Yǒng Quán 湧泉 (KI 1), Rán Gǔ 然谷 (KI 2), and Tài Xī 太谿 (KI 3); Fù Liū 復溜 (KI 7) and Yīn Gǔ 陰谷 (KI 10) are what is suitable for kidneys.

Zhì Yīn 至陰 (UB 67), Tōng Gǔ 通谷 (UB 66), Shù 束 and Jīng Gǔ 京骨 (UB 65 and UB 64); Kūn Lún 崑崙 (UB 60), and Wěi Zhōng 委中 (UB 40) know the urinary bladder.

Zhōng Chōng 中衝 (PC 9) and Láo Gōng 勞宮 (PC 8) are pericardium; Dà Líng 大陵 (PC 7) and Jiān Shǐ 間使 (PC 5) pass on to Qū Zé 曲澤 (PC 3).

Guān Chōng 關衝 (SJ 1), Yè Mén 液門 (SJ 2), and Zhōng Zhǔ 中渚 (SJ 3) are [triple] burner; Yáng Chí 陽池 (SJ 4), Zhī Gōu 支溝 (SJ 6), and Tiān Jǐng 天井 (SJ 10) are bound together.

See that Dà Dūn 大敦 (LV 1), Xíng Jiān 行間 (LV 2), and Tài Chōng 太衝 (LV 3); Zhōng Fēng 中封 (LV 4) and Qū Quán 曲泉 (LV 8) belong to liver.

Qiào Yīn 竅陰 (GB 44), Xiá Xī 俠谿 (GB 43), Lín Qì 臨泣 (GB 41) are gall bladder; Qiū Xū 邱墟 (GB 40), Yáng Fǔ 陽輔 (GB 38), and Yáng Líng Quán 陽陵泉 (GB 34).

井滎俞原經合橫圖 (《聚英》)

Table of the Well, Brook, Stream, Source, River, and Uniting Points (*Gatherings from Eminent Acupuncturists* – Zhēn Jiǔ Jù Yīng[16])

	肺	脾	心	腎	心包絡	肝	
井木	少商	隱白	少衝	湧泉	中衝	大敦	春刺
滎火	魚際	大都	少府	然谷	勞宮	行間	夏刺
俞土	太淵	太白	神門	太谿	大陵	太衝	季夏刺
經金	經渠	商邱	靈道	復溜	間使	中封	秋刺
合水	尺澤	陰陵泉	少海	陰谷	曲澤	曲泉	冬刺

The information in the eighth column comes from the *Nàn Jīng* 《難經》 Classic of Difficulties, 74th Difficult Issue.

	Lung	Spleen	Heart	Kidney	Pericardium	Liver	
Well, wood	Shào Shāng (LU 11)	Yǐn Bái (SP 1)	Shào Chōng (HT 9)	Yǒng Quán (KI 1)	Zhōng Chōng (PC 9)	Dà Dūn (LV 1)	Pierce in the spring
Brook, fire	Yú Jì (LU 10)	Dà Dū (SP 2)	Shào Fǔ (HT 8)	Rán Gǔ (KI 2)	Láo Gōng (PC 8)	Xíng Jiān (LV 2)	Pierce in the summer
Stream, earth	Tài Yuān (LU 9)	Tài Bái (SP 3)	Shén Mén (HT 7)	Tài Xī (KI 3)	Dà Líng (PC 7)	Tài Chōng (LV 3)	Pierce in the last month of summer
River, metal	Jīng Qú (LU 8)	Shāng Qiū (SP 5)	Líng Dào (HT 4)	Fù Liū (KI 7)	Jiān Shǐ (PC 5)	Zhōng Fēng (LV 4)	Pierce in the autumn
Uniting, water	Chǐ Zé (LU 5)	Yīn Líng Quán (SP 9)	Shào Hǎi (HT 3)	Yīn Gǔ (KI 10)	Qū Zé (PC 3)	Qū Quán (LV 8)	Pierce in the winter

16. By Gāo Wǔ 高武, published in 1529 (*Míng*). This table is found in Volume 1.

	大腸	胃	小腸	膀胱	三焦	膽	
井金	商陽	厲兌	少澤	至陰	關衝	竅陰	所出
榮水	二間	內庭	前谷	通谷	液門	俠谿	所溜
俞木	三間	陷谷	後谿	束骨	中渚	臨泣	所注
原	合谷	衝陽	腕骨	京骨	陽池	邱墟	所過
經火	陽谿	解谿	陽谷	崑崙	支溝	陽輔	所行
合土	曲池	三里	小海	委中	天井	陽陵泉	所入

The information in the eighth column comes from *Líng Shū*《靈樞》Magic Pivot, Chapter 1 or the *Nàn Jīng*《難經》Classic of Difficulties, 68th Difficult Issue, except the source point as the place of passing through, which comes from Magic Pivot, Chapter 2. [17]

	Large Intestine	Stomach	Small Intestine	Urinary Bladder	Triple Burner	Gall Bladder	
Well, metal	Shāng Yáng (LI 1)	Lì Duì (ST 45)	Shào Zé (SI 1)	Zhì Yīn (UB 67)	Guān Chōng (SJ 1)	Qiào Yīn (GB 44)	the place of emerging
Brook, water	Èr Jiān (LI 2)	Nèi Tíng (ST 44)	Qián Gǔ (SI 2)	Tōng Gǔ (UB 66)	Yè Mén (SJ 2)	Xiá Xī (GB 43)	the place of flowing
Stream, wood	Sān Jiān (LI 3)	Xiàn Gǔ (ST 43)	Hòu Xī (SI 3)	Shù Gǔ (UB 65)	Zhōng Zhǔ (SJ 3)	Lín Qì (GB 41)	the place of pooling
Source	Hé Gǔ (LI 4)	Chōng Yáng (ST 42)	Wàn Gǔ (SI 4)	Jīng Gǔ (UB 64)	Yáng Chí (SJ 4)	Qiū Xū (GB 40)	the place of passing through
River, fire	Yáng Xī (LI 5)	Jiě Xī (ST 41)	Yáng Gǔ (SI 5)	Kūn Lún (UB 60)	Zhī Gōu (SJ 6)	Yáng Fǔ (GB 38)	the place of traveling
Uniting, earth	Qū Chí (LI 11)	Sān Lǐ (ST 36)	Xiǎo Hǎi (SI 8)	Wěi Zhōng (UB 40)	Tiān Jǐng (SJ 10)	Yáng Líng Quán (GB 34)	the place of entering

Translator's Note:
In different editions, the text that follows is sometimes found above the table, sometimes below it, and sometimes split, partly above and partly below the tables. However, in the two oldest editions available to me, the whole text is below the tables.

---

17. *Magic Pivot* uses *liù* 溜 (a current) while *Classic of Difficulties* uses *liú* 流 (to flow) in the parallel passage. Otherwise, the language of the two texts agrees.

項氏曰：所出為井，井象水之泉。所溜為榮，榮象水之陂。所注為俞，俞象水之窬。所行為經，經象水之流。所入為合，合象水之歸。皆取水義也。

Master Xiàng said: The place of emerging is the well [point]; the image of the well is a spring. The place of flowing is the brook [point]; the image of the brook is a sloped embankment. The place of pooling is the stream [point]; the image of the stream is water [flowing into] a hole. The place of traveling is the river [point]; the image of river is the flowing of water. The place of entering is the uniting [point]; the image of uniting is the return of water. All take on the meaning of water. [18]

又曰：春刺井，井者東方春也，萬物之始生，故言井。冬刺合，合者北方冬也，陽氣入藏，故言合。舉始終而言，榮、俞、經、在其中矣。又曰：諸井肌肉淺薄，瀉井當瀉榮。滑氏曰：補井當補合。

It is also said: In spring, needle the well point. The well [belongs to] the east and spring, the beginning of life for the ten-thousand things; thus it is called the well. In winter, needle the uniting point. The uniting [belongs to] the north and winter, when yáng qì enters into storage; thus it is called uniting. When discussing the beginning [the well points] and end [the uniting points], the brook, stream, and river points are in between. [19]

It is also said: The flesh is shallow and thin at all the well points, so to drain the well you should drain the brook point. [20]

Master Huá said: To supplement the well point, you should supplement the uniting point. [21]

岐伯曰：春刺井者，邪在肝；夏刺榮者，邪在心；季夏刺俞者，邪在脾；秋刺經者，邪在肺；冬刺合者，邪在腎，故也。帝曰：五臟而繫於四時，何以知之？岐伯曰：五臟一病，輒有五驗，假如肝病，色青者肝也。臊臭者肝也，喜酸者肝也，喜呼者肝也，喜泣者肝也。其病眾多，不可盡言也。四臟有驗，並繫於四時者也。針之要紗，在於秋毫。

---

18. The identity of Master Xiàng is unclear. This is a commentary on *Magic Pivot*, Chapter 1 or *Classic of Difficulties*, 68th Difficult Issue.

19. This discusses statements in the *Classic of Difficulties*, 65th and 74th Difficult Issues.

20. This is commentary on the *Classic of Difficulties*, 73rd Difficult Issue. The reason you cannot drain the well point is that there is not enough qì in the shallow flesh to be able to drain it effectively.

21. This refers to Huá Shòu's 滑壽 commentary on the *Classic of Difficulties*, 73rd Difficult Issue, written during the Yuán Dynasty. Some later commentators say that this idea is unfounded.

Qí Bó said: In spring, needle the well points as evil is in the liver. In the summer needle the brook points as evil is in the heart. In the last month of summer, needle the stream points, as the evil is in the spleen. In the autumn, needle the river points, as evil is in the lungs. In the winter, needle the uniting points, as evil is in the kidneys.

The Emperor said: What is the relationship between the five viscera and the four seasons?

Qí Bó said: When the five viscera sicken, there are five expected results. For example, in liver disease, green-blue is the liver. Animal odor is the liver. Preference for sour is the liver. Tendancy to shout is the liver. Frequent tearing is the liver. Its diseases are so numerous they cannot be fully explained. Four of the viscera produce their expected results and are attached to the four seasons.[22] The essential principle of acupuncture is [as subtle as] an autumn hair. [23]

四明陳氏曰：春氣在毛，夏氣在皮，秋氣在分肉，冬氣在骨髓，是淺深之應也。

Master Chén from Sìmíng said: In the spring, qì is in the body hair. In the summer, qì is in the skin. In the autumn, qì is in the divisions of the flesh. In the winter, qì is in the bones [and] marrow. This is the correspondence to depth. [24]

Translator's note:

Now we come to the first section that discusses point selection based on time. More annotations are necessary at this point. See also the appendix on the ten heavenly stems, the twelve earthly branches, and the Chinese calendar. Here I will give a basic explanation of how the open points are calculated before returning to the translation.

The following table shows the ten-day 'week' based on the ten heavenly stems. There is a section in the next poem below describing the open points for each of the ten days. The ten stems and their relevant associations are:[25]

---

22. The spleen is different because it doesn't have a season in the same way as the the other four elements.

23. This is almost an exact quotation of *Classic of Difficulties*, 74th Difficult Issue.

24. Sìmíng 四明 is an ancient name for a place in Zhèjiāng 浙江 province. Chén Zháizhī 陳宅之 and his father Chén Ruìsūn 陳瑞孫, (Yuán 元), lived in the region and wrote *Nàn Jīng Biàn Yí* 《難經辨疑》(Distinguishing Uncertainties about the Classic of Difficulties). Unfortunately, this book has since been lost. It is possible that Sìmíng Chén 四明陳 refers to one of these authors. However, this quote is based on statements in *Magic Pivot*, Chapter 9.

25. These organ associations with the stems (except for triple burner and pericardium) are listed in *Elementary Questions*, Chapter 22.

	Stem		Element	Associated Organ
1	甲	jiǎ	Yáng Wood	Gall Bladder
2	乙	yǐ	Yīn Wood	Liver
3	丙	bǐng	Yáng Fire	Small Intestine
4	丁	dīng	Yīn Fire	Heart
5	戊	wù	Yáng Earth	Stomach
6	己	jǐ	Yīn Earth	Spleen
7	庚	gēng	Yáng Metal	Large Intestine
8	辛	xīn	Yīn Metal	Lungs
9	壬	rén	Yáng Water	Urinary Bladder, Triple Burner
10	癸	guǐ	Yīn Water	Kidneys, Pericardium

The sequence for each day begins with the well point of the channel associated with the day (with the exception of the triple burner and pericardium).

Within each day, there are twelve two-hour time periods. Each time period is associated with one of the twelve branches. The time period associated with a particular branch always occurs at the same time each day. For example, 1:00 to 3:00 a.m. is always associated with the chǒu 丑 branch.

	Branch		Time Period	Element	Associated Organ
1	子	zǐ	11 pm-1 am	Yáng Water	Gall Bladder
2	丑	chǒu	1-3 am	Yīn Earth	Liver
3	寅	yín	3-5 am	Yáng Wood	Lungs
4	卯	mǎo	5-7 am	Yīn Wood	Large Intestine
5	辰	chén	7-9 am	Yáng Earth	Stomach
6	巳	sì	9-11 am	Yīn Fire	Spleen
7	午	wǔ	11 am-1 pm	Yáng Fire	Heart
8	未	wèi	1-3 pm	Yīn Earth	Small Intestine
9	申	shēn	3-5 pm	Yáng Metal	Urinary Bladder
10	酉	yǒu	5-7 pm	Yīn Metal	Kidneys
11	戌	xū	7-9 pm	Yáng Earth	Pericardium
12	亥	hài	9-11 pm	Yīn Water	Triple Burner

Note: Correct for Daylight Savings Time, if necessary.

While the twelve branches are associated with the twelve organs, this relationship is not governed by the five elements (unlike the stems). The organs are not relevant for the next section of the text, but Yáng mentions this correspondence later

Each time-period is also associated with a stem, but since there are twelve time periods in a day and only ten stems, the hour stem pattern does not repeat in a circadian cycle. Stems and branches combine into a cycle of sixty. When applied to the time periods, a stem-branch combination repeats every five days as follows:

The Double-Hour Stems and Branches						
Double-Hour		Day Stem				
Time	Branch	Jiǎ 甲 or Jǐ 己	Yǐ 乙 or Gēng 庚	Bǐng 丙 or Xīn 辛	Dīng 丁 or Rén 壬	Wù 戊 or Guǐ 癸
11 pm-1 am	Zǐ 子	Jiǎ Zǐ 甲子	Bǐng Zǐ 丙子	Wù Zǐ 戊子	Gēng Zǐ 庚子	Rén Zǐ 壬子
1-3 am	Chǒu 丑	Yǐ Chǒu 乙丑	Dīng Chǒu 丁丑	Jǐ Chǒu 己丑	Xīn Chǒu 辛丑	Guǐ Chǒu 癸丑
3-5 am	Yín 寅	Bǐng Yín 丙寅	Wù Yín 戊寅	Gēng Yín 庚寅	Rén Yín 壬寅	Jiǎ Yín 甲寅
5-7 am	Mǎo 卯	Dīng Mǎo 丁卯	Jǐ Mǎo 己卯	Xīn Mǎo 辛卯	Guǐ Mǎo 癸卯	Yǐ Mǎo 乙卯
7-9 am	Chén 辰	Wù Chén 戊辰	Gēng Chén 庚辰	Rén Chén 壬辰	Jiǎ Chén 甲辰	Bǐng Chén 丙辰
9-11 am	Sì 巳	Jǐ Sì 己巳	Xīn Sì 辛巳	Guǐ Sì 癸巳	Yǐ Sì 乙巳	Dīng Sì 丁巳
11 am-1 pm	Wǔ 午	Gēng Wǔ 庚午	Rén Wǔ 壬午	Jiǎ Wǔ 甲午	Bǐng Wǔ 午丙	Wù Wǔ 戊午
1-3 pm	Wèi 未	Xīn Wèi 辛未	Guǐ Wèi 癸未	Yǐ Wèi 乙未	Dīng Wèi 丁未	Jǐ Wèi 己未
3-5pm	Shēn 申	Rén Shēn 壬申	Jiǎ Shēn 甲申	Bǐng Shēn 丙申	Wù Shēn 戊申	Gēng Shēn 庚申
5-7pm	Yǒu 酉	Guǐ Yǒu 癸酉	Yǐ Yǒu 乙酉	Dīng Yǒu 丁酉	Jǐ Yǒu 己酉	Xīn Yǒu 辛酉
7-9pm	Xū 戌	Jiǎ Xū 甲戌	Bǐng Xū 丙戌	Wù Xū 戊戌	Gēng Xū 庚戌	Rén Xū 壬戌
9-11pm	Hài 亥	Yǐ Hài 乙亥	Dīng Hài 丁亥	Jǐ Hài 己亥	Xīn Hài 辛亥	Guǐ Hài 癸亥

Note: Correct for Daylight Savings Time, if necessary.

The pattern below is generally called "Adoping the Stem" (納甲) because each time period is defined by its stem, and the corresponding stem associations with yīn or yáng and an element. The branches are only relevant in that they identify the two-hour time period, not the point to be used at that time. In other words, the stem gives us the point and the branch gives us the time for that point to be used.

The channel associated with the day stem is sometimes called the "on-duty channel." For example, the stem yǐ 乙 is yīn wood and is associated with the liver, so liver is the on-duty channel on yǐ days. Each day starts in the time period that has the same stem as the day. At that time, the well point of the on-duty channel is open.

In the first day of the cycle (jiǎ 甲 stem day), the first time period used is the jiǎ xū 甲戌 hour (7 – 9 pm). The jiǎ zǐ 甲子 hour, which is from 11 pm (of the night before) to 1 am, is skipped over. Since the progression of the jiǎ day starts late in the day, it will spill over into the next (yǐ) day. This spilling over happens throughout the ten-day week.

The Beginning of the Sequence on a Jiǎ Day			
Double-Hour		Day Stem	
Time	Branch	Jiǎ	Notes
11 pm-1 am	Zǐ 子	Jiǎ Zǐ 甲子	This *jiǎ* hour is skipped over.
1-3 am	Chǒu 丑	Yǐ Chǒu 乙丑	
3-5 am	Yín 寅	Bǐng Yín 丙寅	
5-7 am	Mǎo 卯	Dīng Mǎo 丁卯	
7-9 am	Chén 辰	Wù Chén 戊辰	
9-11 am	Sì 巳	Jǐ Sì 己巳	
11 am-1 pm	Wǔ 午	Gēng Wǔ 庚午	
1-3 pm	Wèi 未	Xīn Wèi 辛未	
3-5pm	Shēn 申	Rén Shēn 壬申	
5-7pm	Yǒu 酉	Guǐ Yǒu 癸酉	
7-9pm	Xū 戌	Jiǎ Xū 甲戌	This *jiǎ* hour begins the sequence.
9-11pm	Hài 亥	Yǐ Hài 乙亥	The sequence continues into the next day.

If the day has a yáng stem, only time periods with yáng stems are used. If the day has a yīn stem, only time periods with yīn stems are used. In other words, once a pattern for a day starts, every second time-period is used. In this method, there is no open point on yáng days during yīn time-periods and vice versa.

In the second active time period, the brook point is open. But on which channel? The next channel according to the five elements. However the progression stays with yīn channels for yīn days and yáng channels for yáng days. In two more time periods, we use the stream point of the next channel by element. In two more time periods, we use the river point of the next channel by element. In two more time periods, finally we arrive at the uniting point of the next channel by element.

We can sum this up by saying *a point generates another point* (well to brook to spring to river to uniting points), *a channel generates another channel* (the starting channel depends on the day stem, but it goes in the usual order of wood to fire to earth to metal to water). Here is a table for the pattern so far:

	Time Period	Transport Point	Channel	Example
1	time period with the same stem as the day	well point	channel represented by the day stem (on-duty channel)	Yáng wood: jiǎ 甲 day, jiǎ 甲 hour, Qiào Yīn 竅陰 (GB 44)
	Skip the yīn time period on the yáng day or the yáng time period on the yīn day.			
2	two time periods later	spring point	channel of the next element with same yīn-yáng correspondence	Yáng fire: bǐng 丙 hour (this has flowed into the next day, but is still part of the sequence for the jiǎ 甲 day), Qián Gǔ 前谷 (SI 2)
	Skip the yīn time period on the yáng day or the yáng time period on the yīn day.			
3	two time periods later	stream point	channel of the next element with same yīn-yáng correspondence	Yáng earth: wù 戊 hour, Xiàn Gǔ 陷谷 (ST 43)
	Skip the yīn time period on the yáng day or the yáng time period on the yīn day.			
4	two time periods later	river point	channel of the next element with same yīn-yáng correspondence	Yáng metal: gēng 庚 hour, Yáng Xī 陽谿 (LI 5)
	Skip the yīn time period on the yáng day or the yáng time period on the yīn day.			
5	two time periods later	uniting point	channel of the next element with same yīn-yáng correspondence	Yáng water: rén 壬 hour, Wěi Zhōng 委中 (UB 40)

We still have three more details to work out in this complex pattern:

1. The use of the source point: In the third step of the sequence, two points are open. As described above, one is the stream point of the third channel in the sequence. The other is the source point of the first channel in the sequence. This is called "returning to the root (channel) and coming back to the source (point)."

2. The last time period of the sequence: Two time periods after the uniting point of the sequence, we have the final stage of the pattern. The same hour stem appears twice in one 24 hour day because there are only ten stems to cover twelve time periods. Now we are concerned with the second time period that has the same stem as the day when the sequence started. It is also the same stem as the original time period in the sequence. This is called "the stems meet again."

On yáng days, a triple burner point is open when the stems meet again. This is called. "Qi adopts the triple burner." Choose the point corresponding to the element that feeds the day stem governing this sequence. For example, in the sequence of a jiǎ 甲 day (yáng wood, gall bladder), we pick the water point of the triple burner because water feeds the wood of the gall bladder Yè Mén 液門 (SJ 2). This is because yáng advances or moves forward.

On yīn days, a pericardium point is open when the stems meet again. This is called, "Blood adopts the pericardium." Choose the point corresponding to the element that drains the day stem governing this sequence. For example, in the sequence of a yǐ 乙 day (yīn wood, liver), we pick the fire point of the pericardium, Láo Gōng 勞宮 (PC 8) because fire drains the wood of the liver. This is because yīn retreats or moves backwards.

The appropriate triple burner or pericardium point is called the reunion point because it is when the hour stem reunites with the day stem governing the sequence. Here is the revised pattern, highlighting the additions.

	Time Period	Transport Point	Channel	Example
1	time period with the same stem as the day	well point	channel represented by the day stem (on-duty channel)	Yáng wood: jiǎ 甲 day, jiǎ 甲 hour, Qiào Yīn 竅陰 (GB 44)
	Skip the yīn time period on the yáng day or the yáng time period on the yīn day.			
2	two time periods later	spring point	channel of the next element with same yīn-yáng correspondence	Yáng fire: bǐng 丙 hour (this has flowed into the next day, but is still part of the sequence for the jiǎ 甲 day), Qián Gǔ 前谷 (SI 2)
	Skip the yīn time period on the yáng day or the yáng time period on the yīn day.			
3	two time periods later: return to the root and come back to the source	1. stream point 2. source point (return to the root)	1. channel of the next element with same yīn-yáng correspondence 2. original channel in the sequence	1. Yáng earth: wù 戊 hour, Xiàn Gǔ 陷谷 (ST 43) 2. Qiū Xū 邱墟 (GB 40)
	Skip the yīn time period on the yáng day or the yáng time period on the yīn day.			

4	two time peri-ods later	river point	channel of the next element with same yīn-yáng correspondence	Yáng metal: gēng 庚 hour, Yáng Xī 陽谿 (LI 5)
	Skip the yīn time period on the yáng day or the yáng time period on the yīn day.			
5	two time peri-ods later	uniting point	channel of the next element with same yīn-yáng correspondence	Yáng water: rén 壬 hour, Wěi Zhōng 委中 (UB 40)
	Skip the yīn time period on the yáng day or the yáng time period on the yīn day.			
6	two time peri-ods later: the reunion point	yáng days: the element of the point feeds the day stem yīn days: the element of the point drains the day stem	yáng days: triple burner yīn days: pericardium	jiǎ 甲 hour (return to yáng wood) so Yè Mén 液門 (SJ 2) (water point feeds jiǎ wood)

After the sixth part of the sequence, the very next time period will have the same stem as the day you are now in (the next day), so the sequence starts over. We do not skip a time period here as we do in the rest of the sequence.

3. Rén 壬 and guǐ 癸 days have special circumstances because they are additionally associated with the triple burner and pericardium: Since there are ten stems and twelve channels, these two channels are left over and must share stems with the urinary bladder and kidney channel. The triple burner *lodges with* the rén stem along with the urinary bladder. The pericardium *lodges with* the guǐ stem along with the kidneys.

The word translated as "lodges with" in the above paragraph is *jì* 寄. The translation of this word is a little problematic, yet the word is used relatively frequently. This word has many meanings, primarily to lodge somewhere, to send, to entrust, to deposit, to leave something in someone else's custody. It is often used in phrases that mean a foster mother or a foster child. In effect, the triple burner and pericardium are more like foster family to rén and guǐ whereas the urinary bladder and kidneys are like biological family. This image is also suggested in phrases such as "Qì adopts the triple burner" and "Blood adopts the pericardium."

On rén 壬 days, in the third step of the sequence we return to the root as usual, but we also have a third point open at this time, the source point of the triple burner, Yáng Chí 陽池 (SJ 4).

The sixth and final step of the rén sequence is at the rén zǐ 壬子 hour, with Guān Chōng 關衝 (SJ 1). As usual, the triple burner point corresponds to the element that feeds the day stem: Guān Chōng 關衝 (SJ 1) is the metal point and the rén day corresponds to water.

This rén zǐ 壬子 hour is actually the first time period of the next day, guǐ 癸. However, the guǐ sequence does not begin until the guǐ hài 癸亥 hour, at the end of the day. Ten time periods (20 hours) in a row are left without open points on the guǐ day. Otherwise, once it finally begins, the guǐ sequence continues as expected except for the third step. Similar to the pattern of the rén day, when we return to the root, the stream point of the heart (Shén Mén 神門 – HT 7), the source point of the kidneys (Tài Xī 太谿 – KI 3), and the source point of the pericardium (Dà Líng 大陵 – PC 7) are all open. The guǐ sequence ends as usual, in the guǐ yǒu 癸酉 hour (5-7 pm) of the jiǎ 甲 day (since it has overlapped from guǐ), with Zhōng Chōng 中衝 (PC 9) open. This is the wood point, which drains the water of the guǐ sequence, the appropriate element on a yīn day.

The whole pattern begins again with the jiǎ 甲 day sequence.

This is a complicated calculation, but later, Yáng Jìzhōu provides tables so that the calculation need not be done each time.

徐氏子午流注，逐日按時定穴歌
Master Xú's[26] Midnight-Noon Flowing and Pooling (*Zǐ Wǔ Liú Zhù*)[27] Song to Determine the Point Day by Day According to the Hour

甲日戌時膽竅陰，丙子時中前谷榮，
戊寅陷谷陽明俞，返本邱墟木在寅，
庚辰經注陽谿穴，壬午膀胱委中尋，
甲申時納三焦水，榮合天干取液門。

On a Jiǎ 甲 Day in a xū 戌 hour: gall bladder, Qiào Yīn 竅陰 (GB 44); in the bǐng zǐ 丙子 hour: Qián Gǔ 前谷 (SI 2), the brook point;

Wù yín 戊寅: Xiàn Gǔ 陷谷 (ST 43), the yángmíng stream point; return to the root with Qiū Xū 邱墟 (GB 40), wood in the yín branch hour;

In gēng chén 庚辰, the river pools into Yáng Xī 陽谿 (LI 5); rén wǔ 壬午 seeks Wěi Zhōng 委中 (UB 40) of the urinary bladder;

26. Xú Fèng 徐鳳 published *Zhēn Jiǔ Dà Quán*《針灸大全》(Great Completion of Acupuncture-Moxibustion) in 1439 (*Míng*). This poem is from Volume 3.

27. The name of this method is *Zǐ Wǔ Liú Zhù* 子午流注. *Zǐ* is the two-hour time period that contains midnight. *Wǔ* is the two-hour time period that contains noon. Together, they refer to circadian cycle of time. *Liú* (flowing) refers to the brook point (the place of flowing) and *zhù* (pooling) refers to the stream point (the place of pooling). The term 'flowing and pooling' (*liú zhù*) is often used to refer to the five transport points as a group.

The jiǎ shēn 甲申 hour adopts the triple burner's water point;
the brook point unites with the heavenly stem, so select Yè Mén 液門 (SJ 2).

乙日酉時肝大敦，丁亥時滎少府心，
己丑太白太衝穴，辛卯經渠是肺經，
癸巳腎宮陰谷合，乙未勞宮火穴滎 。

On a Yǐ 乙 Day in a yǒu 酉 hour: liver, Dà Dūn 大敦 (LV 1);
ding hài 丁亥 hour: the brook point, Shào Fǔ 少府 (HT 8), heart;

Ji chǒu 己丑: Tài Bái 太白 (SP 3) and Tài Chōng 太衝 (LV 3) points;
xīn mǎo 辛卯: Jīng Qú 經渠 (LU 8) is the lung river point;

Guǐ sì 癸巳: the kidney palace, Yīn Gǔ 陰谷 (KI 10), the uniting point;
yǐ wèi 乙未: Láo Gōng 勞宮 (PC 8), the fire point, brook.

丙日申時少澤當，戊戌內庭治脹康，
庚子時在三間俞，本原腕骨可袪黃，
壬寅經火崑崙上，甲辰陽陵泉合長，
丙午時受三焦木，中渚之中仔細詳 。

On a Bǐng 丙 Day in a shēn 申 hour, Shào Zé 少澤 (SI 1) is proper;
in wù xū 戊戌, Nèi Tíng 內庭 (ST 44) treats distention for well-being;

The gēng zǐ 庚子 hour is in Sān Jiān 三間 (LI 3), the stream point;
the source of the root is Wàn Gǔ 腕骨 (SI 4) which can dispel jaundice;

Rén yín 壬寅: the river point, fire, Kūn Lún 崑崙 (UB 60) ascends;
jiǎ chén 甲辰: Yáng Líng Quán 陽陵泉 (GB 34), the uniting point is long-lasting;

The bǐng wǔ 丙午 hour receives the wood of the triple burner;
be attentive to the center of Zhōng Zhǔ 中渚 (SJ 3) in particular.

丁日未時心少衝，己酉大都脾土逢，
辛亥太淵神門穴，癸丑復溜腎水通，
乙卯肝經曲泉合，丁巳包絡大陵中 。

On a Dīng 丁 Day in a wèi 未 hour: heart, Shào Chōng 少衝 (HT 9);
jǐ yǒu 己酉 meets Dà Dū 大都 (SP 2), spleen, earth;

Xīn hài 辛亥: Tài Yuān 太淵 (LU 9) and Shén Mén 神門 (HT 7) points;
in **guǐ chǒu** 癸丑, kidney water flows through Fù Liū 復溜 (KI 7);

Yǐ mǎo 乙卯: the liver channel, Qū Quán 曲泉 (LV 8), the uniting point;
dīng sì 丁巳: the pericardium in Dà Líng 大陵 (PC 7).

戊日午時屬兌先，庚申滎穴二間遷，
壬戌膀胱尋束骨，衝陽土穴必還原，
甲子膽經陽輔是，丙寅小海穴安然，
戊辰氣納三焦脈，經穴支溝刺必痊 。

On a Wù 戊 **[Stem] Day in a wǔ** 午 **[branch] hour:** Lì Duì 属兌 (ST 45) is first;
gēng shēn 庚申 moves the brook point, Èr Jiān 二間 (LI 2);

In rén xū 壬戌, the urinary bladder seeks Shù Gǔ 束骨 (UB 65);
Chōng Yáng 衝陽 (ST 42), the earth point, must return to the source;

Jiǎ zǐ 甲子: the gall bladder river point, Yáng Fǔ 陽輔 (GB 38) is it;
in **bǐng yín** 丙寅, the Xiǎo Hǎi 小海 (SI 8) point is tranquil;

In wù chén 戊辰, qì adopts the triple burner vessel;
needling the river point, Zhī Gōu 支溝 (SJ 6), will bring recovery.

己日巳時隱白始，辛未時中魚際取，
癸酉太谿太白原，乙亥中封內踝比，
丁丑時合少海心，己卯間使包絡止 。

On a Jǐ 己 **Day the sì** 巳 **hour begins with** Yǐn Bái 隱白 (SP 1);
in the **xīn wèi** 辛未 hour select Yú Jì 魚際 (LU 10);

Guǐ yǒu 癸酉: Tài Xī 太谿 (KI 3) and Tài Bái 太白 (SP 3), the source points;
yǐ hài 乙亥: Zhōng Fēng 中封 (LV 4) near the medial malleolus;

Dīng chǒu 丁丑 hour: the uniting point, Shào Hǎi 少海 (HT 3), heart;
jǐ mǎo 己卯 stops at Jiān Shǐ 間使 (PC 5), pericardium.

庚日辰時商陽居，壬午膀胱通谷之，
甲申臨泣為俞木，合谷金原返本歸，
丙戌小腸陽谷火，戊子時居三里宜，
庚寅氣納三焦合，天井之中不用疑 。

On a Gēng 庚 Day the chén 辰 hour occupies Shāng Yáng 商陽 (LI 1);
rén wǔ 壬午 goes to the urinary bladder, Tōng Gǔ 通谷 (UB 66);

Jiǎ shēn 甲申: Lín Qì 臨泣 (GB 41) is the stream point, wood;
Hé Gǔ 合谷 (LI 4), the metal source returns to its root;

Bǐng xū 丙戌: small intestine, Yáng Gǔ 陽谷 (SI 5), fire;
the wù zǐ 戊子 hour is suitable to occupy Sān Lǐ 三里 (ST 36);

Gēng yín 庚寅: qì adopts the triple burner uniting point;
the center of Tiān Jǐng 天井 (SJ 10) is not used with any doubt.

辛日卯時少商木，癸巳然谷何須忖，
乙未太衝原太淵，丁酉心經靈道引，
己亥脾合陰陵泉，辛丑曲澤包絡準 。

On a Xīn 辛 Day in a mǎo 卯 hour: Shào Shāng 少商 (LU 11), wood;
in guǐ sì 癸巳, how fortunate to ponder Rán Gǔ 然谷 (KI 2);

Yǐ wèi 乙未: Tài Chōng 太衝 (LV 3), the source point Tài Yuān 太淵 (LU 9);
dīng yǒu 丁酉 guides the heart's river point, Líng Dào 靈道 (HT 4);

Jǐ hài 己亥: spleen uniting point, Yīn Líng Quán 陰陵泉 (SP 9);
xīn chǒu 辛丑: Qū Zé 曲澤 (PC 3), pericardium is the standard.

壬日寅時起至陰，甲辰膽脈俠谿滎，
丙午小腸後谿俞，返求京骨本原尋，
三焦寄有陽池穴，返本還原似的親，
戊申時注解谿胃，大腸庚戌曲池真，
壬子氣納三焦寄，井穴關衝一片金，
關衝屬金壬屬水，子母相生恩義深 。

On a Rén 壬 Day the yín 寅 [branch] hour arises in Zhì Yīn 至陰 (UB 67);
jiǎ chén 甲辰: the gall bladder vessel, Xiá Xī 俠谿 (GB 43), the brook point;

Bǐng wǔ 丙午: the small intestine, Hòu Xī 後谿 (SI 3), stream point;
go back to Jīng Gǔ 京骨 (UB 64), seek its root source;

The triple burner lodging has Yáng Chí 陽池 (SJ 4); it goes back to the root
and returns to the source, like a member of the family;

The wù shēn 戊申 hour pools into Jiě Xī 解谿 (ST 41), stomach;
large intestine, gēng xū 庚戌, **Qū Chí** 曲池 (LI 11) is true;

Rén zǐ 壬子: qì adopts the triple burner lodging; the well point,
Guān Chōng 關衝 (SJ 1), is a flake of gold [metal];

Guān Chōng 關衝 (SJ 1) belongs to metal, rén 壬 belongs to water;
the child and mother engender each other, bound by deep affection.

癸日亥時井湧泉，乙丑行間穴必然，
丁卯俞穴神門是，本尋腎水太谿原，
包絡大陵原並過，己巳商邱內踝邊，
辛未肺經合尺澤，癸酉中衝包絡連，
子午截時安定穴，留傳後學莫忘言。

On a Guǐ 癸 Day in a hài 亥 hour: the well point, **Yǒng Quán** 湧泉 (KI 1);
in yǐ chǒu 乙丑, **Xíng Jiān** 行間 (LV 2) must be like this;

Dīng Mǎo 丁卯: the stream point is **Shén Mén** 神門 (HT 7);
seek its root, kidney water, **Tài Xī** 太谿 (KI 3), the source point;

The pericardium passes through the source, **Dà Líng** 大陵 (PC 7);
jǐ sì 己巳: **Shāng Qiū** 商邱 (SP 5) to the side of the medial malleolus;

Xīn wèi 辛未: the lung channel uniting point, **Chǐ Zé** 尺澤 (LU 5);
guǐ yǒu 癸酉 links with **Zhōng Chōng** 中衝 (PC 9), pericardium.

Midnight and noon (zǐ wǔ 子午) cut the hours in two
and place the points in position.
The teachings are transmitted.
Afterwards study and do not forget the words.

Translator's note:
The table on the following pages summarizes the open points during the ten day cycle. The sequences for yīn days have a grey background. The hour with the same stem as the day begins the sequence. This hour stem has a box around it to highlight its importance.

Note that open points belong to the channel with the same element and yīn-yáng polarity as the stem of its hour. Exceptions to this are the source point in the third step of the sequence and the triple burner or pericardium point in the last step of the sequence.

Yīn hours on yáng day sequences or yáng hours on yīn day sequences have no open point in this system.

As to how one figure out the day stem for a given day, please see the appendix on the Stems, Branches, and the Chinese calendar.

Open Points for the Method of Adopting the Stems										
	Jiǎ 甲 Day		Yǐ 乙 Day		Bǐng 丙 Day		Dīng 丁 Day		Wù 戊 Day	
Time	Hour	Point	Hour	Point	Hour	Point	Hour	Point	Hour	Point
11 pm-1 am	Jiǎ Zǐ 甲子		Bǐng Zǐ 丙子	SI 2	Wù Zǐ 戊子		Gēng Zǐ 庚子	LI 3, SI 4	Rén Zǐ 壬子	
1-3 am	Yǐ Chǒu 乙丑	LV 2	Dīng Chǒu 丁丑		Jǐ Chǒu 己丑	SP 3, LV 3	Xīn Chǒu 辛丑		Guǐ Chǒu 癸丑	KI 7
3-5 am	Bǐng Yín 丙寅		Wù Yín 戊寅	ST 43, GB 40	Gēng Yín 庚寅		Rén Yín 壬寅	UB 60	Jiǎ Yín 甲寅	
5-7 am	Dīng Mǎo 丁卯	HT 7, KI 3, PC 7	Jǐ Mǎo 己卯		Xīn Mǎo 辛卯	LU 8	Guǐ Mǎo 癸卯		Yǐ Mǎo 乙卯	LV 8
7-9 am	Wù Chén 戊辰		Gēng Chén 庚辰	LI 5	Rén Chén 壬辰		Jiǎ Chén 甲辰	GB 34	Bǐng Chén 丙辰	
9-11 am	Jǐ Sì 己巳	SP 5	Xīn Sì 辛巳		Guǐ Sì 癸巳	KI 10	Yǐ Sì 乙巳		Dīng Sì 丁巳	PC 7
11 am-1 pm	Gēng Wǔ 庚午		Rén Wǔ 壬午	UB 40	Jiǎ Wǔ 甲午		Bǐng Wǔ 丙午	SJ 3	Wù Wǔ 戊午	ST 45
1-3 pm	Xīn Wèi 辛未	LU 5	Guǐ Wèi 癸未		Yǐ Wèi 乙未	PC 8	Dīng Wèi 丁未	HT 9	Jǐ Wèi 己未	
3-5 pm	Rén Shēn 壬申		Jiǎ Shēn 甲申	SJ 2	Bǐng Shēn 丙申	SI 1	Wù Shēn 戊申		Gēng Shēn 庚申	LI 2
5-7 pm	Guǐ Yǒu 癸酉	PC 9	Yǐ Yǒu 乙酉	LV 1	Dīng Yǒu 丁酉		Jǐ Yǒu 己酉	SP 2	Xīn Yǒu 辛酉	
7-9 pm	Jiǎ Xū 甲戌	GB 44	Bǐng Xū 丙戌		Wù Xū 戊戌	ST 44	Gēng Xū 庚戌		Rén Xū 壬戌	UB 65, ST 42
9-11 pm	Yǐ Hài 乙亥		Dīng Hài 丁亥	HT 8	Jǐ Hài 己亥		Xīn Hài 辛亥	LU 9	Guǐ Hài 癸亥	

Note: Correct for Daylight Savings Time, if necessary.

Open Points for the Method of Adopting the Stems

Time	Jǐ 己 Day Hour	Point	Gēng 庚 Day Hour	Point	Xīn 辛 Day Hour	Point	Rén 壬 Day Hour	Point	Guǐ 癸 Day Hour	Point
11 pm–1 am	Jiǎ Zǐ 甲子	GB 38	Bǐng Zǐ 丙子		Wù Zǐ 戊子	ST 36	Gēng Zǐ 庚子		Rén Zǐ 壬子	SJ 1
1–3 am	Yǐ Chǒu 乙丑		Dīng Chǒu 丁丑	HT 3	Jǐ Chǒu 己丑		Xīn Chǒu 辛丑	PC 3	Guǐ Chǒu 癸丑	x
3–5 am	Bǐng Yín 丙寅	SI 8	Wù Yín 戊寅		Gēng Yín 庚寅	SJ 10	Rén Yín 壬寅	UB 67	Jiǎ Yín 甲寅	x
5–7 am	Dīng Mǎo 丁卯		Jǐ Mǎo 己卯	PC 5	Xīn Mǎo 辛卯	LU 11	Guǐ Mǎo 癸卯		Yǐ Mǎo 乙卯	x
7–9 am	Wù Chén 戊辰	SJ 6	Gēng Chén 庚辰	LI 1	Rén Chén 壬辰		Jiǎ Chén 甲辰	GB 43	Bǐng Chén 丙辰	x
9–11 am	Jǐ Sì 己巳	SP 1	Xīn Sì 辛巳		Guǐ Sì 癸巳	KI 2	Yǐ Sì 乙巳		Dīng Sì 丁巳	x
11 am–1 pm	Gēng Wǔ 庚午		Rén Wǔ 壬午	UB 66	Jiǎ Wǔ 甲午		Bǐng Wǔ 丙午	SI 3, UB 64, SJ 4	Wù Wǔ 戊午	x
1–3 pm	Xīn Wèi 辛未	LU 10	Guǐ Wèi 癸未		Yǐ Wèi 乙未	LV 3, LU 9	Dīng Wèi 丁未		Jǐ Wèi 己未	x
3–5 pm	Rén Shēn 壬申		Jiǎ Shēn 甲申	GB 41, LI 4	Bǐng Shēn 丙申		Wù Shēn 戊申	ST 41	Gēng Shēn 庚申	x
5–7 pm	Guǐ Yǒu 癸酉	KI 3, SP 3	Yǐ Yǒu 乙酉		Dīng Yǒu 丁酉	HT 4	Jǐ Yǒu 己酉		Xīn Yǒu 辛酉	x
7–9 pm	Jiǎ Xū 甲戌		Bǐng Xū 丙戌	SI 5	Wù Xū 戊戌		Gēng Xū 庚戌	LI 11	Rén Xū 壬戌	x
9–11 pm	Yǐ Hài 乙亥	LV 4	Dīng Hài 丁亥		Jǐ Hài 己亥	SP 9	Xīn Hài 辛亥		Guǐ Hài 癸亥	KI 1

Note: Correct for Daylight Savings Time, if necessary.

針灸大成 · 卷之五

49

十二經納天干歌（以下俱徐氏）
Song of the Twelve Channels Adopting the Heavenly Stems (from here down is all from Master Xú[28])

甲膽乙肝丙小腸，丁心戊胃己脾鄉，
庚屬大腸辛屬肺，壬屬膀胱癸腎藏，
三焦亦向壬中寄，包絡同歸入癸方。

Jiǎ 甲 is gall bladder, yǐ 乙 is liver, bǐng 丙 is small intestine,
Dīng 丁 is heart, wù 戊 is stomach, jǐ 己 is the spleen's home town,
Gēng 庚 belongs to large intestine, xīn 辛 belongs to lungs,
Rén 壬 belongs to urinary bladder, guǐ 癸 is the kidney viscus,
Triple burner also turns into rén 壬 for lodging,
Pericardium similarly returns into the guǐ 癸 direction.

十二經納地支歌
Twelve Channels Appoint the Earthly Branches Song

肺寅大卯胃辰宮，脾巳心午小未中，
申胱酉腎心包戌，亥焦子膽丑肝通。

The lungs are yín 寅 [branch], large [intestine] is mǎo 卯,
stomach is the chén 辰 palace,
The spleen is sì 巳, heart is wǔ 午,
small [intestine] is in wèi 未,
Shēn 申 is bladder, yǒu 酉 is kidneys,
pericardium is xū 戌,
Hài 亥 is [triple] burner, zǐ 子 is gall bladder,
and chǒu 丑 communicates with the liver.

28. Xú Fèng 徐鳳 published *Zhēn Jiǔ Dà Quán* 《針灸大全》(Great Completion of Acupuncture-Moxibustion) in 1439 (*Míng*). This and the next poem are from Volume 3.

針
灸
大
成
·
卷
之
五

腳不過膝手不過肘歌

The Legs Do Not Go Past the Knees; The Arms Do Not Go Past the Elbows Song[29]

陽日陽時氣在前，血在後兮脈在邊，
陰日陰時血在前，氣在後兮脈歸原。
陽日陽時針左轉，先取陽經脈病看，
陰日陰時針右轉，行屬陰經臟腑痊。

**On yáng days at yáng hours, qì exists first;
blood exists after, and the vessels exist on the periphery,
On yīn days at yīn hours, blood exists first;
qì exists after,[30] and the vessels return to the source.
On yáng days at yáng hours, rotate the needle to the left;
first apply treatment to the yáng channel-vessels when disease is seen,
On yīn days at yīn hours, rotate the needle to the right;
this movement belongs to the yīn channels.
The viscera and bowels will recover.**

Translator's notes: In the next section, Yáng mentions a relationship the heavenly stems have with each other. This relationship is called the Five Unities.

The Five Unities (五合)							
This stem		unites with this stem		This stem		unites with this stem	
1	jiǎ 甲	6	jǐ 己	6	jǐ 己	1	jiǎ 甲
2	yǐ 乙	7	gēng 庚	7	gēng 庚	2	yǐ 乙
3	bǐng 丙	8	xīn 辛	8	xīn 辛	3	bǐng 丙
4	dīng 丁	9	rén 壬	9	rén 壬	4	dīng 丁
5	wù 戊	10	guǐ 癸	10	guǐ 癸	5	wù 戊

Note that each stem unites with the stem that is five positions away. This relationship is called the

---

29. From *Zhēn Jiǔ Jù Yīng*《針灸聚英》(Gatherings from Eminent Acupuncturists) by Gāo Wǔ 高武, published in 1529 (*Míng*). This poem is from Volume 4. The title reminds us that the five transport points are all distal to the elbows and knees.

30. Later in this volume, it says, "On yáng days qì moves first and blood follows after it. On yīn days, blood moves first and qì follows after it."

five unities because there are five pairs of stems. In the table above, the last five unities are repeats of the first five. The importance of this relationship will be seen later.

In the section below, all the yáng channels are said to guide the movement of qì. All the yīn channels are said to guide the movement of blood.

Each of the ten days in the 'week' of ten stems is addressed in order. The stem and branch of the time periods with open points are given. Then the text says which point is open, but the point is listed by its category, not its name. It is basically giving the same information as in the table called *"Open Points for the Method of Adopting the Stems,"* above.

流注圖
Flowing and Pooling Diagrams[31]

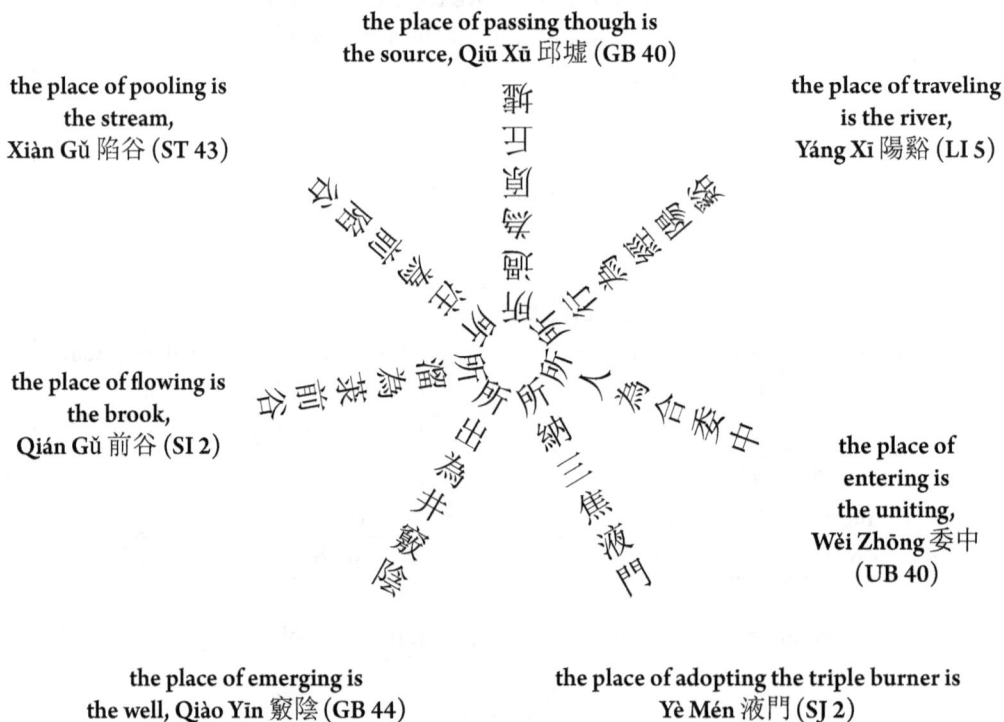

the place of passing though is the source, Qiū Xū 邱墟 (GB 40)

the place of pooling is the stream, Xiàn Gǔ 陷谷 (ST 43)

the place of traveling is the river, Yáng Xī 陽谿 (LI 5)

the place of flowing is the brook, Qián Gǔ 前谷 (SI 2)

the place of entering is the uniting, Wěi Zhōng 委中 (UB 40)

the place of emerging is the well, Qiào Yīn 竅陰 (GB 44)

the place of adopting the triple burner is Yè Mén 液門 (SJ 2)

---

31. This is from Xú Fèng's 徐鳳 *Zhēn Jiǔ Dà Quán* 《針灸大全》(Great Completion of Acu-puncture-Moxibustion). This section is from Volume 3.

足少陽膽之經:甲主,與己合,膽引氣行 。
甲日:甲戌時開膽為井金 。
　　丙子時:小腸滎水 。
　　戊寅時:胃俞木,并過膽原邱墟,木原在寅 。
　　庚辰時:大腸經火 。
　　壬午時:膀胱合土 。
　　甲申時:氣納三焦之滎水,甲屬木,是以水生木,子母相生 。

Foot shàoyáng gall bladder channel: Jiǎ 甲 governs it; jiǎ unites with jǐ 己.
The gall bladder guides the movement of qì.

Jiǎ 甲 *day:* The jiǎ xū 甲戌 hour opens the gall bladder as the well point, metal.

> **Bǐng zǐ** 丙子 hour: small intestine, brook point, water.

> **Wù yín** 戊寅 hour: stomach, stream point, wood; at the same time passing through the gall bladder source point, Qiū Xū 邱墟 (GB 40). The wood source is located in the yín 寅 [branch].

> **Gēng chén** 庚辰 hour: large intestine, river point, fire.

> **Rén wǔ** 壬午 hour: urinary bladder, uniting point, earth.

> **Jiǎ shēn** 甲申 hour: qì adopts the brook point of the triple burner, water. Jiǎ 甲 belongs to wood. This uses water to engender wood. The son and mother engender each other.

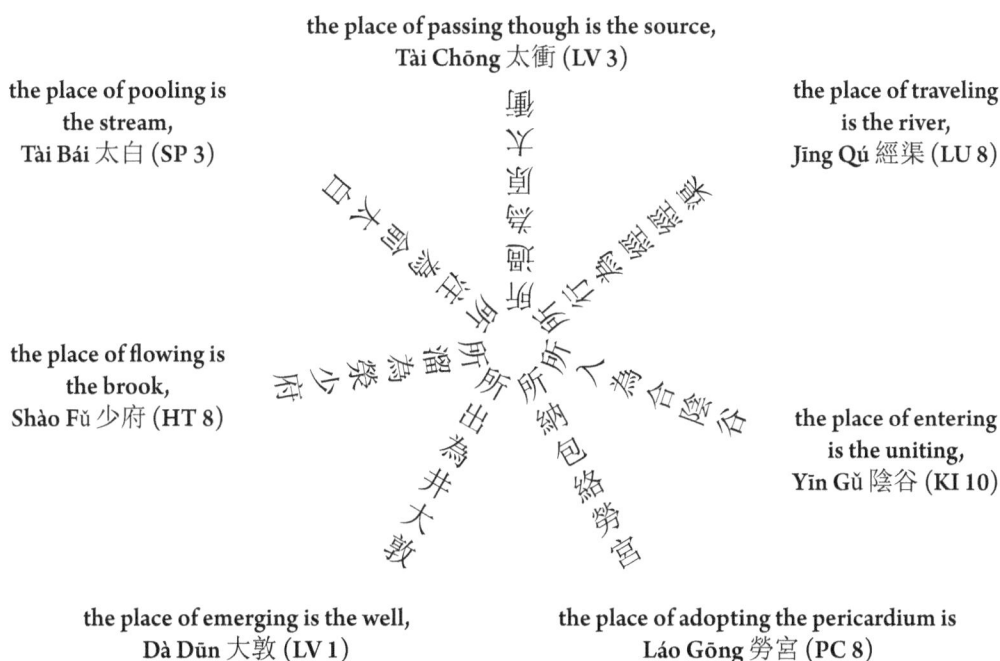

the place of passing though is the source,
Tài Chōng 太衝 (LV 3)

the place of pooling is
the stream,
Tài Bái 太白 (SP 3)

the place of traveling
is the river,
Jīng Qú 經渠 (LU 8)

the place of flowing is
the brook,
Shào Fǔ 少府 (HT 8)

the place of entering
is the uniting,
Yīn Gǔ 陰谷 (KI 10)

the place of emerging is the well,
Dà Dūn 大敦 (LV 1)

the place of adopting the pericardium is
Láo Gōng 勞宮 (PC 8)

足厥陰肝之經：乙主，與庚合，肝引血行 。
乙日：乙酉時開肝為井木 。
　　　丁亥時：心滎火 。
　　　己丑時：脾俞土，并過肝原 。
　　　辛卯時：肺經金 。
　　　癸巳時：腎合水 。
　　　乙未時：血納包絡之滎火，乙屬木，是以木生火也 。

Foot juéyīn liver channel: Yǐ 乙 governs it; yǐ 乙 unites with gēng 庚.
The liver guides the movement of blood.

Yǐ 乙 day: The yǐ yǒu 乙酉 hour opens the liver as the well point, wood.

　　　Dīng hài 丁亥 hour: heart, brook point, fire.
　　　Ji chǒu 己丑 hour: spleen, stream point, earth; at the same time passing
　　　　　through the liver source point.
　　　Xīn mǎo 辛卯 hour: lung, river point, metal.
　　　Guǐ sì 癸巳 hour: kidney, uniting point, water.
　　　Yǐ wèi 乙未 hour: blood adopts the brook point of the pericardium, fire. Yǐ
　　　　　belongs to wood. This uses wood to engender fire.

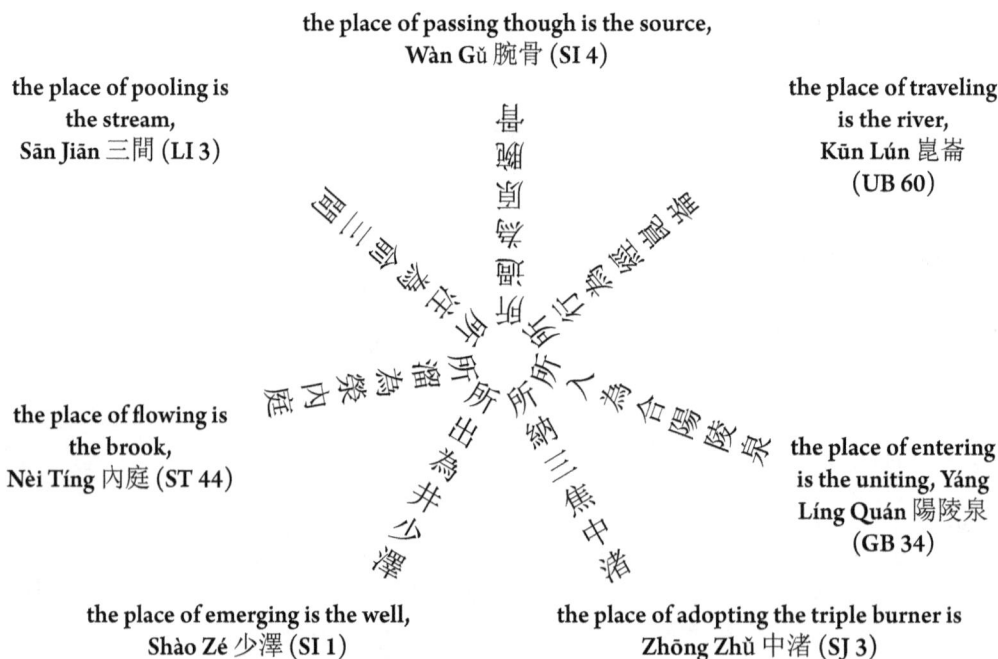

the place of passing though is the source,
Wàn Gǔ 腕骨 (SI 4)

the place of pooling is
the stream,
Sān Jiān 三間 (LI 3)

the place of traveling
is the river,
Kūn Lún 崑崙
(UB 60)

the place of flowing is
the brook,
Nèi Tíng 内庭 (ST 44)

the place of entering
is the uniting, Yáng
Líng Quán 陽陵泉
(GB 34)

the place of emerging is the well,
Shào Zé 少澤 (SI 1)

the place of adopting the triple burner is
Zhōng Zhǔ 中渚 (SJ 3)

手太陽小腸經：丙主，與辛合，小腸引氣行 。
丙日：丙申時開小腸井金 。
　　　戊戌時：胃滎水 。
　　　庚子時：大腸俞木，並過小腸原 。
　　　壬寅時：膀胱經火 。
　　　甲辰時：膽合土 。
　　　丙午時：氣納三焦之俞木，丙屬火，是以木生火也 。

Hand tàiyáng small intestine channel: Bǐng 丙 governs it; bǐng unites with xīn 辛. The small intestine guides the movement of qì.

Bǐng 丙 *day:* The bǐng shēn 丙申 hour opens the small intestine as the well point, metal.

　　　Wù xū 戊戌 hour: stomach, brook point, water.
　　　Gēng zǐ 庚子 hour: large intestine, stream point, wood; at the same time passing through the small intestine source point.
　　　Rén yín 壬寅 hour: urinary bladder, river point, fire.
　　　Jiǎ chén 甲辰 hour: gall bladder, uniting point, earth.
　　　Bǐng wǔ 丙午 hour: qì adopts the stream point of the triple burner, wood. Bǐng belongs to fire. This uses wood to engender fire.

the place of passing though is the source,
Shén Mén 神門 (HT 7)

the place of pooling is
the stream,
Tài Yuān 太淵 (LU 9)

the place of traveling
is the river,
Fù Liū 復溜 (KI 7)

the place of flowing is
the brook,
Dà Dū 大都 (SP 2)

the place of entering
is the uniting,
Qū Quán 曲泉
(LV 8)

the place of emerging is the well,
Shào Chōng 少衝 (HT 9)

the place of adopting the pericardium is
Dà Líng 大陵 (PC 7)

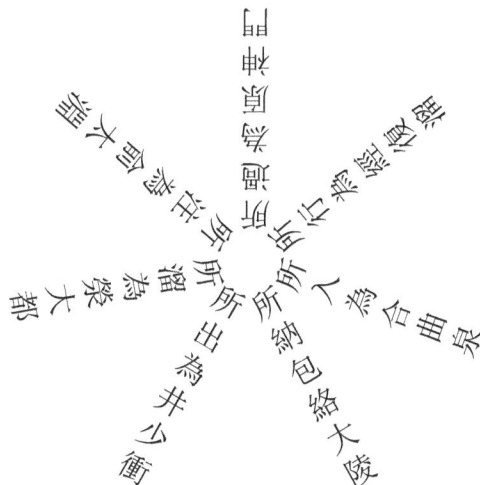

手少陰心之經：丁主，與壬合，心引血行。
丁日：丁未時開心為井木。
　　己酉時：脾滎火。
　　辛亥時：肺俞土，并過心原。
　　癸丑時：腎經金。
　　乙卯時：肝合水。
　　丁巳時：血納包絡之俞土，丁屬火，是以火生土也。

Hand shàoyīn heart channel: Dīng 丁 governs it; dīng unites with rén 壬.
The heart guides the movement of blood.

> Dīng 丁 day: The dīng wèi 丁未 hour opens the heart as the well point, wood.
> Jǐ yǒu 己酉 hour: spleen, brook point, fire.
> Xīn hài 辛亥 hour: lung, stream point, earth; at the same time passing
> 　　through the heart source point.
> Guǐ chǒu 癸丑 hour: kidney, river point, metal
> Yǐ mǎo 乙卯 hour: liver, uniting point, water.
> Dīng sì 丁巳 hour: blood adopts the stream point of the pericardium, earth.
> 　　Dīng belongs to fire. This uses fire to engender earth.

the place of passing though is the source,
Chōng Yáng 衝陽 (ST 42)

the place of pooling is
the stream,
Shù Gǔ 束骨 (UB 65)

the place of traveling
is the river,
Yáng Fǔ 陽輔
(GB 38)

the place of flowing is
the brook,
Èr Jiān 二間 (LI 2)

the place of entering
is the uniting,
Xiǎo Hǎi 小海 (SI 8)

the place of emerging is the well,
Lì Duì 厲兌 (ST 45)

the place of adopting the triple burner is
Zhī Gōu 支溝 (SJ 6)

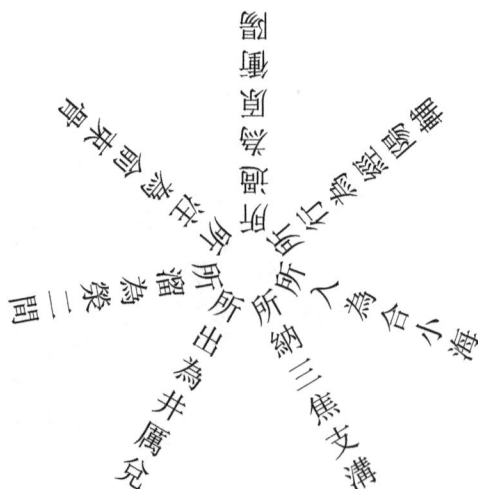

56

足陽明胃之經：戊主，與癸合，胃引氣行 。
戊日：戊午時開胃為井金 。
　　庚申時：大腸滎水 。
　　壬戌時：膀胱俞木，并過胃原 。
　　甲子時：膽經火 。
　　丙寅時：小腸合土 。
　　戊辰時：氣納三焦之經火，戊屬土，是以火生土也 。

Foot yángmíng stomach channel: **Wù** 戊 governs it; **wù** unites with **guǐ** 癸.
The stomach guides the movement of **qì**.

Wù day: The **wù wǔ** 戊午 hour opens the stomach as the well point, metal.
　　Gēng shēn 庚申 hour: large intestine, brook point, water.
　　Rén xū 壬戌 hour: urinary bladder, stream point, wood; at the same time
　　　　passing through the stomach source point.
　　Jiǎ zǐ 甲子 hour: gall bladder, river point, fire.
　　Bǐng yín 丙寅 hour: small intestine, uniting point, earth.
　　Wù chén 戊辰 hour: **qì** adopts the river point of the triple burner, fire. **Wù** 戊
　　　　[stem] belongs to earth. This uses fire to engender earth.

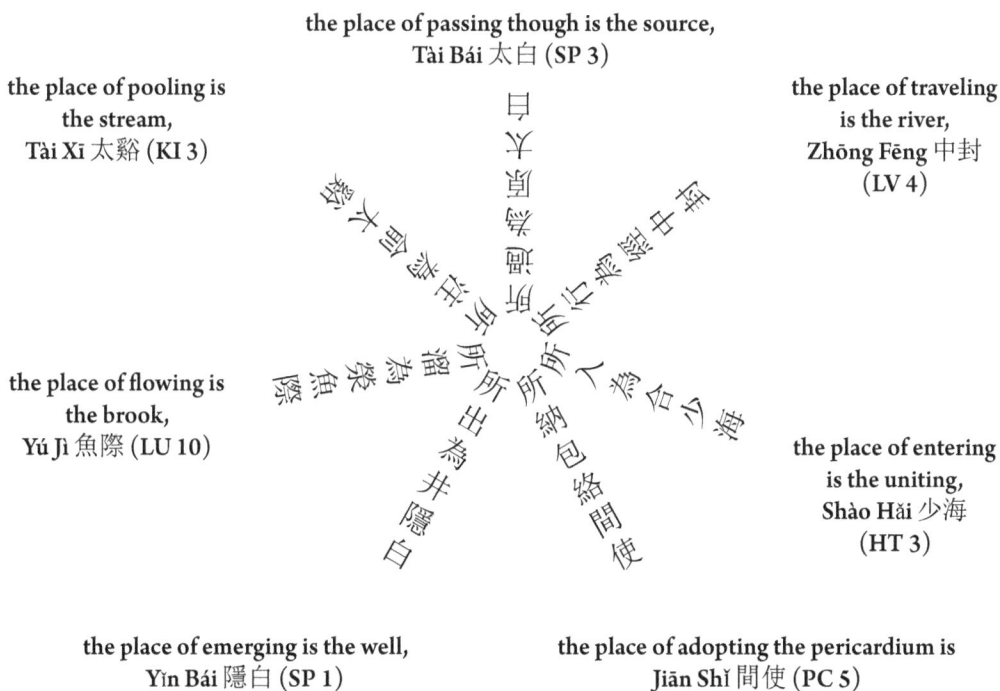

the place of passing though is the source,
Tài Bái 太白 (SP 3)

the place of pooling is
the stream,
Tài Xī 太谿 (KI 3)

the place of traveling
is the river,
Zhōng Fēng 中封
(LV 4)

the place of flowing is
the brook,
Yú Jì 魚際 (LU 10)

the place of entering
is the uniting,
Shào Hǎi 少海
(HT 3)

the place of emerging is the well,
Yǐn Bái 隱白 (SP 1)

the place of adopting the pericardium is
Jiān Shǐ 間使 (PC 5)

足太陰脾之經：己主，與甲合，脾引血行 。
己日：己巳時開脾為井木 。
　　　辛未時：肺滎火 。
　　　癸酉時：腎俞土，并過脾原 。
　　　乙亥時：肝經金 。
　　　丁丑時：心合水 。
　　　己卯時：血納包絡之經金，己屬土，是以土生金也 。

Foot tàiyīn spleen channel: Jǐ 己 governs it; jǐ unites with jiǎ 甲.
The spleen guides the movement of blood.

Ji day: The jǐ sì 己巳 hour opens the spleen as the well point, wood.
　　　Xīn wèi 辛未 hour: lung, brook point, fire.
　　　Guǐ yǒu 癸酉 hour: kidney, stream point, earth; at the same time passing
　　　　　through the spleen source point.
　　　Yǐ hài 乙亥 hour: liver, river point, metal.
　　　Dīng chǒu 丁丑 hour: heart, uniting point, water.
　　　Jǐ mǎo 己卯 hour: blood adopts the river point of the pericardium, metal. Jǐ
　　　　　belongs to earth. This uses earth to engender metal.

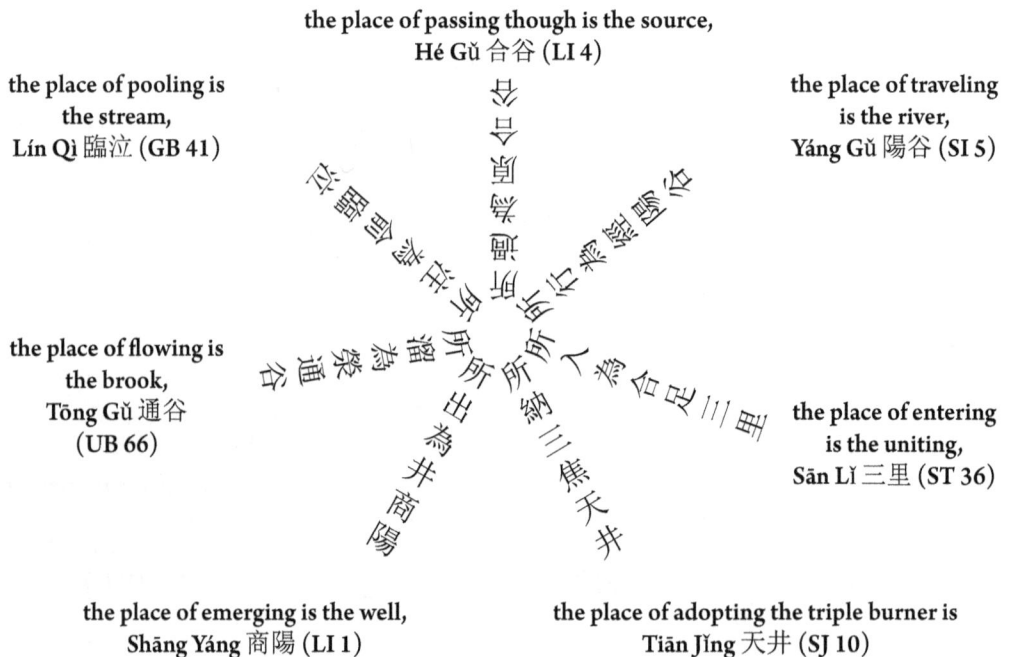

the place of passing though is the source,
Hé Gǔ 合谷 (LI 4)

the place of pooling is
the stream,
Lín Qì 臨泣 (GB 41)

the place of traveling
is the river,
Yáng Gǔ 陽谷 (SI 5)

the place of flowing is
the brook,
Tōng Gǔ 通谷
(UB 66)

the place of entering
is the uniting,
Sān Lǐ 三里 (ST 36)

the place of emerging is the well,
Shāng Yáng 商陽 (LI 1)

the place of adopting the triple burner is
Tiān Jǐng 天井 (SJ 10)

58

手陽明大腸經:庚主，與乙合，大腸引氣行。

庚日:庚辰時開大腸井金。

　　壬午時:膀胱滎水。

　　甲申時:膽俞木，並過大腸原。

　　丙戌時:小腸經火。

　　戊子時:胃合土。

　　庚寅時:氣納三焦之合土，庚屬金，是以土生金也。

Hand yángmíng large intestine channel: Gēng 庚 governs it; gēng unites with yǐ 乙. The large intestine guides the movement of qì.

Gēng 庚 *day*: The gēng chén 庚辰 hour opens the large intestine well point, metal.

　　Rén wǔ 壬午 hour: urinary bladder, brook point, water.

　　Jiǎ shēn 甲申 hour: gall bladder, stream point, wood; at the same time
　　　　passing through the large intestine source point.

　　Bǐng xū 丙戌 hour: small intestine, river point, fire.

　　Wù zǐ 戊子 hour: stomach, uniting point, earth.

　　Gēng yín 庚寅 hour: qì adopts the uniting point of the triple burner, earth.
　　　　Gēng belongs to metal. This uses earth to engender metal.

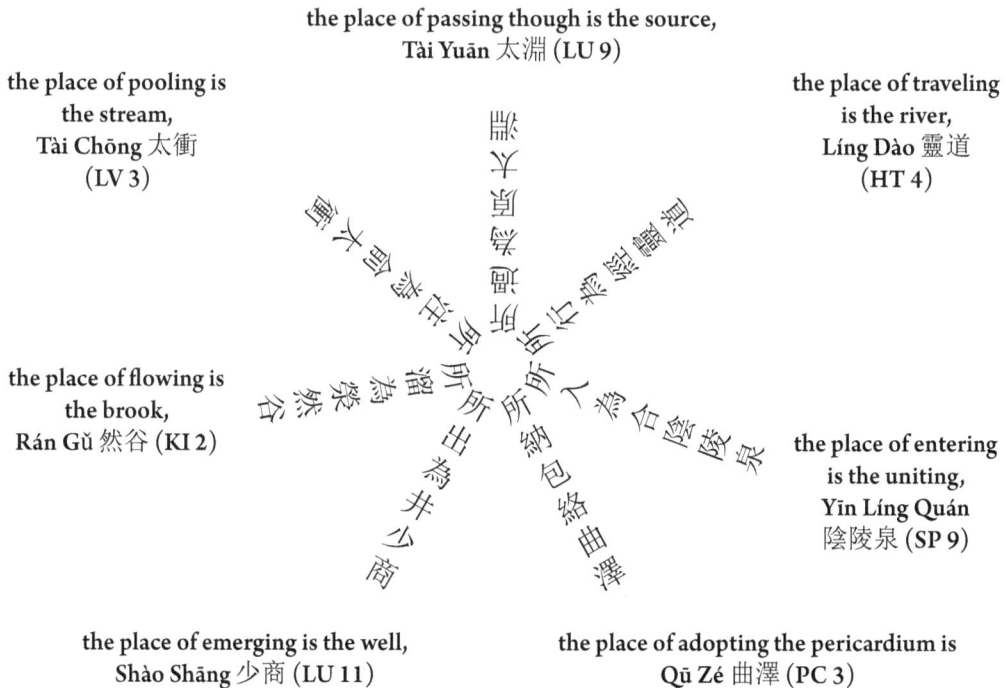

the place of passing though is the source,
Tài Yuān 太淵 (LU 9)

the place of pooling is
the stream,
Tài Chōng 太衝
(LV 3)

the place of traveling
is the river,
Líng Dào 靈道
(HT 4)

the place of flowing is
the brook,
Rán Gǔ 然谷 (KI 2)

the place of entering
is the uniting,
Yīn Líng Quán
陰陵泉 (SP 9)

the place of emerging is the well,
Shào Shāng 少商 (LU 11)

the place of adopting the pericardium is
Qū Zé 曲澤 (PC 3)

手太陰肺之經：辛主，與丙合，肺引血行 。
辛日：辛卯時開肺為井木 。
　　癸巳時：腎滎火 。
　　己未時：肝俞土，并過肺原 。
　　丁酉時：心經金 。
　　己亥時：脾合水 。
　　辛丑時：血納包絡之合水，辛屬金，是以金生水也 。

Hand tàiyīn lung channel: Xīn 辛 governs it; xīn unites with bǐng 丙.
The lungs guide the movement of blood.

Xīn 辛 *day:* The xīn mǎo 辛卯 hour opens the lungs as the well point, wood.

　　Guǐ sì 癸巳 hour: kidney, brook point, fire.

　　Jǐ wèi 己未 hour: liver, stream point, earth; at the same time passing through
　　　　the lung source point.

　　Dīng yǒu 丁酉 hour: heart, river point, metal.

　　Jǐ hài 己亥 hour: spleen, uniting point, water.

　　Xīn chǒu 辛丑 hour: blood adopts the uniting point of the pericardium,
　　　　water. Xīn belongs to metal. This uses metal to engender water.

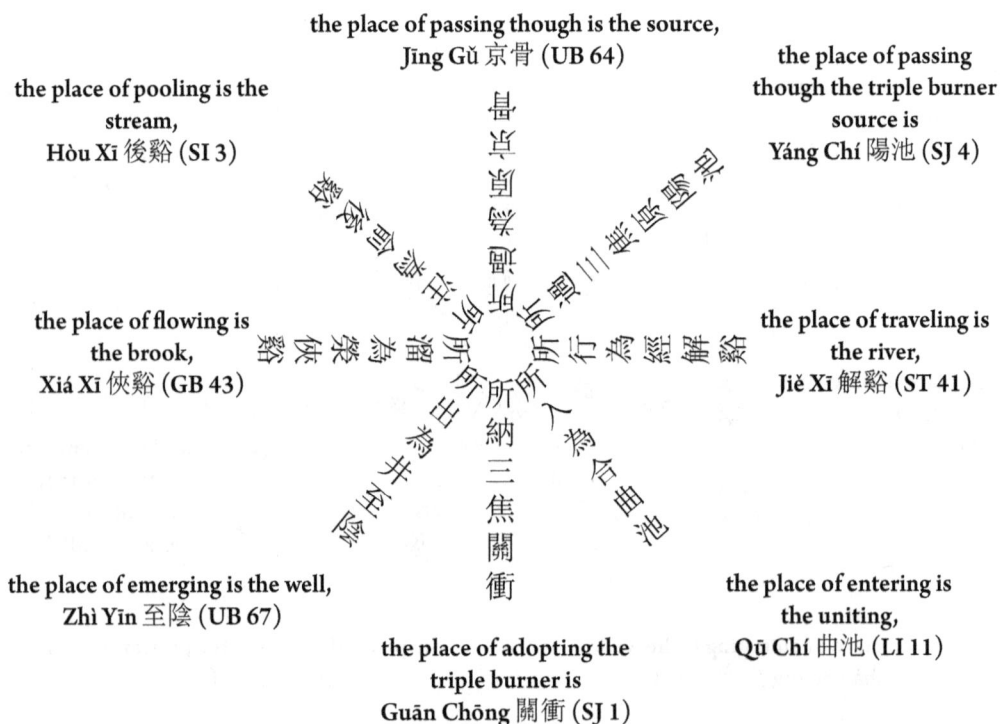

the place of passing though is the source,
Jīng Gǔ 京骨 (UB 64)

the place of passing though the triple burner source is
Yáng Chí 陽池 (SJ 4)

the place of pooling is the stream,
Hòu Xī 後谿 (SI 3)

the place of flowing is the brook,
Xiá Xī 俠谿 (GB 43)

the place of traveling is the river,
Jiě Xī 解谿 (ST 41)

the place of emerging is the well,
Zhì Yīn 至陰 (UB 67)

the place of entering is the uniting,
Qū Chí 曲池 (LI 11)

the place of adopting the triple burner is
Guān Chōng 關衝 (SJ 1)

針灸大成 · 卷之五

足太陽膀胱經:壬主,與丁合,膀胱引氣行。
壬日:壬寅時開膀胱井金。
　　甲辰時:膽滎水。
　　丙午時:小腸俞木,所過本原京骨,本原在午,水入火鄉。故壬丙子
　　午相交也。兼過三焦之原陽池。
　　戊申時:胃經火。
　　庚戌時:大腸合土。
　　壬子時:氣納三焦井金。

Foot tàiyáng urinary bladder channel: Rén 壬 governs it; rén unites with dīng 丁. The urinary bladder guides the movement of qì.

Rén 壬 day: The rén yín 壬寅 hour opens the urinary bladder well point, metal.

> Jiǎ chén 甲辰 hour: gall bladder, brook point, water.

> Bǐng wǔ 丙午 hour: small intestine, stream point, wood. The place of passing through is the root [channel's] source point, Jīng Gǔ 京骨 (UB 64). The root [channel] source [point] is located in the wǔ 午 hour.[32] Water enters fire's homeland.[33] Thus rén 壬, bǐng 丙, zǐ 子, and wǔ 午 meet each other.[34] At the same time, the source point of the triple burner, Yáng Chí 陽池 (SJ 4) passes through. [35]

> Wù shēn 戊申 hour: stomach, river point, fire.

> Gēng xū 庚戌 hour: large intestine, uniting point, earth.

> Rén zǐ 壬子 hour: qì adopts the well point of the triple burner, metal.

---

32. "本原在午 The root [channel] source [point] is located in the wǔ 午 hour." The source text for this section, the *Great Completion of Acupuncture-Moxibustion* has instead "水原在午 The water source [point] is located in the wǔ hour." Here water refers to the urinary bladder channel. Other editions of the *Great Compendium* have "木原在午 The wood source [point] is located in the wǔ hour," but this must be an error.

33. Water enters fire's homeland: both bǐng 丙 and wù 戊 (the time period stem and branch) are yáng fire. The urinary bladder source point is used at this time, the source point of the yáng water channel.

34. Thus rén 壬, bǐng 丙, zǐ 子, and wù 午 meet each other: Bǐng and wù (branch) are both yáng fire. Rén and zǐ are both yáng water. This is a bǐng wù 丙午 hour on a rén 壬 day. The urinary bladder is yáng water, just like the zǐ branch. In addition, later, the last time period of the rén day sequence is the rén zǐ 壬子 hour. The meeting of the fire and water stems and branches is stressed because the communication of fire and water has the image of harmony between yīn and yáng.

35. Rén 壬 and guǐ 癸 are associated with the urinary bladder and kidneys by element. However, they also are associated with the triple burner and pericardium respectively. Therefore, an additional source point opens at this time on rén and guǐ days.

the place of passing though is the source,
Tài Xī 太谿 (KI 3)

the place of pooling is
the stream,
Shén Mén 神門 (HT 7)

the place of passing
through the pericardium
source is
Dà Líng 大陵 (PC 7)

the place of flowing is
the brook,
Xíng Jiān 行間 (LV 2)

the place of traveling is
the river,
Shāng Qiū 商邱 (SP 5)

the place of emerging is the well,
Yǒng Quán 湧泉 (KI 1)

the place of entering is
the uniting,
Chǐ Zé 尺澤 (LU 5)

the place of adopting the
pericardium is
Zhōng Chōng 中衝 (PC 9)

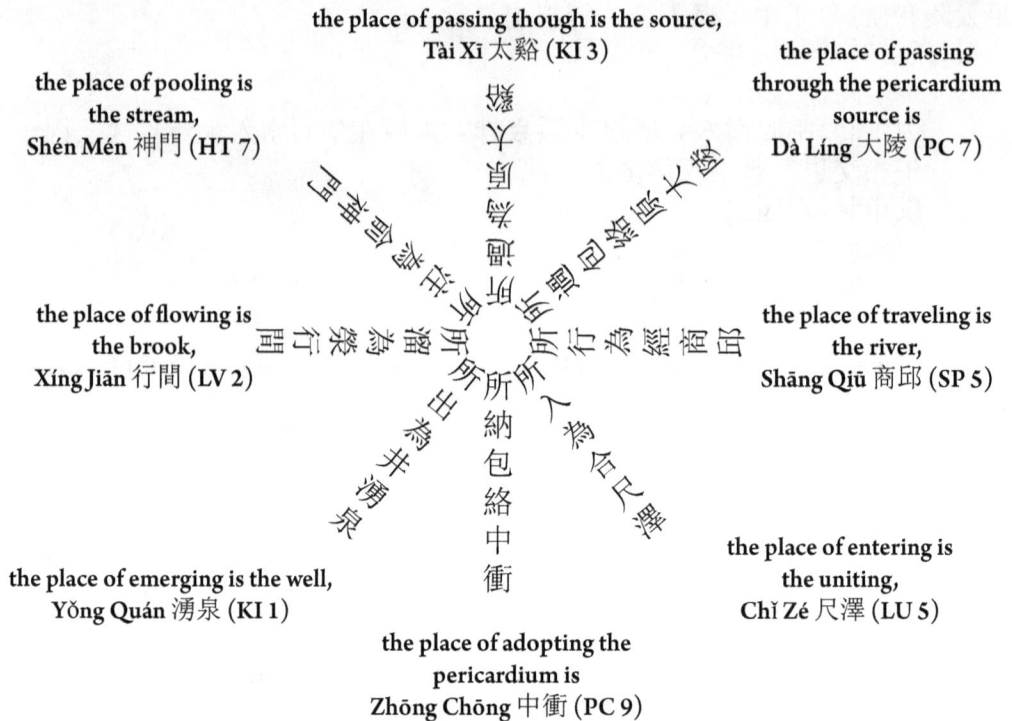

足少陰腎之經：癸主，與戊合，腎引血行。
癸日：癸亥時開腎為井木。
　　　乙丑時：肝滎火。
　　　丁卯時：心俞土，并過腎原太谿，又過包絡原大陵。
　　　己巳時：脾經金。
　　　辛未時：肺合水。
　　　癸酉時：血納包絡之井木，謂水生木也。

Foot shàoyīn kidney channel: Guǐ 癸 governs it; guǐ unites with wù 戊.
The kidneys guide the movement of blood.

Guǐ 癸 day: The guǐ hài 癸亥 hour opens the kidney as the well point, wood.
　　　Yǐ chǒu 乙丑 hour: liver, brook point, fire.
　　　Dīng mǎo 丁卯 hour: heart, stream point, earth; at the same time passing
　　　　　through the kidney source point, Tài Xī 太谿 (KI 3). It also
　　　　　passes through the pericardium source point, Dà Líng 大陵 (PC 7).
　　　Jǐ sì 己巳 hour: spleen, river point, metal.
　　　Xīn wèi 辛未 hour: lungs, uniting point, water.
　　　Guǐ yǒu 癸酉 hour: blood adopts the well point of the pericardium, wood.
　　　This is called water engendering wood.

針灸大成・卷之五

論子午流注法（徐氏）
Discussion of Midnight-Noon Flowing and Pooling Method (Master Xú[36])

子午流注者，謂剛柔相配，陰陽相合，氣血循環，時穴開闔也。何以子午言之？曰：子時一刻，乃一陽之生；至午時一刻，乃一陰之生，故以子午分之，而得乎中也。流者往也。注者住也。

Midnight-noon (*zǐ-wǔ* 子午) flowing and pooling is called hard and soft matching up, yīn and yáng uniting, qì and blood following in a ring, hours and points opening and shutting.

How do we explain zǐ (midnight) and wǔ (noon)? It is said: The zǐ hour is the birth of the first yáng. The arrival of the wǔ hour is the birth of the first yīn. This is why zǐ and wǔ divide it [the day] and result in the center.

Flowing (*liú* 流) means to depart. Pooling (*zhù* 注) means to dwell.

天干有十，經有十二，甲膽、乙肝、丙小腸、丁心、戊胃、己脾、庚大腸、辛肺、壬膀胱、癸腎、餘兩經三焦、包絡也。三焦乃陽氣之父，包絡乃陰血之母。此二經雖寄於壬癸，亦分派於十干，每經之中，有井滎俞經合，以配金水木火土。是故陰井木而陽井金，陰滎火而陽滎水，陰俞土而陽俞木，陰經金而陽經火，陰合水而陽合土。

There are ten heavenly stems. There are twelve channels. Jiǎ 甲 is gall bladder. Yǐ 乙 is liver. Bǐng 丙 is small intestine. Dīng 丁 is heart. Wù 戊 is stomach. Jǐ 己 is spleen. Gēng 庚 is large intestine. Xīn 辛 is lungs. Rén 壬 is urinary bladder. Guǐ 癸 is kidneys. There are two more channels: triple burner and pericardium. Triple burner is the father of yáng qì. Pericardium is the mother of yīn blood. Although these two channels lodge in rén and guǐ, they are also assigned to [all] ten stems.

Within each channel, there are well, brook, stream, river, and uniting points. These are matched with metal, water, wood, fire, and earth. Thus the yīn well point is wood

---

36. Xú Fèng 徐鳳 published *Zhēn Jiǔ Dà Quán*《針灸大全》(Great Completion of Acupuncture-Moxibustion) in 1439 (*Míng*). This is from Volume 3.

and the yáng well point is metal. The yīn brook point is fire and the yáng brook point is water. The yīn stream point is earth and the yáng stream point is wood. The yīn river point is metal and the yáng river point is fire. The yīn uniting point is water and the yáng uniting point is earth.

經中有返本還元者，乃十二經出入之門也。陽經有原，遇俞穴并過之，陰經無原，以俞穴即代之，是以甲出邱墟、乙太衝之例。又按《千金》云：六陰經亦有原穴，乙中都、丁通里、己公孫、辛列缺、癸水泉、包絡內關是也。

Within the channels there is [the principle of] "go back to the root and return to the origin." This is the door of exiting and entering for the twelve channels. Yáng channels have a source point, [found one position] past the stream point. Yīn channels do not have [an additional] source point. They use the stream point to take its place. This uses, for example, jiǎ 甲 going out to Qiū Xū 邱墟 (GB 40) and yǐ 乙 to Tài Chōng 太衝 (LV 3). But note that *Thousand Pieces of Gold*[37] says: The six yīn channels also have source points. Yǐ 乙 is Zhōng Dū 中都 (LV 6). Dīng 丁 is Tōng Lǐ 通里 (HT 5). Jǐ 己 is Gōng Sūn 公孫 (SP 4). Xīn 辛 is Liè Quē 列缺 (LU 7). Guǐ 癸 is Shuǐ Quán 水泉 (KI 5). Pericardium is Nèi Guān 內關 (PC 6).

故陽日氣先行，而血後隨也。陰日血先行，而氣後隨也。得時為之開，失時為之闔。陽干注腑，甲丙戊庚壬而重見者，氣納三焦；陰干注臟，乙丁己辛癸而重見者，血納包絡。如甲日甲戌時，以開膽井，至戊寅時正當胃俞，而又并過膽原，重見甲申時，氣納三焦，滎穴屬水，甲屬木，是以水生木。謂甲合還元化本。

Thus, on yáng days qì moves first and blood follows after it. On yīn days, blood moves first and qì follows after it. When you obtain the [proper] time, regard it as open. When you lose the [proper] time, regard it as closed.

Yáng stems pool in the bowels. When you see jiǎ 甲, bǐng 丙, wù 戊, gēng 庚, or rén 壬 repeat,[38] qì adopts the triple burner. Yīn stems pool in the viscera. When you see yǐ 乙, dīng 丁, jǐ 己, xīn 辛, or guǐ 癸 repeat, blood adopts the pericardium.

---

37. In Volume 29. However, for yǐ (liver), *Thousand Pieces of Gold* lists Zhōng Fēng 中封 (LV 4) not Zhōng Dū 中都 (LV 6).

38. This is referring to the last step in the Midnight-Noon sequence when the stem associated with the day shows up for a second time as the hour stem.

For example, on a jiǎ 甲 day in the jiǎ xū 甲戌 hour, the gall bladder well point is open. When you arrive at the wù yín 戊寅 hour, it is the time for the stomach stream point, and it also passes through the gall bladder source point at the same time. When you see the jiǎ shēn 甲申 hour repeated,[39] qì adopts the triple burner. The brook point belongs to water. Jiǎ 甲 belongs to wood. This uses water to engender wood. This is called jiǎ 甲 uniting to return to the origin and transform the root.

又如乙日乙酉時，以開肝井，至己丑時當脾之俞，並過肝原，重見乙未時，血納包絡榮穴屬火，乙屬木，是以木生火也。餘倣此。俱以子午相生，陰陽相濟也。

Another example: On an yǐ 乙 day in the yǐ yǒu 乙酉 hour, the liver well point is open. When the jǐ chǒu 己丑 hour arrives, it is matched with the stream point of the spleen, and passes though the source point of the liver at the same time. When you see the yǐ wèi 乙未 time repeat, blood adopts the pericardium's brook point, belonging to fire. Yǐ belongs to wood. This uses wood to generate fire.

The rest copies this [pattern]. All of it uses the mutual engenderment of midnight and noon and the mutual aid of yīn and yáng.

陽日無陰時，陰日無陽時。故甲與己合，乙與庚合，丙與辛合，丁與壬合，戊與癸合也。何謂甲與己合？曰：中央戊己屬土，畏東方甲乙之木所剋。戊乃陽為兄，己屬陰為妹，戊兄遂將己妹，嫁與木家，與甲為妻，庶得陰陽和合，而不相傷，所以甲與己合。餘皆然。子午之法，盡於此矣！

Yáng days do not have [open points during] yīn hours. Yīn days do not have [open points during] yáng hours. Because of this [we can use the following:] jiǎ 甲 unites with jǐ 己. Yǐ 乙 unites with gēng 庚. Bǐng 丙 unites with xīn 辛. Dīng 丁 unites with rén 壬. Wù 戊 unites with guǐ 癸.

What does it mean, jiǎ 甲 unites with jǐ 己? It is said: The center, wù 戊 and jǐ 己, belong to earth. They fear the wood of the east, jiǎ 甲 and yǐ 乙, which restrains them. Wù 戊 is yáng so it is the elder brother. Jǐ 己 belongs to yīn so it is the younger sister. The older brother wù 戊 consequently marries out the younger sister jǐ 己 into the wood family to be a wife to jiǎ 甲. This is so that a harmonious union of yīn and yáng

---

39. Here, the jiǎ 甲 stem is repeated, but the shēn 申 branch isn't. However, in this method, point selection is determined by the stem. The branch only represents the time of day.

is obtained and they do not injure each other. Therefore jiǎ 甲 unites with jǐ 己. The rest are like this. The method of midnight and noon is expressed to the utmost in this.

Translator's note:

The Five Unities (五合) have already been introduced. This is how Yáng explains the uniting of jiǎ 甲 (yáng wood) and jǐ 己 (yīn earth): Normally the earth family is afraid of the wood family because wood controls earth according to five element theory. Wù 戊 (the yáng earth stem and therefore the older brother of jǐ 己, the yīn earth stem) makes a deal with jiǎ (the yáng wood stem, and therefore male) in order to prevent trouble. Wù 戊 marries off his younger sister jǐ 己 to jiǎ 甲. This solidifies family ties so that jiǎ 甲 will no longer threaten the wood family.

What is the significance of this? Since jiǎ 甲 and jǐ 己 are now family, you can borrow jiǎ's 甲 points on jǐ 己 days and vice versa. This is important because every yīn time period is empty on yáng days and every yáng time period is empty on yīn days. Since jiǎ 甲 is yáng and jǐ 己 is yīn, this mutual utilization fills in many of the empty time periods. Unfortunately, there are still twelve time periods without any open points, and many of these are during business hours.

Besides this, notice that the sixty time-period cycle of stem-branch combinations repeats every five days. So another way of looking at this is that there are two cycles of sixty in one ten-day week of stems, and now points that were calculated for a specific time-period can be used in the other time-period of the ten-day cycle that has the same stem-branch hour combination.

We can now revise the table for usable points as follows:

針灸大成・卷之五

Open Points for the Method of Mutual Utilization									
	Jiǎ 甲 or Jǐ 己 Day		Yǐ 乙 or Gēng 庚 Day		Bǐng 丙 or Xīn 辛 Day		Dīng 丁 or Rén 壬 Day		Wù 戊 or Guǐ 癸 Day	
Time	Hour	Point	Hour	Point	Hour	Point	Hour	Point	Hour	Point
11 pm- 1 am	Jiǎ Zǐ 甲子	GB 38	Bǐng Zǐ 丙子	SI 2	Wù Zǐ 戊子	ST 36	Gēng Zǐ 庚子	LI 3, SI4	Rén Zǐ 壬子	SJ 1
1-3 am	Yǐ Chǒu 乙丑	LV 2	Dīng Chǒu 丁丑	HT 3	Jǐ Chǒu 己丑	SP 3, LV 3	Xīn Chǒu 辛丑	PC 3	Guǐ Chǒu 癸丑	KI 7
3-5 am	Bǐng Yín 丙寅	SI 8	Wù Yín 戊寅	ST 43, GB 40	Gēng Yín 庚寅	SJ 10	Rén Yín 壬寅	UB 60 or UB 67	Jiǎ Yín 甲寅	
5-7 am	Dīng Mǎo 丁卯	HT 7, KI 3, PC 7	Jǐ Mǎo 己卯	PC 5	Xīn Mǎo 辛卯	LU 8 or LU 11	Guǐ Mǎo 癸卯		Yǐ Mǎo 乙卯	LV 8
7-9 am	Wù Chén 戊辰	SJ 6	Gēng Chén 庚辰	LI 5 or LI 1	Rén Chén 壬辰		Jiǎ Chén 甲辰	GB 34 or GB 43	Bǐng Chén 丙辰	
9-11 am	Jǐ Sì 己巳	SP 5 or SP 1	Xīn Sì 辛巳		Guǐ Sì 癸巳	KI 10 or KI 2	Yǐ Sì 乙巳		Dīng Sì 丁巳	PC 7
11 am- 1 pm	Gēng Wǔ 庚午		Rén Wǔ 壬午	UB 40 or UB 66	Jiǎ Wǔ 甲午		Bǐng Wǔ 丙午	SJ 3 or SI 3, UB 64, SJ 4	Wù Wǔ 戊午	ST 45
1-3 pm	Xīn Wèi 辛未	LU 5 or LU 10	Guǐ Wèi 癸未		Yǐ Wèi 乙未	PC 8 or LV 3, LU 9	Dīng Wèi 丁未	HT 9	Jǐ Wèi 己未	
3-5 pm	Rén Shēn 壬申		Jiǎ Shēn 甲申	SJ 2 or GB 41, LI 4	Bǐng Shēn 丙申	SI 1	Wù Shēn 戊申	ST 41	Gēng Shēn 庚申	LI 2
5-7 pm	Guǐ Yǒu 癸酉	PC 9 or KI 3, SP 3	Yǐ Yǒu 乙酉	LV 1	Dīng Yǒu 丁酉	HT 4	Jǐ Yǒu 己酉	SP 2	Xīn Yǒu 辛酉	
7-9 pm	Jiǎ Xū 甲戌	GB 44	Bǐng Xū 丙戌	SI 5	Wù Xū 戊戌	ST 44	Gēng Xū 庚戌	LI 11	Rén Xū 壬戌	UB 65, ST 42
9-11 pm	Yǐ Hài 乙亥	LV 4	Dīng Hài 丁亥	HT 8	Jǐ Hài 己亥	SP 9	Xīn Hài 辛亥	LU 9	Guǐ Hài 癸亥	KI 1

Note: Correct for Daylight Savings Time, if necessary.

流注開闔 (《醫學入門》)

Flowing and Pooling, Opening and Shutting (*Entering the Gate of Medicine – Yī Xué Rù Mén*[40])

人每日一身，週流六十六穴，每時週流五穴。

Each day a circuit flows through the 66 points of the whole human body.[41] Each time period, the circuit flows through five points.

> 除六原穴，乃過經之所。
>
> Not counting the six source points which are the place of passing through the channel.

相生相合者為開，則刺之。相剋者為闔，則不刺。

When there is mutual engendering or mutual uniting [the points] are open so you can needle them. When there is mutual restraint they are shut so you should not needle them.

> 陽生陰死，陰生陽死。如甲木死於午，生於亥；乙木死於亥，生於午。丙火生於寅，死於酉；丁火生於酉，死於寅。戊土生於寅，死於酉；己土生於酉，死於寅。庚金生於巳，死於子；辛金生於子，死於巳。壬水生於申，死於卯；癸水生於卯，死於申。
>
> When yáng is born, yīn dies. When yīn is born, yáng dies.
>
> For example, jiǎ 甲 wood dies in wǔ 午 [branch] but is born in hài 亥; yǐ 乙 wood dies in hài 亥 but is born in wǔ 午 [branch].
>
> Bǐng 丙 fire is born in yín 寅 [branch] but dies in yǒu 酉; dīng 丁 fire is born

---

40. By Lǐ Chān 李梴, published in 1575 (*Míng*). This is from Volume 1. This consists of original text and commentary. The commentary is indented. Both original text and commentary are from *Entering the Gate* and are simply passed on by Yáng.

41. Five transport points times twelve channels makes 60. The source points of the yáng channels bring the total to 66.

in yǒu 酉 but dies in yín 寅.

Wù 戊 earth is born in yín 寅 but dies in yǒu 酉; **jǐ** 己 earth is born in yǒu 酉 but dies in yín 寅.

Gēng 庚 metal is born in sì 巳 but dies in zǐ 子; **xīn** 辛 metal is born in zǐ 子 but dies in sì 巳.

Rén 壬 water is born in shēn 申 but dies in mǎo 卯; **guǐ** 癸 water is born in mǎo 卯 but dies in shēn 申.

Translator's notes:

According to the above paragraphs we can make the following diagrams.[42] Note that if we consider the branches in terms of months, yín 寅, mǎo 卯, and chén 辰 belong to spring. Sì 巳, wǔ 午, and wèi 未 make up summer. Shēn 申, yǒu 酉, and xū 戌 correspond to autumn. Hài 亥, zǐ 子, and chǒu 丑 are the winter months. This relationship is called the Three Meetings (sān huì 三會).

Besides this, the four corners are yín 寅, sì 巳, shēn 申, and hài 亥. The reason is obvious if you examine their location in the diagram below. The four directions are zǐ 子 (north), wǔ 午 (south), mǎo 卯 (east), and yǒu 酉 (west).

gēng 庚 is born sì 巳 branch	jiǎ 甲 dies wǔ 午 branch	wèi 未 branch	rén 壬 is born shēn 申 branch
chén 辰 branch	**Yáng Stems**		bǐng 丙 and wù 戊 die yǒu 酉 branch
rén 壬 dies mǎo 卯 branch			xū 戌 branch
bǐng 丙 and wù 戊 are born yín 寅 branch	chǒu 丑 branch	gēng 庚 dies zǐ 子 branch	jiǎ 甲 is born hài 亥 branch

Yáng stems are born in the four corners and die in the four directions.

- They are born in the corner before their season (not the corner at the beginning of their season). This is generally associated with the element that gives birth to the season.
- They die in the direction that comes after their season. This is generally associated with the

---

42. These relationships are quite similar to a pattern called the Five-Element Long Life Spirits (五行長生神), commonly used in Chinese metaphysics (玄學). Describing this, though, would take us far afield.

element that drains it.
- Earth doesn't have its own season, so wù 戊 (yáng earth) goes with bǐng 丙 (yáng fire).

xīn 辛 dies sì 巳 branch	yǐ 乙 is born wǔ 午 branch	wèi 未 branch	guǐ 癸 dies shēn 申 branch
chén 辰 branch	**Yīn Stems**		dīng 丁 and jǐ 己 are born yǒu 酉 branch
guǐ 癸 is born mǎo 卯 branch			xū 戌 branch
dīng 丁 and jǐ 己 die yín 寅 branch	chǒu 丑 branch	xīn 辛 is born zǐ 子 branch	yǐ 乙 dies hài 亥 branch

Yīn stems are born in the four directions and die in the four corners.
- They are born in the direction after their season. This is generally associated with the element that drains it.
- They die in the corner that comes before their season (not the corner at the beginning of their season). This is generally associated with the element that gives birth to it.
- Earth doesn't have its own season, so jǐ 己 (yīn earth) goes with dīng 丁 (yīn fire).

The yīn and yáng stems of the same element are born and die in the same two palaces, but where the yīn stem is born, the yáng stem dies, and vice versa. This is related to the principle that yáng advances and yīn retreats.

Let's continue on with the commentary from *Entering the Gate of Medicine*.

凡值生我我生，及相合者，乃氣血生旺之時，故可辨虛實刺之。剋我我剋，及闔閉時穴，氣血正值衰絕，非氣行未至，則氣行已過，誤刺妄引邪氣，壞亂真氣，實實虛虛，其害非小。

Overall, when the on-duty entity gives birth to me, I give birth to it, or we unite with each other, it is the time-period when qì and blood are born (*shēng* 生) or effulgent (*wàng* 旺). Thus, you can differentiate vacuity or repletion and needle it.

In the time-period when I am restrained, when I restrain, and when it is a closed time period for points, qì and blood of the main on-duty entity are debilitated (*shuāi* 衰) or exhausted (*jué* 絕). If the circulating qì hasn't yet arrived, then the circulating qì has already passed. It is an error to needle it and rashly guide the evil qì, to spoil and disorder true qì, to replenish repletion and evacuate vacuity. The harm is not small.

針灸大成 • 卷之五

Translator's notes:

The practical application of these sentences is not fully explained in the *Great Compendium*. However, *Entering the Gate of Medicine* goes on with more explanation which is summarized here: In this context, "the on-duty entity" refers to the open point in a time period, for example on a jiǎ 甲 day in the jiǎ xū 甲戌 time period, Qiào Yīn 竅陰 (GB 44) is open. The words "I" or "me" refer to the on-duty (open) point.

In a time period, you can combine the open point with other points of the same category. For example, if a well point is open during a certain time period, you can pair it with other appropriate well points. If the brook point is open, you can pair it with other appropriate brook points, and so forth. But what other points of the same category are appropriate?

Relationship	Example: jiǎ 甲, Gall Bladder (yáng wood)		Outcome	
Gives birth to me	Water: rén 壬 (UB) and guǐ 癸 (KI)	Use to supplement (water engenders wood)	birth (*shēng* 生) or effulgence (*wàng* 旺)	Can be needled
I give birth to	Fire: bǐng 丙 (SI) and dīng 丁 (HT)	Use to drain (fire drains wood)		
Unite with each other	Yīn earth: jǐ 己 (SP)	When wood attacks earth	five unities (jiǎ 甲 and jǐ 己 unite with each other)	
I am restrained	Metal: gēng 庚 (LI) and xīn 辛 (LU)	Cannot use	debilitation (*shuāi* 衰) or exhaustion (*jué* 絕)	Erroneous to needle
I restrain	Yáng Earth: wù 戊 (ST)			

According to the above table, any time a gall bladder point is open, you could combine it with a kidney or urinary bladder point of the same category to supplement the gall bladder. You could combine it with a small intestine or heart point of the same caegory to drain the gall bladder. You could also use a spleen point because of the five unities relationship. In all these cases, it would be a point of the same category as the gall bladder point.

"Thus, you can differentiate vacuity or repletion and needle it." In other words, pick the point from the channel with the element that drains or supplements the gall bladder according to the pattern of the patient.

However, you should avoid lung, large intestine, or stomach points as these are inharmonious and may cause harm.

The four designations of birth (shēng 生), effulgence (wàng 旺), debilitation (shuāi 衰), and exhaustion (jué 絕) (or death – sǐ 死) are commonly used in Chinese metaphysics. They are used as a measure of how strong or beneficial something is.

Below, one more aspect of the Five Unities is added. The two stems that unite with each other transform into one of the five elements as follows:[43]

The Five Unities (五合)				
When these stems unite with each other				they transform into
1	jiǎ 甲	6	jǐ 己	earth
2	yǐ 乙	7	gēng 庚	metal
3	bǐng 丙	8	xīn 辛	water
4	dīng 丁	9	rén 壬	wood
5	wù 戊	10	guǐ 癸	fire

流注時日
Flowing and Pooling of the Hour and Day[44]

陽日陽時陽穴，陰日陰時陰穴，陽以陰為闔，陰以陽為闔，闔者閉也。閉則以本時天干，與某穴相合者針之。

On a yáng day at a yáng hour, use a yáng point. On a yīn day at yīn hour, use a yīn point. Yáng regards yīn as closed. Yīn regards yáng as closed. Closed means shut. When [an hour is] closed, needle the specific point united with heavenly stem of the current hour.

> 陽日遇陰時，陰日遇陽時，則前穴已閉。取其合穴針之，合者，甲與己合化土，乙與庚合化金，丙與辛合化水，丁與壬合化木，戊與癸合化火，五門十變，此之謂也。

---

43. The reason each pair transforms into their corresponding element has to do with Chinese cosmology and the observation of streaks of color in the sky from the region of one stem to the other.

44. This section is also from *Entering the Gate of Medicine*, Volume 1. As with the previous section, it contains original text and commentary. The commentary is indented.

When a yáng day meets a yīn hour or when a yīn day meets a yáng hour, the previous point is already closed. Select the united point and needle it. "United" means jiǎ 甲 unites with jǐ 己 and transforms into earth. Yǐ 乙 unites with gēng 庚 and transforms into metal. Bǐng 丙 unites with xīn 辛 and transforms into water. Dīng 丁 unites with rén 壬 and transforms into wood. Wù 戊 unites with guǐ 癸 and transforms into fire. This is called the five gates and ten mutations.

其所以然者，陽日注腑，則氣先至而後血行，陰日注臟，則血先至而後氣行，順陰陽者，所以順氣血也。

That being so, when yáng days pool in the bowels, qì arrives first and blood moves after it. When yīn days pool in the viscera, blood arrives first and qì moves after it. The proper flow of yīn-yáng is therefore the proper flow of qì and blood.

陽日六腑值日者引氣，陰日五臟值日者引血。

On yáng days, the six bowels that are on duty for the day guide qì. On yīn days, the five viscera that are on duty for the day guide blood.

或曰：陽日陽時已過，陰日陰時已過，遇有急疾，奈何？曰：夫妻子母互用，必適其病為貴耳！

Someone said: What should you do when you come across an acute disease on a yáng day when the yáng hour has already passed, or on a yīn day when the yīn hour has already passed? I say: The husband and wife, the son and mother can be used for each other. They are surely suitable for the disease and are regarded as precious!

妻閉則針其夫，夫閉則針其妻，子閉針其母，母閉針其子，必穴與病相宜，乃可針也。

If the wife is closed, needle her husband. If the husband is closed, needle his wife. If the child is closed, needle his mother. If the mother is closed, needle her child. The point will certainly be suitable for the disease, so you can needle it.

噫！用穴則先主而後客，用時則棄主而從賓。

Ah! When using points, first use the host and afterwards the guests. When using the hour, abandon the host and follow the visitors.

假如甲日膽經為主，他穴為客，針必先主後客，其甲戌等時主穴不
開，則針客穴。

**For example, on a jiǎ 甲 day the gall bladder channel is the host. Other points
are the guests. You must first needle the host and afterwards the guests. During the jiǎ xū 甲戌 sequence of hours, when the host points are not open,
needle the guest points.**

按日起時，循經尋穴，時上有穴，穴上有時，分明實落，不必數上衍數 。此
所以甯守子午而舍爾靈龜也 。

**The hour arises according to the day [stem]. Seek points according to channel. In the
hour, there are points [that are open]; in the point, there are hours [when the point
is open]. There is a clearly marked target to hit. You need not count up superfluous
numbers. Therefore it is better to attend to Midnight-Noon and set aside this Mystical Tortoise.**

靈龜八法，專為奇經八穴而設，（ 其圖具後 ），但子午法，其理易
明，其穴亦肘膝內穴，豈能逃子午之流注哉！

**The Eight Methods of the Mystical Tortoise are established especially for the
eight points of the extraordinary channels (this is illustrated below). Yet, the
rationale of the Midnight-Noon Method is easier to understand. Its points
are also inside the elbow and knees. How could anyone run away from of
Midnight-Noon Flowing and Pooling!**

Translator's Notes:

This section restates that you can use the five unities to select points during times when there are
no open points. For details, see above. The original authors of the text and the commentary express
a strong preference for Midnight-Noon Flowing and Pooling over the Eight Methods of the Mystical Tortoise. Yáng Jìzhōu, by including this text, is also expressing a preference, although he goes on
to include a lengthy discussion of the Mystical Tortoise.

臟腑井滎俞經合主治（《聚英》）

Viscera and Bowels Well, Brook, Transport, River, and Uniting Point Indications (*Gatherings from Eminent Acupuncturists* – Zhēn Jiǔ Jù Yīng[45])

假令得弦脈，病人善潔（膽為清淨之府故耳），面青善怒，此膽病也。若心下滿，當刺竅陰（井），身熱當刺俠谿（滎），體重節痛刺臨泣（俞），喘嗽寒熱刺陽輔（經），逆氣而泄刺陽陵泉（合），又總刺邱墟（原）。

Suppose you obtain a bowstring pulse, the patient tends toward cleanliness (the reason is that the gall bladder is the mansion of the clear and clean), the face is green-blue, and he frequently angers. This is gall bladder disease. If there is fullness below the heart, you should needle Qiào Yīn 竅陰 (GB 44) (well point). If the body is hot, needle Xiá Xī 俠谿 (GB 43) (brook point). If the body feels heavy and there is joint pain, needle Lín Qì 臨泣 (GB 41) (stream point). If there is panting and cough, and sensations of cold and heat, needle Yáng Fǔ 陽輔 (GB 38) (river point). If there is counterflow qì and diarrhea, needle Yáng Líng Quán 陽陵泉 (GB 34) (uniting point). Also in general, needle Qiū Xū 邱墟 (GB 40) (source point).

假令得弦脈，病人淋溲，便難，轉筋，四支滿閉，臍左有動氣，此肝病也。若心下滿刺大敦（井），身熱刺行間（滎），體重節痛刺太衝（俞），喘嗽寒熱刺中封（經），逆氣而泄刺曲泉（合）。

Suppose you obtain a bowstring pulse, the patient has dribbling urination, difficult defecation, cramping, and heaviness and blockage of the four limbs. There is stirring qì to the left of the umbilicus. This is liver disease. If there is fullness below the heart, needle Dà Dūn 大敦 (LV 1) (well point). If the body is hot, needle Xíng Jiān 行間 (LV 2) (brook point). If the body feels heavy and there is joint pain, needle Tài Chōng 太衝 (LV 3) (stream point). If there is panting and cough, and sensations of cold and heat, needle Zhōng Fēng 中封 (LV 4) (river point). If there is counterflow qì and diarrhea, needle Qū Quán 曲泉 (LV 8) (uniting point).

---

45. From *Zhēn Jiǔ Jù Yīng*《針灸聚英》(Gatherings from Eminent Acupuncturists) by Gāo Wǔ 高武, published in 1529 (*Míng*). This is from Volume 2. The symptoms listed come from the *Classic of Difficulties*, 16th Difficulty. The functions of the five transport points come from the 68th Difficulty.

假令得浮洪脈，病人面赤，口乾喜笑，此小腸病也。若心下滿刺少澤（ 井 ），身熱刺前谷（ 滎 ），體重節痛刺後谿（ 俞 ），喘嗽寒熱刺陽谷（ 經 ），逆氣而泄刺少海（ 合 ），又總刺腕骨（ 原 ）。

Suppose you obtain a floating surging pulse, the patient has a red face, dry mouth, and tends to laugh. This is small intestine disease. If there is fullness below the heart, needle Shào Zé 少澤 (SI 1) (well point). If the body is hot, needle Qián Gǔ 前谷 (SI 2) (brook point). If the body feels heavy and there is joint pain, needle Hòu Xī 後谿 (SI 3) (stream point). If there is panting and cough, and sensations of cold and heat, needle Yáng Gǔ 陽谷 (SI 5) (river point). If there is counterflow qì and diarrhea, needle Shào Hǎi 少海 (SI 8) (uniting point). Also in general, needle Wàn Gǔ 腕骨 (SI 4) (source point).

假令得浮洪脈，病人煩心，心痛，掌中熱而呃，臍上有動氣，此心病也。若心下滿刺少衝（ 井 ），身熱刺少府（ 滎 ），體重節痛刺神門（ 俞 ），喘嗽寒熱刺靈道（ 經 ），逆氣而泄刺少海（ 合 ）。

Suppose you obtain a floating surging pulse, the patient has heart vexation, heart pain, and the centers of the palms are hot, with dry retching. There is stirring qì above the umbilicus. This is heart disease. If there is fullness below the heart, needle Shào Chōng 少衝 (HT 9) (well point). If the body is hot, needle Shào Fǔ 少府 (HT 8) (brook point). If the body feels heavy and there is joint pain, needle Shén Mén 神門 (HT 7) (stream point). If there is panting and cough, and sensations of cold and heat, needle Líng Dào 靈道 (HT 4) (river point). If there is counterflow qì and diarrhea, needle Shào Hǎi 少海 (HT 3) (uniting point).

假令得浮緩脈，病人面黃，善噫，善思，善沬，此胃病也。若心下滿刺厲兌（ 井 ），身熱刺內庭（ 滎 ），體重節痛刺陷谷（ 俞 ），喘嗽寒熱刺解谿（ 經 ），逆氣而泄刺三里（ 合 ），又總刺衝陽（ 原 ）。

Suppose you obtain a floating moderate pulse, the patient has a yellow face, tends to belch, is susceptible to [excessive] thought, and likes tasty food. This is stomach disease. If there is fullness below the heart, needle Lì Duì 厲兌 (ST 45) (well point). If the body is hot, needle Nèi Tíng 內庭 (ST 44) (brook point). If the body feels heavy and there is joint pain, needle Xiàn Gǔ 陷谷 (ST 43) (stream point). If there is panting and cough, and sensations of cold and heat, needle Jiě Xī 解谿 (ST 41) (river point). If there is counterflow qì and diarrhea, needle Sān Lǐ 三里 (ST 36) (uniting point). Also, in general, needle Chōng Yáng 衝陽 (ST 42) (source point).

假令得浮緩脈，病人腹脹滿，食不消，體重節痛，怠惰嗜臥，四肢不收，當臍有動氣，按之牢苦痛，此脾病也。若心下滿刺隱白（井），身熱刺大都（滎），體重節痛刺太白（俞），喘嗽寒熱刺商邱（經），逆氣而泄刺陰陵泉（合）。

Suppose you obtain a floating moderate pulse, the patient has abdominal distention and fullness, non-transformation of food, the body feels heavy with joint pain, fatigue and somnolence, and loss of use of the limbs. There is stirring qì right at the umbilicus and when you press, it is firm with bitter pain. This is spleen disease. If there is fullness below the heart, needle Yīn Bái 隱白 (SP 1) (well point). If the body is hot, needle Dà Dū 大都 (SP 2) (brook point). If the body feels heavy and there is joint pain, needle Tài Bái 太白 (SP 3) (stream point). If there is panting and cough, and sensations of cold and heat, needle Shāng Qiū 商邱 (SP 5) (river point). If there is counterflow qì and diarrhea, needle Yīn Líng Quán 陰陵泉 (SP 9) (uniting point).

假令得浮脈，病人面白，善嚏，悲愁不樂欲哭，此大腸病也。若心下滿刺商陽（井），身熱刺二間（滎），體重節痛刺三間（俞），喘嗽寒熱刺陽谿（經），逆氣而泄刺曲池（合），又總刺合谷（原）。

Suppose you obtain a floating pulse, the patient has a white face and tends to sneeze. He has sorrow and sadness; he is unhappy and wants to cry. This is large intestine disease. If there is fullness below the heart, needle Shāng Yáng 商陽 (LI 1) (well point). If the body is hot, needle Èr Jiān 二間 (LI 2) (brook point). If the body feels heavy and there is joint pain, needle Sān Jiān 三間 (LI 3) (stream point). If there is panting and cough, and sensations of cold and heat, needle Yáng Xī 陽谿 (LI 5) (river point). If there is counterflow qì and diarrhea, needle Qū Chí 曲池 (LI 11) (uniting point). Also, in general, needle Hé Gǔ 合谷 (LI 4) (source point).

假令得浮脈，病人喘嗽，洒淅寒熱，臍右有動氣，按之牢痛，此肺病也。若心下滿刺少商（井），身熱刺魚際（滎），體重節痛刺太淵（俞），喘嗽寒熱刺經渠（經），逆氣而泄刺尺澤（合）。

Suppose you obtain a floating pulse, the patient has panting and cough, and sensations of cold and heat as if after a soaking. There is stirring qì to the right of the umbilicus and when you press, it is firm with bitter pain. This is lung disease. If there is fullness below the heart, needle Shào Shāng 少商 (LU 11) (well point). If the body is hot, needle Yú Jì 魚際 (LU 10) (brook point). If the body feels heavy and there is joint pain, needle Tài Yuān 太淵 (LU 9) (stream point). If there is panting and cough, and sensations of cold and heat, needle Jīng Qú 經渠 (LU 8) (river point). If there is counterflow qì and diarrhea, needle Chǐ Zé 尺澤 (LU 5) (uniting point).

假令得沉遲脈，病人面黑，善恐欠，此膀胱病也。若心下滿刺至陰（井），身熱刺通谷（滎），體重節痛刺束骨（俞），喘嗽寒熱刺崑崙（經），逆氣而泄刺委中（合），又總刺京骨（原）。

Suppose you obtain a deep slow pulse, the patient has a black face, susceptibility to fear and frequent yawning. This is urinary bladder disease. If there is fullness below the heart, needle Zhì Yīn 至陰 (UB 67) (well point). If the body is hot, needle Tōng Gǔ 通谷 (UB 66) (brook point). If the body feels heavy and there is joint pain, needle Shù Gǔ 束骨 (UB 65) (stream point). If there is panting and cough, and sensations of cold and heat, needle Kūn Lún 崑崙 (UB 60) (river point). If there is counterflow qì and diarrhea, needle Wěi Zhōng 委中 (UB 40) (uniting point). Also, in general, needle Jīng Gǔ 京骨 (UB 64) (source point).

假令得沉遲脈，病人逆氣，小腹急痛，泄如下重，足脛寒而逆，臍下有動氣，按之牢若痛，此腎病也。若心下滿刺湧泉（井），身熱刺然谷（滎），體重節痛刺太谿（俞），喘嗽寒熱刺復溜（經），逆氣而泄刺陰谷（合）。

Suppose you obtain a deep slow pulse, the patient has counterflow qì, tight pain in the smaller abdomen, diarrhea like something heavy moving downward, and counterflow cold of the feet and shins. There is stirring qì below the umbilicus and when you press, it is firm with bitter[46] pain. This is kidney disease. If there is fullness below the heart, needle Yǒng Quán 湧泉 (KI 1) (well point). If the body is hot, needle Rán Gǔ 然谷 (KI 2) (brook point). If the body feels heavy and there is joint pain, needle Tài Xī 太谿 (KI 3) (stream point). If there is panting and cough, and sensations of cold and heat, needle Fù Liū 復溜 (KI 7) (river point). If there is counterflow qì and diarrhea, needle Yīn Gǔ 陰谷 (KI 10) (uniting point).

---

46. Above, the text has kǔ 苦 "bitter," while here it has ruò 若 "as if." This is probably a typo.

針
灸
大
成
・
卷
之
五

總論
General Summary

紀氏曰：井之所治，不以五臟六腑，皆主心下滿。滎之所治，不以五臟六腑，皆主身熱。俞之所治，不以五臟六腑，皆主體重節痛。經之所治，不以五臟六腑，皆主喘嗽寒熱。合之所治，不以五臟六腑，皆主逆氣而泄。

Master Jì[47] said: What well points treat is not the five viscera and six bowels; all of them govern fullness below the heart. What brook points treat is not the five viscera and six bowels; all of them govern heat in the body. What stream points treat is not the five viscera and six bowels; all of them govern the feeling of heaviness in the body and joint pain. What river points treat is not the five viscera and six bowels; all of them govern panting and cough and sensations of cold and heat. What uniting points treat is not the five viscera and six bowels; all of them govern counterflow qì and diarrhea.

十二經是動所生病補瀉迎隨（《聚英》）
The Twelve Channels, Stirring and Engendered Disease, Supplementing and Draining, Facing and Following (*Gatherings from Eminent Acupuncturists – Zhēn Jiǔ Jù Yīng*[48])

《內經》曰：十二經病，盛則瀉之，虛則補之，熱則疾之，寒則留之，不盛不虛，以經取之。又曰：迎而奪之，隨而濟之。又曰：虛則補其母，實則瀉其子。

《難經》曰：經脈行血氣，通陰陽，以榮於其身者也。其始（平旦）從中焦，注手太陰（肺寅）、陽明（大腸卯），陽明注足陽明（胃辰）、太陰（脾巳），太陰注手少陰（心午）、太陽（小腸未），太陽注足太陽（膀胱申）、少陰（腎酉），少陰注手厥陰（包絡戌）、少陽（三焦亥），少陽注足少陽（膽子）、厥陰（肝丑），厥陰復注於手太陰（明日寅時），如環無端，轉相灌溉。

又曰：迎隨者，知榮衛流行，經脈往來，隨其順逆而取之也。

---

47. Probably Jì Tiānxī 紀天錫, 12th century.

48. From *Zhēn Jiǔ Jù Yīng*《針灸聚英》(Gatherings from Eminent Acupuncturists) by Gāo Wǔ 高武, published in 1529 (*Míng*). This is from Volume 2.

The *Inner Classic* says:[49] Diseases of the twelve channels: When exuberant, drain it; when vacuous, supplement it; when hot, [needle] it quickly; when cold, retain it;[50] if it is not exuberant and not vacuous, use the channels to treat it.

It also says:[51] Face and seize it; follow and aid it.[52]

It also says:[53] In vacuity, supplement the mother; in repletion, drain the son.

The *Classic of Difficulties* says:[54] The channel-vessels circulate blood and qì and pass freely through yīn and yáng in order to make the body flourish. They begin (at dawn) from the middle burner and pool into the hand tàiyīn (lung, yín 寅 hour) and yáng-míng channels (large intestine, mǎo 卯 hour). The yángmíng pools into the foot yángmíng (stomach, chén 辰 hour) and tàiyīn channels (spleen, sì 巳 hour). The tàiyīn pools into the hand shàoyīn (heart, wǔ 午 hour) and tàiyáng channels (small intestine, wèi 未 hour). The tàiyáng pools into the foot tàiyáng (urinary bladder, shēn 申 hour) and shàoyīn channels (kidney, yǒu 酉 hour). The shàoyīn pools into the hand juéyīn (pericardium, xū 戌 hour) and shàoyáng channels (triple burner, hài 亥 hour). The shàoyáng pools into the foot shàoyáng (gall bladder, zǐ 子 hour) and juéyīn channels (liver, chǒu 丑 hour). The juéyīn goes back to pool into the hand tàiyīn channel (next day, yín 寅 hour). It is like a ring without end, passing on, each [channel] irrigating another.

It also says:[55] Facing and following means knowing the flowing and movement of construction and defense and the going and coming in the channel-vessels. Apply treatment based on going with or against the flow.

---

49. In 《靈樞·經脈第十》 *Magic Pivot*, Chapter 10.

50. "When hot, [needle] it quickly; when cold, retain it." In other words, do not retain the needle in heat patterns; retain the needle in cold patterns.

51. This is not an exact quote but there is a very similar statement in 《靈樞·九鍼十二原第一》 *Magic Pivot*, Chapter 1 and 《靈樞·小鍼解第三》 Chapter 3.

52. This is taken to mean, to drain, needle against the direction of flow in the channel; to supplement, needle with the direction of flow in the channel. It is also used in the timing of treatment, below. Treat repletion of an organ in its own time-period. This is 'facing it' directly. Treat a vacuity of an organ in the time-period immediately after the organ's time. This is following it.

53. This statement is not in *Magic Pivot* or *Elementary Questions*. It is stated in the *Classic of Difficulties*, Chapter 69. 《難經·六十九難》

54. This is from 《難經·二十三難》 the *Classic of Difficulties*, Chapter 23.

55. This is from 《難經·七十二難》 the *Classic of Difficulties*, Chapter 72.

十二經之原歌
Song of the Source Points of the Twelve Channels[56]

甲出邱墟乙太衝，丙居腕骨是原中，
丁出神門原內過，戊胃衝陽氣可通，
己出太白庚合谷，辛原本出太淵同，
壬歸京骨陽池穴，癸出太谿大陵中。

三焦行于諸陽，故置一俞曰原。又曰：三焦者，水谷之道路，原氣之別使
也。主通行三氣，經歷五臟六腑。原者，三焦之尊號。故所止輒為原也。
按《難經》云：五臟六腑之有病者，皆取其原。
王海藏曰：假令補肝經，於本經原穴補一針，（太衝穴是），如瀉肝經，於
本經原穴亦瀉一針，餘倣此。

Jiǎ 甲 emerges in Qiū Xū 邱墟 (GB 40); yǐ 乙 in Tài Chōng 太衝 (LV 3); bǐng 丙 resides in Wàn Gǔ 腕骨 (SI 4); these are within the source.

Dīng 丁 emerges in Shén Mén 神門 (HT 7), the source passes through the interior; wù 戊 stem is stomach, Chōng Yáng 衝陽 (ST 42), where qì can flow.

Jǐ 己 emerges in Tài Bái 太白 (SP 3); gēng 庚 in Hé Gǔ 合谷 (LI 4); xīn's 辛 source root emerges in Tài Yuān 太淵 (LU 9) in the same way.

Rén 壬 returns to Jīng Gǔ 京骨 (UB 64) and Yáng Chí 陽池 (SJ 4); guǐ 癸 emerges in Tài Xī 太谿 (KI 3) and in Dà Líng 大陵 (PC 7).

The triple burner circulates in all yáng [regions of the body]. Thus an [additional] transport point is is established [on the yáng channels] called the source point. [57]

It also says:[58] The triple burner is the pathway of water and grains, the unique envoy of source qì. It governs the free circulation of the three qì, passing though the five viscera and six bowels. "Source" is a venerated name of the triple burner. That is why the place where it stops is consequently regarded as the source.

---

56. From *Zhēn Jiǔ Jù Yīng*《針灸聚英》(Gatherings from Eminent Acupuncturists) by Gāo Wǔ 高武, published in 1529 (*Míng*). This is from Volume 4. The notes after the poem are also from *Gatherings*, but they are found near the end of Volume 1.

57. This is from《難經‧六十二難》the *Classic of Difficulties*, Chapter 62.

58. In《難經‧六十六難》the *Classic of Difficulties*, Chapter 66.

Note that the *Classic of Difficulties* says:[59] For all those who have diseases of the five viscera and six bowels, apply treatment to the source point.

Wáng Hǎicáng[60] said: In the case of supplementing the liver channel, supplement with a needle in the source point of its own channel (this is Tài Chōng 太衝, LV 3). If draining the liver channel, also drain with a needle in the source point of its own channel. The rest are also like this.

十二經病井滎俞經合補瀉虛實
Diseases of the Twelve Channels, the Well, Brook, Stream, River, and Uniting Points, Supplementing Vacuity and Draining Repletion[61]

Translator's notes:

1. *Gatherings from Eminent Acupuncturists* largely took this section from 《黃帝内經·靈樞·經脈第十》 *Magic Pivot*, Chapter 10. Yáng Jìzhōu passed on Gāo Wǔ's rendering unchanged. In it, the phrases 是動病 ("disease when this [channel] stirs") and 所生病 ("disease which is engendered") are repeated for each channel. They are shortened from 是動則病 (when this [channel] stirs, it sickens with...) and 是主脾所生病 (this indicates the spleen [or whatever organ or substance] which engender the sickness of...). Gāo Wǔ stated (and Yáng Jìzhōu agreed, since he passed the text along) that disease when the channel stirs is due to qì and the disease which is engendered is due to blood. All twelve channels follow the same basic format.

2. Dòng 動 means movement, but often signifies pathological movement as opposed to free flowing in the channels. Wiseman glosses this term as "to stir."

Ancient books did not use punctuation, one factor that gives rise to differences in interpretation. In this section of *Magic Pivot*, Chapter 10, most frequently you see 是主脾所生病 (this indicates the spleen which engenders the sickness of...) as one sentence. However, Gāo Wǔ and Yáng have 是主脾 (This indicates the spleen) at the end of one paragraph and 所生病 (The disease which is engendered...) at the beginning of the next paragraph. Arranging the words like this affects the meaning significantly in some cases.

---

59. This is also from 《難經·六十六難》 the *Classic of Difficulties*, Chapter 66.

60. Wáng Hǎicáng was also known as Wáng Hàogǔ 王好古. He was a 13th century (*Yuán*) author and physician.

61. From *Zhēn Jiǔ Jù Yīng* 《針灸聚英》 (Gatherings from Eminent Acupuncturists) by Gāo Wǔ 高武, published in 1529 (*Míng*). This is from Volume 2.

手太陰肺經，屬辛金。起中府，終少商，多氣少血，寅時注此。

The hand tàiyīn lung channel belongs to xīn 辛 metal. It arises in Zhōng Fǔ 中府 (LU 1) and ends in Shào Shāng 少商 (LU 11). It contains copious qì and scant blood which pool into it during the yín 寅 hour [3-5 am].

是動病（ 邪在氣，氣留而不行，為是動病 ）：肺脹膨膨而喘咳，缺盆中痛。甚則交兩手而瞀，是謂臂厥 。（ 瞀音茂 ）

Disease when this [channel] stirs (Evil is located in qì. Qì lodges and does not move. This is regarded as the disease when this [channel] stirs): The lungs are distended and cannot diffuse with panting and cough, and pain in the supraclavicular fossa (Quē Pén 缺盆, ST 12). If it is severe, the patient crosses his two arms over his chest and has visual distortion. This is called reversal cold in the arms. [There is a note here on the pronounciation of *mào* 瞀, visual distortion.][62]

所生病（ 邪在血，血壅而不濡，為所生病 ）：咳喘上氣，喘渴煩心，胸滿，臑臂內前廉痛，掌中熱 。

Disease which is engendered (Evil is located in the blood. Blood congests and does not moisten. This is regarded as disease which is engendered.): Cough and panting with ascending qì, panting and thirst, vexation of the heart, chest fullness, pain on the medial anterior aspect of the arms, heat in the center of the palms.

氣盛有餘，則肩背痛，風寒（ 疑寒字衍 ），汗出中風，小便數而欠，寸口大三倍於人迎 。

When qì is exuberant and superabundant, there is pain in the shoulders and upper back, wind cold (I suspect the 'cold' character is superfluous[63]) sweating, wind-stroke, frequent but scant urination. The inch opening [*cùn kǒu* 寸口] is quadruple the size of [the pulse at] man's prognosis (*rén yíng* 人迎). [64]

---

62. Since Chinese is not phonetic in the same way as English, the pronunciation of a word that is not commonly used is described by saying it sounds like another more common word. This section has many such instances, but they will be omitted in the translation from now on.

63. This note is from Gāo Wǔ. He thinks the word "cold" should not be there. The word "cold" is not in Volume 1 of the *Mài Jīng* 脈經 (Pulse Classic).

64. According to Deng in his *Practical Diagnosis in Traditional Chinese Medicine*, (page 85) man's prognosis governs the exterior and reflects yáng. The inch opening governs the interior and reflects yīn. In this passage of text, when a viscera has repletion, the inch opening is bigger. When it has vacuity, the inch opening is smaller. When a bowel has repletion, man's prognosis is bigger.

虛則肩背痛寒，少氣不足以息，溺色變，卒遺矢無度，寸口反小於人迎也 。

In vacuity, there is pain and coldness of the shoulders and upper back, scant qì insufficient for breathing, color changes in the urine, sudden unrestrained fecal incontinence. The inch opening retreats to become smaller than man's prognosis.

補（ 虛則補之 ）：用卯時（ 隨而濟之 ）。太淵為俞土，土生金，為母 。
《 經 》曰：虛則補其母 。

Supplement (In vacuity, supplement it.): Use the mǎo 卯 hour [5-7 am] (follow and aid it).[65] Tài Yuān 太淵 (LU 9) is the stream point, earth. Earth engenders metal so it is the mother. The *Classic* says: In vacuity, supplement its mother.

瀉（ 盛則瀉之 ）：用寅時（ 迎而奪之 ）。尺澤為合水，金生水，為子 。實則瀉其子 。

Drain (In exuberance, drain it.): Use the yín 寅 hour [3-5 am] (face and seize it).[66] Chǐ Zé 尺澤 (LU 5) is the uniting point, water. Metal engenders water so it is the son. In repletion, drain its son.

手陽明大腸經，為庚金 。起商陽，終迎香，氣血俱多，卯時氣血注此 。

The hand yángmíng large intestine channel is gēng 庚 metal. It arises in Shāng Yáng 商陽 (LI 1) and ends in Yíng Xiāng 迎香 (LI 20). Both qì and blood are copious. Qì

When it has vacuity, man's prognosis is smaller. According to *Magic Pivot*, when there is repletion in the juéyīn and tàiyáng channels, the relevant pulse is one time bigger (twice the size). In the shàoyīn and tàiyáng channels, the relevant pulse is two times bigger (meaning triple the size). In the tàiyīn and yángmíng channels, the relevant pulse is three times bigger (meaning quadruple the size). Most sources say man's prognosis is the pulse located by the point called Rén Yíng 人迎 (ST 9) and the inch opening is the pulse at the radial artery. Some believe that the left radial pulse is man's prognosis and right radial pulse is the inch opening. In any case, in these passages, yīn channels focus on the inch opening and yáng channels focus on man's prognosis. This style of pulse diagnosis was discussed in the *Inner Canon*, but is not practiced by many today. Most follow a variation of the style of pulse diagnosis first described in the *Classic of Difficulties*, focusing only on the radial pulse. This was also true during the Míng dynasty.

65. "Follow and aid it." In vacuity, supplement the mother point during the time period following the affected channel's time period.

66. "Face and seize it." In repletion, drain the son point during the affected channel's own time period.

and blood pool into it during the mǎo 卯 hour [5-7 am].

是動病：齒痛，頄腫，是主津 。（ 頄音拙 ）

Disease when this [channel] stirs: Toothache and swelling of the facial prominence. [67] This indicates the liquids [*jīn* 津, thin body fluids].

所生病：目黃，口乾，鼽衄，喉痹，肩前臑痛，大指次指不用 。

Disease which is engendered: Yellow eyes, dry mouth, sniveling and nosebleed, throat impediment (*bì* 痹), pain in the anterior shoulder and upper arm, and loss of function of the index finger.

氣有餘則當脈所過者熱腫，人迎大三倍於寸口；虛則寒慄不復，人迎反小於寸口也 。（ 鼽音求 ）

When qì is superabundant, there is heat and swelling where the vessel [meaning channel] passes. The pulse at man's prognosis is quadruple the size of the inch opening.

In vacuity [the patient has] cold shudders and doesn't recover. Man's prognosis retreats to become smaller than the inch opening.

補：用辰時 。曲池為合土 。土生金，虛則補其母 。

Supplement: Use the chén 辰 hour [7-9 am]. Qū Chí 曲池 (LI 11) is the uniting point, earth. Earth engenders metal. In vacuity, supplement its mother.

瀉：用卯時 。二間為滎水 。金生水，實則瀉其子 。

Drain: Use the mǎo 卯 hour [5-7 am]. Èr Jiān 二間 (LI 2) is the brook point, water. Metal engenders water. In repletion, drain its son.

足陽明胃經，屬戊土 。起頭維，終屬兌，氣血俱多，辰時注此 。

The foot yángmíng stomach channel belongs to the wù 戊 stem, earth. It arises in Tóu Wéi 頭維 (ST 8) and ends in Lì Duì 厲兌 (ST 45). Both qì and blood are copious

---

67. The facial prominence is the region of the cheekbones below the eyes. Some commentators feel this should read the neck, instead.

and pool into it during the chén 辰 hour [7-9 am].

是動病：洒洒然振寒，善呻，數欠，顏黑，病至惡人與火。聞木音則惕然而
驚（心動欲獨）閉戶牖而處。甚則欲登高而歌，棄衣而走。賁嚮腹脹，是謂
骭厥，主血。（骭音幹）

Disease when this [channel] stirs: **Quivering with cold as if sprinkled with water, ten-
dency to groan, frequent yawning, and black forehead. The disease reaches the extent
of aversion to people and fire [heat]. When [the patient] hears a sound associated
with wood, he becomes fearful and frightened (when the heart stirs, there is desire to
be alone), blocks the doors and stays inside. When severe, he desires to climb to high
places and sing, throw off his clothes and run around. There is abdominal gurgling
and distention. This is tibia reversal[68] and indicates the blood.**

所生病：狂瘧溫淫，汗出，鼽衄，口喎，唇裂，喉痹，大腹水腫，膝臏腫
痛，循胸乳，氣膺伏兔，骺外廉，足跗上皆痛，中指不用。

Disease which is engendered: **Mania, malaria, warm excesses, sweating, sniveling and
nosebleeds, deviated mouth, cracked lips, throat impediment (*bì* 痹), water swelling
of the greater abdomen, swelling and pain of the patella; pain affecting the chest and
breast, the path of qì [or Qì Jiē 氣街 (ST 30)],[69] Fú Tù 伏兔 (ST 32), outer aspect of
the shin, and dorsum of the foot; loss of function of the middle toe.**

氣盛則身以前皆熱，其有餘於胃，則消穀善飢，溺色黃。人迎大三倍於寸
口；氣不足則身已前皆寒慄，胃中寒則脹滿，人迎反小於寸口也。（骺音
杭）

When qì is exuberant, the whole front of the body is hot. When its superabudance is
in the stomach, there is swift digestion and tendancy to hunger with yellow colored
urine. The pulse at man's prognosis is is quadruple the size of the inch opening.

When qì is insufficient, the whole front of the body is cold and shudders. When there
is cold in the stomach, there is distention and fullness. Man's prognosis retreats to
become smaller than the inch opening.

補：用巳時。解谿為經火。火生土，虛則補其母。

---

68. This is tibia reversal because qì is ascending up the stomach channel which traverses the tibia.

69. The *Great Compendium* has *qì yīng* 氣膺, which seems to be in error. *Magic Pivot* and *Gatherings from Eminent Acupuncturists* have Qì Jiē 氣街, the path of qì, also a name for ST 30.

Supplement: Use the sì 巳 hour [9-11 am]. Jiě Xī 解谿 (ST 41) is the river point, fire. Fire engenders earth. In vacuity, supplement its mother.

瀉：用辰時 。屬兌為井金 。土生金，實則瀉其子 。

Drain: Use the chén 辰 hour [7-9 am]. Lì Duì 厲兌 (ST 45) is the well point, metal. Earth engenders metal. In repletion, drain its son.

足太陰脾經，屬己土 。起隱白，終大包，多氣少血，巳時注此 。

The foot tàiyīn spleen channel belongs to jǐ 己 earth. It arises in Yǐn Bái 隱白 (SP 1) and ends in Dà Bāo 大包 (SP 21). It contains copious qì and scant blood which pools into it during the sì 巳 hour [9-11 am].

是動病：舌本強，食則嘔，胃脘痛，腹脹善噫，得後出與氣則快然如衰，身體皆重，是主脾 。

Disease when this [channel] stirs: The root of the tongue is stiff, with vomiting after eating, epigastric pain, abdominal distention, and frequent belching. A bowel movement expels the surplus qì[70] [but the patient] is debilitated and his whole body is heavy. This indicates the spleen.

所生病：舌本痛，體不能動搖，食不下，煩心，心下急痛，寒瘧，溏瀉泄水，身黃疸，不能臥，強立股膝內腫厥，足大指不用 。

Disease which is engendered: Pain at the root of the tongue, the body is unable to sway from side to side, difficulty swallowing, vexation of the heart, acute pain below the heart, cold malaria, sloppy diarrhea like water, jaundiced body, unable to sleep, barely able to stand, swelling and reversal of the medial thigh and knees, and loss of function of the big toe.

盛者寸口大三倍於人迎；虛者寸口小三倍於人迎也 。

When exuberant, the inch opening is is quadruple the size of man's prognosis.

---

70. *Líng Shū*, Chapter 10 says 得後與氣. A parallel passage in *Tài Sù*, Volume 8 《 太素・卷八 》 has 得後出餘氣. This translation is based on the *Tài Sù* and Yáng Shàngshàn's 楊上善 comments. The "surplus qì" means intestinal gas.

In vacuity, the inch opening is three times smaller than man's prognosis. [71]

補：用午時。大都為滎火。火生土，虛則補其母。

Supplement: Use the wǔ 午 hour [11 am – 1 pm]. Dà Dū 大都 (SP 2) is the brook point, fire. Fire engenders earth. In vacuity, supplement its mother.

瀉：用巳時。商邱為經金。土生金，實則瀉其子。

Drain: Use the sì 巳 hour [9-11 am]. Shāng Qiū 商丘 (SP 5) is the river point, metal. Earth engenders metal. In repletion, drain its son.

手少陰心經，屬丁火。起極泉，終少衝，多氣少血，午時注此。

The hand shàoyīn heart channel belongs to dīng 丁 fire. It arises in Jí Quán 極泉 (HT 1) and ends in Shào Chōng 少衝 (HT 9). It contains copious qì and scant blood which pools into it during the wǔ 午 hour [11 am – 1 pm].

是動病：咽乾心痛，渴而欲飲，是為臂厥，主心。

Disease when this [channel] stirs: Dry throat, heart pain, thirst with desire to drink. This is arm reversal and indicates the heart.

所生病：目黃，舌痛，臑臂內後廉痛、厥，掌中熱。

Disease which is engendered: Yellow eyes, painful tongue, pain of the medial posterior aspect of the upper arm and arm, reversal, and heat in the center of the palms.

盛者寸口大再倍於人迎；虛者寸口反小於人迎也。（臑音鐃）

In exuberance, the inch opening is triple the size of man's prognosis.

In vacuity, the inch opening retreats to become smaller than man's prognosis.

補：用未時。少衝為井木。木生火，虛則補其母。

Supplement: Use the wèi 未 hour [1-3 pm]. Shào Chōng 少衝 (HT 9) is the well

71. *Líng Shū*, Chapter 10 says "In vacuity, the inch opening retreats to become smaller than man's prognosis."

88

point, wood. Wood engenders fire. In vacuity, supplement its mother.

瀉：用午時 。神門為俞土 。火生土，實則瀉其子 。

Drain: Use the wǔ 午 hour [11 am – 1 pm]. Shén Mén 神門 (HT 7) is the stream point, earth. Fire engenders earth. In repletion, drain its son.

手太陽小腸經，屬丙火 。起少澤，終聽宮，多血少氣，未時注此 。

The hand tàiyáng small intestine channel belongs to bǐng 丙 fire. It arises in Shào Zé 少澤 (SI 1) and ends in Tīng Gōng 聽宮 (SI 19). It contains copious blood and scant qì which pool into it during the wèi 未 hour [1-3 pm].

是動病：嗌痛頷腫，不可回顧，肩似拔，臑似折，是主液 。

Disease when this [channel] stirs: Throat pain, submandibular swelling, and inability to turn the neck. The shoulder feels like it is dislocated; the upper arm feels like it is broken. This indicates the humors [yè 液, thick fluids].

所生病：耳聾目黃，頰腫，頸頷肩臑肘臂外後廉痛 。

Disease which is engendered: Deafness, yellow eyes, swollen cheeks; and pain in the lateral posterior aspect of the neck, chin, shoulder, upper arm, elbow, and forearm.

盛者人迎大再倍於寸口；虛者人迎反小於寸口也 。

In exuberance, man's prognosis is triple the size of the inch opening.

In vacuity, man's prognosis retreats to become smaller than the inch opening.

補：用申時 。後谿為俞木 。木生火，虛則補其母 。

Supplement: Use the shēn hour 申 [3-5 pm]. Hòu Xī 後谿 (SI 3) is the stream point, wood. Wood engenders fire. In vacuity, supplement its mother.

瀉：用未時 。小海為合土 。火生土，實則瀉其子 。

Drain: Use the wèi 未 hour [1-3 pm]. Xiǎo Hǎi 小海 (SI 8) is the uniting point, earth. Fire engenders earth. In repletion, drain its son.

足太陽膀胱經，屬壬水。起睛明，終至陰，多血少氣，申時注此。

The foot tàiyáng urinary bladder channel belongs to rén 壬 water. It arises in Jīng Míng 睛明 (UB 1) and ends in Zhì Yīn 至陰 (UB 67). It contains copious blood and scant qì which pool into it during the shēn 申 hour [3-5 pm].

是動病：頭痛，目似脫，項似拔，脊痛，腰似折，髀不可以曲，膕如結，腨似裂，是為踝厥，是主筋。（膕音國、腨音善）

Disease when this [channel] stirs: Headache and the eyes feel fit to burst from their sockets. The nape feels dislocated, with pain of the spine, and the low back feels like it is broken. The thighs cannot bend, the popliteal fossa feels like it is bound up, and the calves feel like they are ripped open. This is ankle reversal. This indicates the sinews.

所生病：痔瘧狂顛，頭顖頂痛，目黃淚出，衂衄，項背腰尻膕腨腳皆痛，小指不用。

Disease which is engendered: Hemorrhoids, malaria, mania, withdrawal; pain of the head, cheek, and vertex; yellow eyes, tearing, snivelling and nosebleeds. The nape, upper back, lower back, sacrum and coccyx, popliteal fossa, and calf are all painful; and loss of function of the little toe.

盛者人迎大再倍於寸口；虛者人迎反小於寸口也。

In exuberance, man's prognosis is triple the size of the inch opening.

In vacuity, man's prognosis retreats to become smaller than the inch opening.

補：用酉時。至陰為井金。金生水，虛則補其母。

Supplement: Use the yǒu 酉 hour [5-7 pm]. Zhì Yīn 至陰 (UB 67) is the well point, metal. Metal engenders water. In vacuity, supplement its mother.

瀉：用申時。束骨為俞水。水生木，實則瀉其子。

Drain: Use the shēn 申 hour [3-5 pm]. Shù Gǔ 束骨 (UB 65) is the stream point, water. Water engenders wood. In repletion, drain its son.

足少陰腎經，屬癸水。起湧泉，終俞府，多氣少血，酉時注此。

The foot shàoyīn kidney channel belongs to guǐ 癸 water. It arises in Yǒng Quán 湧泉 (KI 1) and ends in Shū Fǔ 俞府 (KI 27). It contains copious qì and scant blood which pool into it during the yǒu 酉 hour [5-7 pm].

是動病：飢不欲食，而黑如炭色，咳唾則有血，嗚嗚而喘，坐而欲起，目䀮䀮然，如無所見，心懸如飢狀，氣不足則善恐，心惕然如人將捕之，是謂骨厥，是主腎。

Disease when this [channel] stirs: No desire to eat despite hunger, and complexion black like charcoal, coughing or spitting blood, rales and panting, desire to get up when sitting, dim vision as if there is nothing on which to focus, the heart is suspended as if famished,[72] fearful when qì is insufficient, and the heart is apprehensive as if about to be arrested. This is bone reversal and indicates the kidneys.

所生病：口熱，舌乾咽腫，上氣嗌乾及痛，煩心，心痛，黃疸，腸澼，脊股內後廉痛，痿厥，嗜臥，足下熱而痛。

Disease which is engendered: Hot mouth, dry tongue, swollen throat, ascending qì, dry painful throat, vexed heart, heart pain, yellow jaundice, intestinal afflux (*pì* 澼) , pain in the spine and medial posterior aspect of the thighs, wilting reversal, somnolence, and hot painful soles of the feet.

盛者寸口大再倍於人迎；虛者寸口反小於人迎也。

In exuberance, the inch opening is triple the size of man's prognosis.

In vacuity, the inch opening retreats to become smaller than man's prognosis.

補：用戌時。復溜為經金。金生水，虛則補其母。

Supplement: Use the xū 戌 hour [7-9 pm]. Fù Liū 復溜 (KI 7) is the river, metal. Metal engenders water. In vacuity, supplement its mother.

瀉：用酉時。湧泉為井木。水生木，實則瀉其子。

---

72. Zhāng Jièbīn 張介賓 commented in the *Categorized Classic*: "When the heart and kidneys do not communicate, essence and spirit separate and scatter. Thus the heart is suspended. When there is yīn vacuity, the interior is hungry, so it is constantly as if it were famished."

Drain: Use the yǒu hour 酉 [5-7 pm]. Yǒng Quán 湧泉 (KI 1) is the well, wood. Water engenders wood. In repletion, drain its son.

手厥陰心包絡經，配腎（屬相火）。起天池，終中衝，多血少氣，戌時注此。

The hand juéyīn pericardium channel matches up with the kidneys (and belongs to minister fire). It arises in Tiān Chí 天池 (PC 1) and ends in Zhōng Chōng 中衝 (PC 9). It contains copious blood and scant qì which pool into it during the xū 戌 hour [7-9 pm].

是動病：手心熱，肘臂攣痛，腋下腫，甚則胸脅支滿，心中澹澹或大動，面赤目黃，善笑不休，是主心包絡。

Disease when this [channel] stirs: Heat in the heart of the hands, hypertonicity and pain of the elbows and arms, and swelling below the axilla. When it is severe, propping fullness of the chest and rib-sides, the heart [beating] "dan! dan! (澹澹)," sometimes stirring greatly, red face, yellow eyes, frequent laughter without rest. This indicates the pericardium.

所生病：煩心，心痛，掌中熱。

Disease which is engendered: Vexation of the heart, heart pain, and heat in the center of the palms.

盛者寸口大三倍於人迎；虛者寸口反小於人迎也。

In exuberance, the inch opening is quadruple the size of man's prognosis. [73]

In vacuity, the inch opening retreats to become smaller than man's prognosis.

補：用亥時。中衝為井木。木生火，虛則補其母。

Supplement: Use the hài 亥 hour [9-11 pm]. Zhōng Chōng 中衝 (PC 9) is the well point, wood. Wood engenders fire. In vacuity, supplement its mother.

瀉：用戌時。大陵為俞土。火生土，實則瀉其子。

---

73. *Magic Pivot*, Chapter 10 says, "In exuberance, the inch opening is double the size of man's prognosis."

Drain: Use the xū 戌 hour [7-9 pm]. Dà Líng 大陵 (PC 7) **is the stream point, earth. Fire engenders earth. In repletion, drain its son.**

手少陽三焦經，配心包絡，（ 屬相火 ）。起關衝，終耳門，多氣少血，亥時注此 。

The hand shàoyáng triple burner channel **matches up with the pericardium (and belongs to minister fire). It arises in Guān Chōng** 關衝 **(SJ 1) and ends in Ěr Mén** 耳門 **(SJ 21).[74] It contains copious qì and scant blood which pool into it during the hài** 亥 **hour [9-11 pm].**

是動病：耳聾，渾渾焞焞，咽腫喉痹，是主氣 。（ 焞音吞 ）

Disease when this [channel] stirs: **Deafness, sounds are garbled, swollen throat, throat impediment (***bì*** 痹). This indicates qì.**

所生病：汗出，目銳眥痛，頰痛，耳後肩臑肘臂外皆痛，小指次指不用 。

Disease which is engendered: **Sweating, pain at the outer canthus, cheek pain; pain all behind the ears and on the outside of the shoulders, upper arms, elbows, and forearms; loss of function in the ring finger.**

盛者人迎大一倍於寸口；虛者人迎反小於寸口也 。

In exuberance, man's prognosis is double the size of the inch opening.

In vacuity, man's prognosis retreats to become smaller than the inch opening.

補：用子時 。中渚為俞木 。木生火，虛則補其母 。

Supplement: **Use the zǐ** 子 **hour [11 pm – 1 am]. Zhōng Zhǔ** 中渚 **(SJ 3) is the stream point, wood. Wood engenders fire. In vacuity, supplement its mother.**

瀉：用亥時 。天井為合土 。火生土，實則瀉其子 。

Drain: **Use the hài** 亥 **hour [9-11 pm]. Tiān Jǐng** 天井 **(SJ 10) is the uniting point,**

---

74. According to most sources, there are 23 points on the Triple Burner Channel. Later, in Volume 7, Yáng continues to list Ěr Mén 耳門 (SJ 21) as the last point on the Triple Burner Channel.

earth. Fire engenders earth. In repletion, drain its son.

足少陽膽經，屬甲木。起瞳子髎，終竅陰，多氣少血，子時注此。（髎音僚）

The foot shàoyáng gall bladder channel belongs to jiǎ 甲 wood. It arises in Tóng Zǐ Liáo 瞳子髎 (GB 1) and ends in Qiào Yīn 竅陰 (GB 44). It contains copious qì and scant blood which pool into it during the zǐ 子 hour [11 pm – 1 am].

是動病：口苦，善太息，心脅痛，不能轉側，甚則面微有塵，體無膏澤，足外反熱，是為陽厥，是主骨。

Disease when this [channel] stirs: Bitter mouth, frequent sighing, pain of the heart and rib-sides, and inability to turn to the sides. When severe, the facial complexion is slightly dusty, the body lacks oil and luster, and heat returns up the outside of the legs. This is yáng reversal. This indicates the bones.

所生病：頭角頷痛，目銳眥痛，缺盆中腫痛，腋下腫，馬刀挾癭，汗出，振寒瘧，胸中脅肋髀膝外，至脛絕骨外踝前，乃諸節皆痛，小指次指不用。

Disease which is engendered: Pain at the corners of the head and the submandibular region, pain of the outer canthus, swelling and pain in the supraclavicular fossa (Quē Pén 缺盆 – ST 12), swelling below the axilla, saber and pearl-string lumps,[75] sweating, quivering with cold from malaria; pain in all the joints from the center of the chest and rib-sides, to the lateral thighs and knees, reaching the lower leg at Jué Gǔ 絕骨 (GB 39), anterior to the lateral malleolus; and loss of function of the fourth toe.

盛者人迎大三倍於寸口；虛者人迎反小於寸口也。

In exuberance, man's prognosis is quadruple the size of the inch opening. [76]

In vacuity, man's prognosis retreats to become smaller than the inch opening.

補：用丑時。俠谿為滎水。水生木，虛則補其母。邱墟，為原皆取之。

Supplement: Use the chǒu 丑 hour [1-3 am]. Xiá Xī 俠谿 (GB 43) is the brook point,

---

75. Forms of scrofula.

76. *Magic Pivot*, Chapter 10 says, "In exuberance, man's prognosis is is double the size of the inch opening."

water. Water engenders wood. In vacuity, supplement its mother. Qiū Xū 邱墟 (GB 40) is the source point. Apply treatment to both.

瀉：用子時 。陽輔為經火 。木生火，實則瀉其子 。

Drain: Use the zǐ 子 hour [11 pm – 1 am]. Yáng Fǔ 陽輔 (GB 38) is the river point, fire. Wood engenders fire. In repletion, drain its son.

足厥陰肝經，屬乙木 。起大敦，終期門，多血少氣，丑時注此 。

The foot juéyīn liver channel belongs to yǐ 乙 wood. It arises in Dà Dūn 大敦 (LV 1) and ends in Qī Mén 期門 (LV 14). It contains copious blood and scant qì which pool into it during the chǒu 丑 hour [1-3 am].

是動病：腰痛不可俛仰，丈夫癩疝，婦人小腹腫，甚則咽乾，面塵脫色，是主肝 。

Disease when this [channel] stirs: Low back pain, inability to bend forward and backward, males have bulging mounting [*tuí shàn* 癩疝], and females have swelling in the lower abdomen. When it is severe, there is dry throat and a dusty sloughing facial complexion. This indicates the liver.

所生病：胸滿嘔逆，洞泄，狐疝，遺溺癃閉 。

Disease which is engendered: Chest fullness, vomiting counterflow, throughflux diarrhea, foxy mounting [*hú shàn* 狐疝], incontinence of urine, and dribbling urinary block.

盛者寸口脈大一倍於人迎；虛者寸口脈反小於人迎也 。

In exuberance, the inch opening pulse is double the size of man's prognosis.

In vacuity, the inch opening pulse retreats to become smaller than man's prognosis.

補：用寅時 。曲泉為合水 。水生木，虛則補其母 。

Supplement: Use the yín 寅 hour [3-5 am]. Qū Quán 曲泉 (LV 8) is the uniting point, water. Water engenders wood. In vacuity, supplement its mother.

瀉：用丑時 。行間為滎火 。木生火，實則瀉其子 。

Drain: Use the chǒu 丑 hour [1-3 am]. Xíng Jiān 行間 (LV 2) is the brook point, fire. Wood engenders fire. In repletion, drain its son.

十二經氣血多少歌
Twelve Channels[77] Amounts of Qì and Blood Song[78]

多氣多血經須記，大腸手經足經胃，
少血多氣有六經，三焦膽腎心脾肺，
多血少氣心包絡，膀胱小腸肝所異 。

**The channels with copious qì and copious blood must be recorded:
large intestine is the hand channel, and the foot channel is stomach.**

**There are six channels with scant blood and copious qì:
triple burner, gall bladder, kidney, heart, spleen, and lung.**

**Copious blood and scant qì:
it is pericardium; urinary bladder, small intestine, and liver that differ.**

---

77. Some editions have "Twelve Hours" (十二時) and others have "Twelve Channels" (十二經).

78. This poem isn't from any of the sources Yáng used in this chapter. Perhaps he wrote it himself.

針灸大成 · 卷之五

十二經治症主客原絡圖 （楊氏）
The Twelve Channels Treat Patterns, Using Host-Guest, Source and Luo Points, with Illustrations (Master Yáng)[79]

肺之主大腸客
Lungs as the Host, Large Intestine as the Guest

太陰多氣而少血，心胸氣脹掌發熱，
喘咳缺盆痛莫禁，咽腫喉乾身汗越，
肩內前廉兩乳疼，痰結膈中氣如缺，
所生病者何穴求，太淵偏歷與君說 。

Tàiyīn has copious qì and scant blood;
qì distention of the heart and chest, feverish palms,
No one can avoid panting and cough,
pain in the supraclavicular fossa;
swollen or dry throat, body sweating more and more,
Pain in the medial anterior shoulder and the two breasts;
phlegm binding the diaphragm, qì is lacking,
What points should we seek for disease which is engendered?
Speak with a gentleman about Tài Yuān 太淵 (LU 9)
and Piān Lì 偏歷 (LI 6).

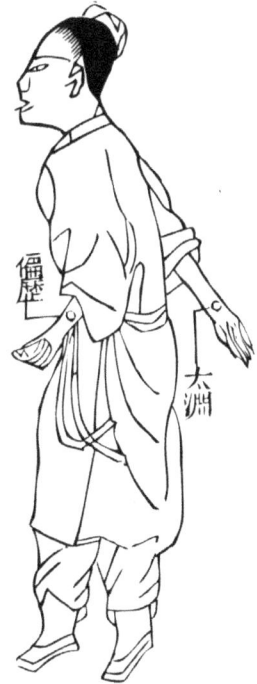

可刺手太陰肺經原（ 原者太淵穴，肺脈所過為原 。掌後內側橫紋頭，動脈相應寸口是 ）。

You can needle the source point of the hand tàiyīn lung channel. (The source point is Tài Yuān 太淵 - LU 9; the source point is "the place of passing through" on the lung vessel. It is proximal to the inner aspect of the palm, at the end of the horizontal crease. This is the stirring vessel that corresponds to the inch opening.)

Fig. 5.13

復刺手陽明大腸絡（ 絡者偏歷穴，去腕三寸，別走太陰 ）。

---

79. Many of the symptoms listed are from *Magic Pivot*, Chapter 10 or *Elementary Questions*, Chapter 63. For each channel there is a poem. Then there are two formulaic sentences that are repeated after each poem, changing only the names of the channels and the points, and describing the point location.

Also needle the network point of the hand yángmíng large intestine channel. (The network point is Piān Lì 偏歷 - LI 6, three *cùn* from the wrist. [The network vessel] diverges [from this point] to run over to the tàiyīn channel.)

大腸主肺之客
Large Intestine as the Host, Lungs as the Guest

陽明大腸俠鼻孔，面痛齒疼腮頰腫，
生疾目黃口亦乾，鼻流清涕及血湧，
喉痹肩前痛莫當，大指次指為一統，
合谷列缺取為奇，二穴針之居病總 。

Yángmíng large intestine channel passes by
both sides of the nostrils:
facial pain, toothache, and swollen cheeks,
Engendered disease: yellow eyes, the mouth is also dry;
runny nose with clear snivel as well as blood gushing,
Throat impediment (*bì* 痹), pain in the anterior shoulder,
none of this should be;
the index finger is part of the whole [pattern],
Applying treatment to Hé Gǔ 合谷 (LI 4)
and Liè Quē 列缺 (LU 7) is extraordinary;
needling the two points manages disease overall.

可刺手陽明大腸原（ 原者合谷穴，大腸脈所過為原，歧骨間 ）。

You can needle the source point of the hand yángmíng large intestine channel. (The source point is Hé Gǔ 合谷 – LI 4; the source point is "the place of passing through" on the large intestine vessel. It is between the forking bones.)

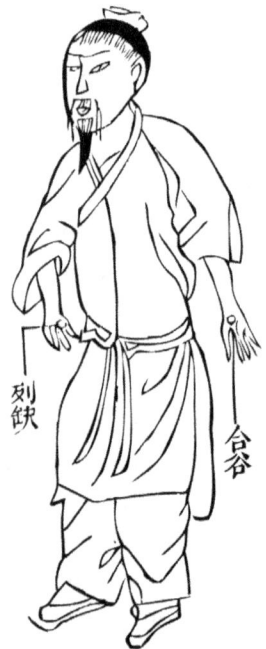

Fig. 5.14

復刺手太陰肺經絡（ 絡者列缺穴，去腕側上寸半，交叉食指盡處是，別走陽明 ）。

Also needle the network point of the hand tàiyīn lung channel. (The network point is Liè Quē 列缺 – LU 7, one and a half *cùn* above the side of the wrist. Make the forks [between the thumbs and the index fingers] meet. It is at the end of the index finger. [The network vessel] diverges [from this point] to run to the yángmíng channel.)

脾主胃客
Spleen as the Host, Stomach as the Guest

脾經為病舌本強，嘔吐胃翻痛腹臟，
陰氣上衝噫難瘳，體重脾搖心事妄，
瘧生振慄兼體羸，秘結疸黃手執杖，
股膝內腫厥而疼，太白豐隆取為尚。

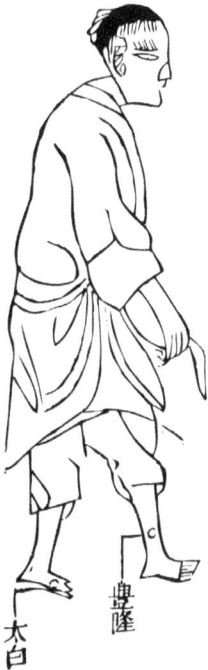

The spleen channel sickens with a stiff root of the tongue;
vomiting, stomach reflux, diseases of the abdominal viscera, [80]
Yīn qì surges upward, with belching that is difficult to heal;
the body is heavy, the spleen shakes,
the affairs of the heart are frenetic,
Malaria is engendered, shivering,
and at the same time emaciation;
bound up stool, yellow jaundice, the hands grasp a cane,
The inside of the thighs and knees is swollen,
with reversal [cold] and pain;
applying treatment to Tài Bái 太白 (SP 3)
and Fēng Lóng 豐隆 (ST 40) is valuable.

可刺足太陰脾經原（ 原者太白穴，脾脈所過為原，足大
指內踝前，核骨下陷中 ）。

Fig. 5.15

You can needle the source point of the foot tàiyīn spleen
channel. (The source point is Tài Bái 太白 – SP 3; the source
point is "the place of passing through" on the spleen vessel. It is in a depression on
the big toe anterior to the medial malleolus, below the node bone.)[81]

復刺足陽明胃經絡（ 絡者豐隆穴，去踝八寸，別走太陰 ）。

Also needle the network point of the foot yángmíng stomach channel. (The network
point is Fēng Lóng 豐隆 – ST 40, eight *cùn* from the malleolus. [The network vessel]
diverges [from this point] to run to the tàiyīn channel.)

---

80. *Magic Pivot* has *zhàng* 脹 (distention) instead of *zàng* 臟 (viscera) in Chapter 10.

81. Node bone: the first metatarsophalangeal joint.

胃主脾客
Stomach as the Host, Spleen as the Guest

腹填心悶意悽愴，惡人惡火惡燈光，
耳聞響動心中惕，鼻衄唇喎瘧又傷，
棄衣驟步身中熱，痰多足痛與瘡瘍，
氣蠱胸腿疼難止，衝陽公孫一刺康 。

Abdominal fullness, heart oppression, reflection and sorrow;
aversion to people, aversion to fire, aversion to light,
When the ear hears sounds stirring,
there is apprehension in the heart;
nosebleeds, deviated lips, and malaria also damages,
Casting off clothes and running around, heat in the body;
copious phlegm, foot pain, and sores,
Qì (*gǔ* 蠱), [82] chest and leg pain that is difficult to stop;
as soon as Chōng Yáng 衝陽 (ST 42)
and Gōng Sūn 公孫 (SP 4) are needled, there is well-being.

可刺足陽明胃經原（ 原者衝陽穴，胃脈所過為原，足跗上五寸，骨間動脈 ）。

You can needle the source point of the foot yángmíng stomach channel. (The source point is Chōng Yáng 衝陽 – ST 42; the source point is "the place of passing through" on the stomach vessel. It is five *cùn* above the instep of the foot at the stirring vessel between the bones.)

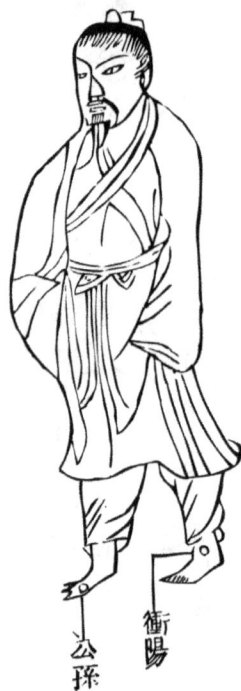

Fig. 5.16

復刺足太陰脾經絡（ 絡者公孫穴，去足大指本節後一寸，內踝前，別走陽明 ）。

Also needle the network point of the foot tàiyīn spleen channel. (The network point is Gōng Sūn 公孫 – SP 4, one *cùn* behind the root joint of the big toe, in front of the medial malleolus. [The network vessel] diverges [from this point] to run to the yángmíng channel.)

---

82. *Gǔ* 蠱 is a toxin that is said to be from various insects and reptiles. It affects the liver and speen and can result in drum distention. There are various kinds of *gǔ* 蠱. This one affects qì.

真心主小腸客
True Heart as the Host, Small Intestine as the Guest

少陰心痛并乾嗌，渴欲飲分為臂厥，
生病目黃口亦乾，脅臂疼分掌發熱，
若人欲治勿差求，專在醫人心審察，
驚悸嘔血及怔忡，神門支正何堪缺。

Shàoyīn heart pain and dry throat;
thirst and desire to eat, these are arm reversal,
Engendered disease: yellow eyes, the mouth is also dry;
rib-side and arm pain, feverish palms,
If the patient desires treatment, do not seek after error;
the doctor must concentrate his
heart for careful examination,
Fright palpitations, vomiting blood and fearful throbbing;
how can Shén Mén 神門 (HT 7)
and Zhī Zhèng 支正 (SI 7) be lacking!

可刺手少陰心經原（原者神門穴，心脈所過為原，手掌後銳骨端陷中）。

You can needle the source point of the hand shàoyīn heart channel. (The source point is Shén Mén 神門 – HT 7; the source point is "the place of passing through" on the heart vessel. It is in a depression behind the palm at the end of the styloid process of the ulna.)

Fig. 5.17

復刺手太陽小腸絡（絡者支正穴，腕上五寸，別走少陰）。

Also needle the network point of the hand tàiyáng small intestine channel. (The network point is Zhī Zhèng 支正 – SI 7, five *cùn* above the wrist. [The network vessel] diverges [from this point] to run to the shàoyīn channel.)

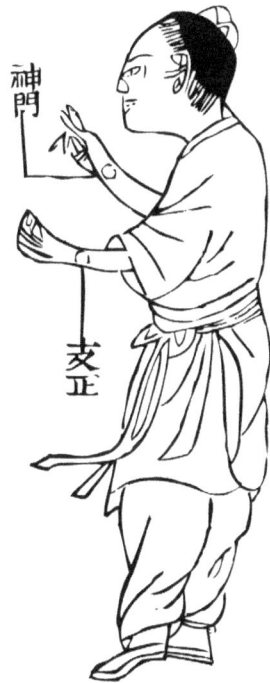

小腸主真心客
Small Intestine as the Host, True Heart as the Guest

小腸之病豈為良，頰腫肩疼兩臂旁，
項頸強疼難轉側，嗌頷腫痛甚非常，
肩似拔兮臑似折，生病耳聾及目黃，
臑肘臂外後廉痛，腕骨通里取為詳 。

How can you improve diseases of the small intestine?
Swollen cheeks, shoulder pain, the sides of the two arms,
Stiffness and pain of the neck,
difficulty turning to the side;
swollen painful throat and submandibular region,
this is quite abnormal,
Shoulders seem dislocated, upper arms seem broken;
engendered disease: deafness and yellow eyes,
For pain in the lateral posterior aspect of the upper arm,
elbow, and forearm; select Wàn Gǔ 腕骨 (SI 4)
and Tōng Lǐ 通里 (HT 5) in particular.

可刺手太陽小腸原（ 原者腕骨穴，小腸脈所過為
原，手外側腕前起骨下陷中 ）。

You can needle the source point of the hand tàiyáng small
intestine channel. (The source point is Wàn Gǔ 腕骨 –
SI 4; the source point is "the place of passing through"
on the small intestine vessel. It is in a depression on the
lateral aspect of the arm, in front of the wrist, below the place where the bone arises.)

Fig. 5.18

復刺手少陰心經絡（ 絡者通里穴，去腕一寸，別走太陽 ）。

Also needle the network point of the hand shàoyīn heart channel. (The network
point is Tōng Lǐ 通里 – HT 5, one *cùn* away from the wrist. [The network vessel]
diverges [from this point] to run to the tàiyáng channel.)

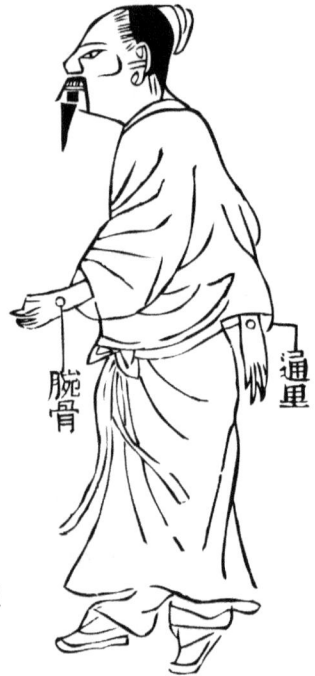

腎之主膀胱客
Kidneys as the Host, Urinary Bladder as the Guest

臉黑嗜臥不欲粮，目不明兮發熱狂，
腰痛足疼步難履，若人捕獲難躲藏，
心膽戰兢氣不足，更兼胸結與身黃，
若欲除之無更法，太谿飛揚取最良。

Black shanks of the legs, somnolence, no desire for food; the
eyes are not bright, fever, and mania,
Low back pain, leg pain, difficulty walking;
the person acts like he is about to be captured,
having difficulty hiding,
Heart and gall bladder trembling with fear, qì insufficiency;
in addition, bound up chest and yellow body,
If you desire to eliminate it, there is no better method;
applying treatment to Tài Xī 太谿 (KI 3)
and Fēi Yáng 飛揚 (UB 58) is the best.

可刺足少陰腎經原（原者太谿穴，腎脈所過為原，內踝
下後跟骨上，動脈陷中，屈五指乃得穴）。

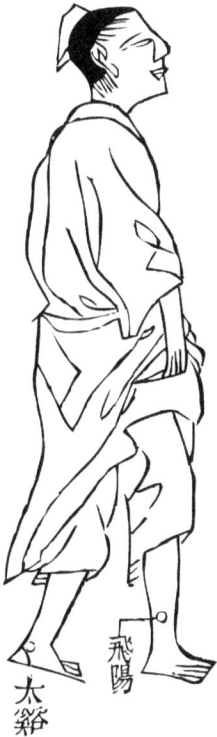
Fig. 5.19

You can needle the source point of the foot shàoyīn kidney
channel. (The source point is Tài Xī 太谿 – KI 3; the source
point is "the place of passing through" on the kidney vessel.
It is below and behind the medial malleolus, above the heel
bone in a depression at the stirring vessel. Bend the five toes
to locate the point.)

復刺足太陽膀胱絡（絡者飛揚穴，外踝上七寸，別走少陰）。

Also needle the network point of the foot tàiyáng urinary bladder channel. (The
network point is Fēi Yáng 飛揚 – UB 58, seven *cùn* above the lateral malleolus. [The
network vessel] diverges [from this point] to run to the shàoyīn channel.)

膀胱主腎之客
Urinary Bladder as the Host, Kidneys as the Guest

膀胱頸病目中疼，項腰足腿痛難行，
痢瘧狂顛心膽熱，背弓反手額眉稜，
鼻衄目黃筋骨縮，脫肛痔漏腹心膨，
若要除之無別法，京骨大鍾任顯能 。

Urinary bladder neck pain, pain in the eyes;
nape, low back, feet, and leg pain, difficult to walk,
Dysentery, malaria, mania and withdrawal,
heat in the heart and gall bladder;
upper back arched, arms to the back,
forehead and eyebrows ridged,
Nosebleeds, yellow eyes, contracted sinews and bones;
prolapse of the rectum, hemorrhoids and fistulas,
inflated abdomen and heart region,
If it is important to eliminate it,
do not diverge from this method;
Jīng Gǔ 京骨 (UB 64) and
Dà Zhōng 大鍾 (KI 4) show obvious ability.

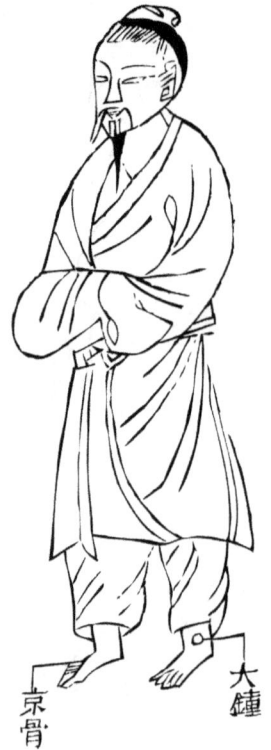

Fig. 5.20

可刺足太陽膀胱原（ 原者京骨穴，膀胱脈所過為原，
足小指大骨下，赤白肉際陷中 ）。

You can needle the source point of the foot tàiyáng urinary
bladder channel. (The source point is Jīng Gǔ 京骨 – UB
64; the source point is "the place of passing through" on the
urinary bladder vessel. It is below the large bone of the little
toe in a depression at the junction of the red and white skin.)

復刺足少陰腎經絡（ 絡者大鍾穴，當踝後繞跟，別走太陽 ）。

Also needle the network point of the foot shàoyīn kidney channel. (The network
point is Dà Zhōng 大鍾 – KI 4, right behind the malleolus skirting around the heel.
[The network vessel] diverges [from this point] to run to the tàiyáng channel.)

三焦主包絡客
Triple Burner as the Host, Pericardium as the Guest

三焦為病耳中聾，喉痹咽乾目腫紅，
耳後肘疼并出汗，脊間心後痛相從，
肩背風生連膊肘，大便堅閉及遺癃，
前病治之何穴愈，陽池內關理法同。

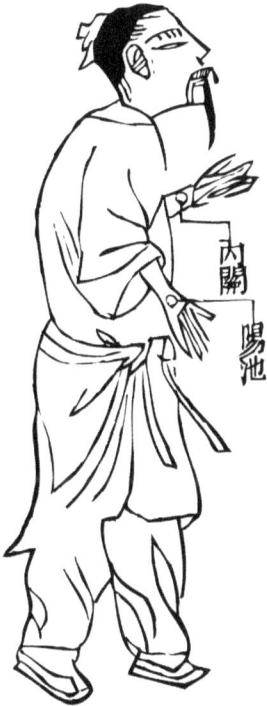

**When the three burners become diseased:
deafness in the ears; throat impediment (*bì* 痹),
dry throat, swollen red eyes,
Pain behind the ears and in the elbows with sweating;
pain travels between the spine and the back of the heart,
Wind is engendered in the shoulders
and upper back radiating to the arm and elbows;
stool is hard and blocked,
as well as incontinence [of urine] or dribbling blockage,
To treat the previous diseases, which points will cure?
Yáng Chí 陽池 (SJ 4) and Nèi Guān 內關 (PC 6)
together are the method of rectification.**

可刺手少陽三焦經原（ 原者陽池穴，三焦脈所過為
原，手表腕上橫斷處陷中 ）。

**You can needle the source point of the hand shàoyáng
triple burner channel. (The source point is Yáng Chí 陽
池 – SJ 4; the source point is "the place of passing through"
on the triple burner vessel. It is in a depression on the exterior wrist at the site of the
horizontal break.)**

復刺手厥陰心包經絡（ 絡者內關穴，去掌二寸兩筋間，別走少陽 ）。

**Also needle the network point of the hand juéyīn pericardium channel. (The net-
work point is Nèi Guān 內關 – PC 6, two *cùn* away from the palm between the two
sinews. [The network vessel] diverges [from this point] to run to the shàoyáng channel.)**

包絡主三焦客
Pericardium as the Host, Triple Burner as the Guest

包絡為病手攣急，臂不能伸痛如屈，
胸膺脅滿腋腫平，心中淡淡面色赤，
目黃善笑不肯休，心煩心痛掌熱極，
良醫達士細推詳，大陵外關病消釋。

When the pericardium becomes diseased,
there is hypertonicity of the hands;
the arms are unable to extend,
and are painful if they are bent,
Fullness of the chest, breasts, and rib-sides,
swollen axilla [until] level;
the heart is agitated and the facial complexion is red,
Yellow eyes, frequent laughter, cannot rest;
heart vexation, heart pain, palms extremely hot,
A good doctor or penetrating scholar
carefully infers the details;
Dà Líng 大陵 (PC 7) and Wài Guān 外關 (SJ 5)
disperse and dispel disease.

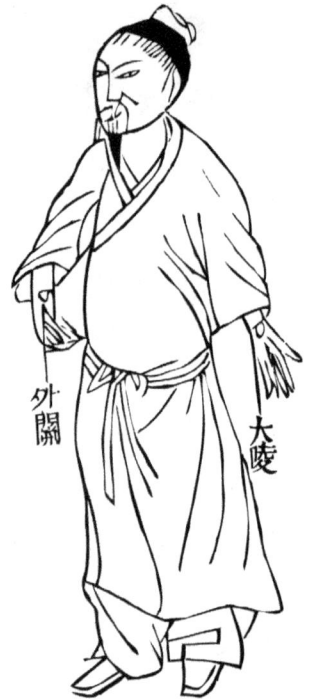

可刺手厥陰心包經原（ 原者大陵穴，包絡脈所過為
原，掌後橫紋中 ）。

You can needle the source point of the hand juéyīn pericardium channel. (The source point is Dà Líng 大陵 – PC
7; the source point is "the place of passing through" on the
pericardium vessel. It is proximal to the palm in the center of the horizontal crease.)

復刺手少陽三焦經絡（ 絡者外關穴，去腕二寸，別走厥陰 ）。

Also needle the network point of the hand shàoyáng triple burner channel. (The
network point is Wài Guān 外關 – SJ 5, two *cùn* away from the wrist. [The network
vessel] diverges [from this point] to run to the juéyīn channel.)

肝主膽客
Liver as the Host, Gall Bladder as the Guest

氣少血多肝之經，丈夫潰散苦腰疼，
婦人腹膨小腹腫，甚則咽乾面脫塵，
所生病者胸滿嘔，腹中泄瀉痛無停，
癃閉遺溺疝瘕痛，太光二穴即安甯 。
（ 潰散虛憊 ）

The liver channel has scant qì and copious blood;
males are dispersed and scattered,[83] suffering low back pain,
Females have abdominal inflation,
swelling of the lower abdomen;
when it is severe: dry throat, the facial complexion
is sloughing and dusty,
Engendered disease: chest fullness and vomiting;
in the abdomen, diarrhea and pain that does not stop,
Dribbling urinary block or incontinence of urine,
shàn 疝 (mounting), conglomerations (jiǎ 瘕), and pain;
the two points Tài Chōng 太衝 (LV 3)
and Guāng Míng 光明 (GB 37) mean health and tranquility.
("dispersed and scattered" means vacuity fatigue)

可刺足厥陰肝之原（ 原者太衝穴，肝脈所過為原，足大
指節後二寸，動脈陷是 ）。

You can needle the source point of the foot juéyīn liver channel.
(The source point is Tài Chōng 太衝 – LV 3; the source point is
"the place of passing through" on the liver vessel. It is two *cùn*
behind the joint of the big toe in the depression with the stirring vessel.)

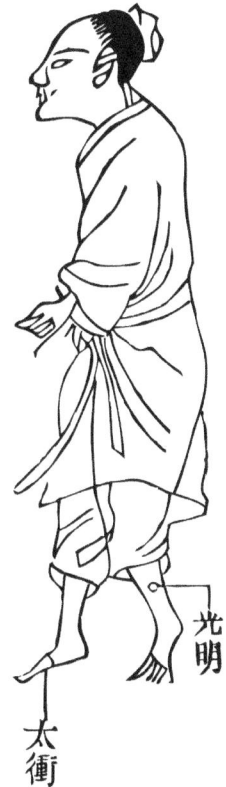

Fig. 5.23

復刺足少陽膽經絡（ 絡者光明穴，去外踝五寸，別走厥陰 ）。

Also needle the network point of the foot shàoyáng gall bladder channel. (The network point is Guāng Míng 光明 – GB 37, five *cùn* away from the lateral malleolus.
[The network vessel] diverges [from this point] to run to the juéyīn channel.)

---

83. Some editions have *tuí shàn* 癀疝 (prominent mounting) instead of *kuì sǎn* 潰散 (dispersed
and scattered). However, there is also a note in the editions that have *kuì sǎn* 潰散 that it means
"vacuity fatigue."

膽主肝客
Gall Bladder as the Host, Liver as the Guest

膽經之穴何病主？胸脅肋疼足不舉，
面體不澤頭目疼，缺盆腋腫汗如雨，
頸項瘻瘤堅似鐵，瘧生寒熱連骨髓，
以上病症欲除之，須向邱墟蠡溝取 。

What diseases are indicated for points
of the gall bladder channel?
Pain of the chest and rib-sides, the feet cannot be lifted,
The face and body have no sheen, pain of the head and eyes;
swelling of the supraclavicular fossa and axilla,
sweating like rain,
Goiter and tumors on the neck, hard like iron;
malaria engendering cold and heat,
connected to the bone and marrow,
If you desire to eliminate the above disease patterns;
you must apply treatment toward
Qiū Xū 邱墟 (GB 40) and Zhī Gōu 支溝 (LV 5).

可刺足少陽膽經原（ 原者邱墟穴，膽脈所過為原，足
外踝下從前陷中，去臨泣三寸 ）。

You can needle the source point point of the foot shàoyáng
gall bladder channel. (The source point is Qiū Xū 邱墟 – GB
40; the source is "the place of passing through" on the gall
bladder vessel. It is below the lateral malleolus, in the anterior depression, three *cùn* from Lín Qì 臨泣 – GB 41.)

復刺足厥陰肝經絡（ 絡者蠡溝穴，去內踝五寸，別走
少陽 ）。

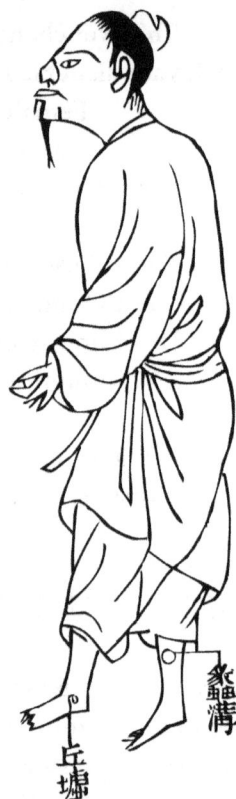

Fig. 5.24

Also needle the network point of the foot juéyīn liver channel. (The network point is
Lǐ Gōu 蠡溝 – LV 5, five *cùn* from the medial malleolus. [The network vessel] diverges [from this point] to run to the shàoyáng channel.)

靈龜取法飛騰針圖 (徐氏)

Mystical Tortoise Selection Method and Flying and Soaring Acupuncture Diagram (Master Xú[84])

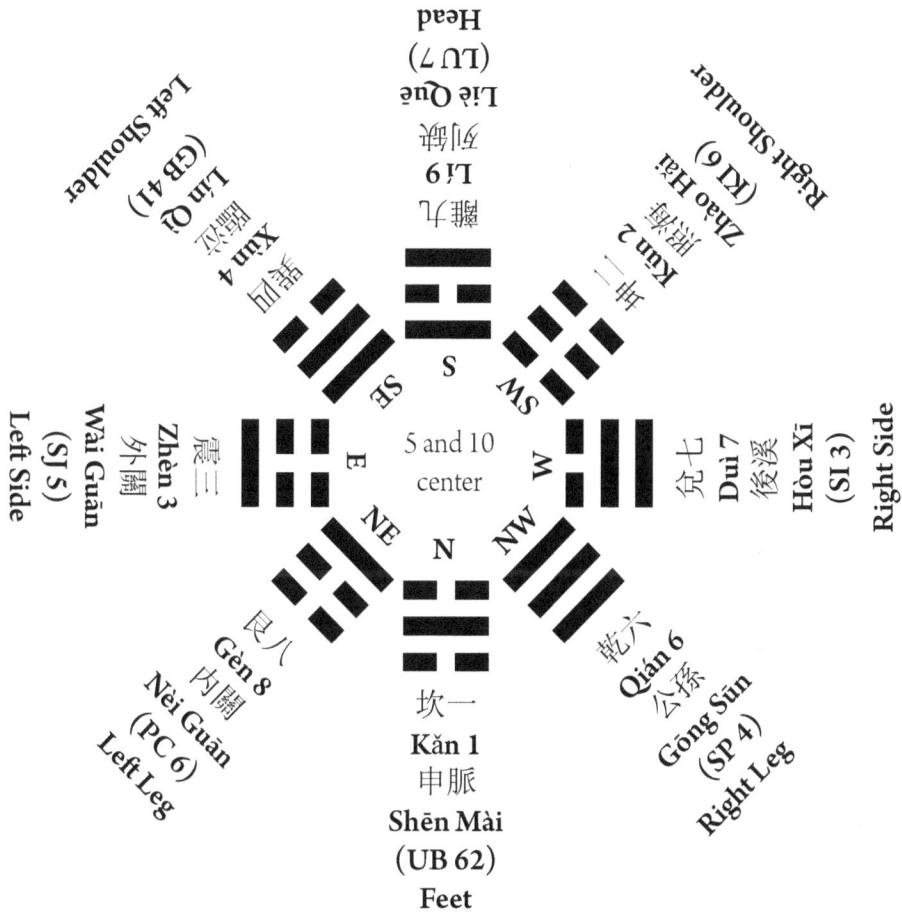

84. Xú Fèng 徐鳳 published *Zhēn Jiǔ Dà Quán*《針灸大全》(the Great Completion of Acupuncture-Moxibustion) in 1439 (*Míng*). This and the following sections come from Volume 4.

九宮歌
Song of the Nine Palaces

戴九履一，左三右七，
二四為肩，八六為足，
五十居中，寄於坤局。

**Wear nine on the head, tread on one; left is three, right is seven,
Two and four are the shoulders; eight and six are the legs,
Five and ten reside in the center; they lodge in the office of kūn.**

Translator's note:

These numbers refer to the *Luò Shū* 洛書 and its related diagram, the magic square of three. The concept of this poem belongs to the image and number theories of the *Yì Jīng* 《 易經 》 Book of Changes. The layout described in the poem can be seen in the following diagram:

Southeast Xùn 4 left shoulder	South Lí 9 head	Southwest Kūn 2 right shoulder
East Zhèn 3 left side	5 and 10 center	West Duì 7 right side
Northeast Gèn 8 left leg	North Kǎn 1 feet	Northwest Qián 6 right leg

This short poem had been passed down for centuries before Yáng included it in his book. It connects certain body parts with the numbers of the *Luò Shū*. For example, "wear nine on the head" refers to the position of nine in the center top. It states "two and four are the shoulders" because two and four are on the upper sides of the diagram.

"Five and ten reside in the center; they are sent to the office of kūn" needs a little explanation. Five is in the center of the *Luò Shū* and Magic Square but ten is usually not included because the *Luò Shū* and Magic Square only contain nine numbers. However, five and ten are both in the center of the Hé Tú 河圖, another diagram associated with the *Book of Changes*. The center belongs to earth as does the southwest kūn (☷) direction. Since the center does not have its own trigram, the earth element of the center is given to the earth trigram: kūn guà 坤卦.

八法歌
Eight Methods Song[85]

坎一聯申脈，照海坤二五 。
震三屬外關，巽四臨泣數 。
乾六是公孫，兌七後谿府 。
艮八繫內關，離九列缺主 。

Kǎn-one (☵) is an ally of Shēn Mài 申脈 (UB 62).
Zhào Hǎi 照海 (KI 6) and kūn (☷) are two and five.
Zhèn-three (☳) belongs to Wài Guān 外關 (SJ 5).
Xùn-four (☴) is the number of Lín Qì 臨泣 (GB 41).
Qián-six (☰) is Gōng Sūn 公孫 (SP 4).
Duì-seven (☱) is the mansion of Hòu Xī 後谿 (SI 3).
Gèn-eight (☶) is attached to Nèi Guān 內關 (PC 6).
Lí-nine (☲) is the host of Liè Quē 列缺 (LU 7).

按靈龜飛騰圖有二，人莫適從，今取其效驗者錄之耳 。

Note: There are two diagrams for Mystical Tortoise and Flying and Soaring. No one agrees which one to follow. Now I have selected the effective one and recorded it.[86]

Translator's note:
This poem assigns the confluence points of the eight extraordinary vessels to the numbers of the *Luò Shū* 洛書 and trigrams of the *Yì Jīng* 《 易經 》. Later, Yáng will describe a calculation for selecting these points based on the time and date. The number resulting from the calculation will define which point is to be used during this time and date.

Kǎn and the number 1 correspond to each other. So when the poem says "kǎn-one" it is essentially referring to the same thing. This also goes for kūn-two, zhèn-three, etc.

There are two point diagrams related to the *Luò Shū* and the eight extraordinary vessels: one for the Mystical Tortoise Method and another for the Flying and Soaring Method. Although both use the confluence points of the eight extraordinary vessels, these are two separate methods with different calculations and different point correspondences with the eight trigrams. Yáng states here that there

---

85. From *Zhēn Jiǔ Dà Quán* 《 針灸大全 》 (Great Completion of Acupuncture-Moxibustion), Volume 4.

86. This note was not in the *Great Completion of Acupuncture-Moxibustion*. It was probably added by Yáng.

is only one correct method. He describes the Method of the Mystical Tortoise and ignores Flying and Soaring. The following table lays out which books up to and including the *Great Compendium* describe these two methods.

Book	Mystical Tortoise	Flying And Soaring*
Zhen Jiu Yù Lóng Jīng《針灸玉龍經》by Wáng Guóruì 王國瑞, *Yuán* Dynasty	no	used day and hour, stem and branch
Zhēn Jiǔ Dà Quán《針灸大全》by Xú Fèng 徐鳳, *Míng* Dynasty	yes	used hour stem, but the author preferred Mystical Tortoise Method
Zhēn Jiǔ Jù Yīng《針灸聚英》by Gāo Wǔ 高武, *Míng* Dynasty	no	used hour stem
This book: *Zhēn Jiǔ Dà Chéng*《針灸大成》by Yáng Jìzhōu 楊繼洲, *Míng* Dynasty	yes	no

* While the association of points with trigrams is the same for both methods of Flying and Soaring, there are two different ways of calculating which trigram (and therefore which point) is associated with a particular hour. However, this does not affect the information in Yáng's *Great Compendium*, since only the Method of the Mystical Tortoise is discussed there.

Since Yáng felt that the Mystical Tortoise is the correct method, he mostly cited *Zhēn Jiǔ Dà Quán* below, the only earlier book to discuss the Method of the Mystical Tortoise.

八法交會八脈
The Eight Methods Confluence of the Eight Vessels[87]

公孫二穴，父，通衝脈	合於心胸胃
內關二穴，母，通陰維脈	
後谿二穴，夫，通督脈	合於目內眥頸項耳肩膊小腸膀胱
申脈二穴，妻，通陽蹻脈	
臨泣二穴，男，通帶脈	合於目銳眥耳後頰頸肩
外關二穴，女，通陽維脈	

---

87. Yáng seems to have taken this whole section from the *Zhēn Jiǔ Dà Quán*《針灸大全》(Great Completion of Acupuncture-Moxibustion), Volume 4. However, this particular diagram was first published in *Zhēn Jīng Zhǐ Nán*《針經指南》(Compass for the Acupuncture Classic) by Dòu Hànqīng 竇漢卿 during the *Yuán* Dynasty.

列缺二穴，主，通任脈	合於肺系咽喉胸膈
照海二穴，客，通陰蹻脈	

The two points of Gōng Sūn 公孫 (SP 4) are the father. They communicate with the Chòng Mài 衝脈.	These unite in the heart, chest, and stomach
The two points of Nèi Guān 內關 (PC 6) are the mother. They communicate with the Yīn Wéi Mài 陰維脈.	
The two points of Hòu Xī 後谿 (SI 3) are the husband. They communicate with the Dū Mài 督脈.	These unite in the inner canthus, neck, nape, ears, shoulders, arms, small intestine, and urinary bladder
The two points of Shēn Mài 申脈 (UB 62) are the wife. They communicate with the Yáng Qiāo Mài 陽蹻脈.	
The two points of Lín Qì 臨泣 (GB 41) are the male. They communicate with the Dài Mài 帶脈.	These unite in the outer canthus, behind the ears, cheeks, neck, and shoulders
The two points of Wài Guān 外關 (SJ 5) are the female. They communicate with the Yáng Wéi Mài 陽維脈.	
The two points of Liè Quē 列缺 (LU 7) are the host. They communicate with the Rèn Mài 任脈.	These unite in the lung tie, throat, chest, and diaphragm
The two points of Zhào Hǎi 照海 (KI 6) are the guest. They communicate with the Yīn Qiāo Mài 陰蹻脈.	

八法交會歌
The Song of the Eight Methods Confluence[88]

內關相應是公孫，外關臨泣總相同，
列缺交經通照海，後谿申脈亦相從 。

Nèi Guān 內關 (PC 6) and Gōng Sūn 公孫 (SP 4) respond to each other;

---

88. No prior source was found for this poem so Yáng probably wrote it himself.

113

Wài Guān 外關 (SJ 5) and Lín Qì 臨泣 (GB 41) gather together,
Liè Quē 列缺 (LU 7) intersects the channels
to communicate with Zhào Hǎi 照海 (KI 6);
Hòu Xī 後谿 (SI 3) and Shēn Mài 申脈 (UB 62) also follow each other.

八脈交會八穴歌
Eight Vessels Confluence Eight Points Song[89]

公孫衝脈胃心胸，內關陰維下總同，
臨泣膽經連帶脈，陽維目銳外關逢 。
後谿督脈內眥頸，申脈陽蹻絡亦通，
列缺任脈行肺系，陰蹻照海膈喉嚨 。

Gōng Sūn 公孫 (SP 4) and Chòng Mài 衝脈: stomach, heart, chest;
Nèi Guān 內關 (PC 6) and Yīn Wéi 陰維 descend to gather together
[with Gōng Sūn 公孫 and the Chòng Mài 衝脈],
Lín Qì 臨泣 (GB 41) and the gall bladder channel connect with the Dài Mài 帶脈;
Yáng Wéi 陽維 and the outer canthus meet with Wài Guān 外關 (SJ 5),
Hòu Xī 後谿 (SI 3) and the Dū Mài 督脈: inner canthus and neck; they also
communicate with Shēn Mài 申脈 (UB 62) and the Yáng Qiāo 陽蹻 network,
Liè Quē 列缺 (LU 7) and Rèn Mài 任脈 move through the lung tie;
Yīn Qiāo 陰蹻 and Zhào Hǎi 照海 (KI 6): diaphragm and throat.

八脈配八卦歌
Song to Match the Eight Vessels with the Eight Trigrams[90]

乾屬公孫艮內關，巽臨震位外關還，
離居列缺坤照海，後谿兌坎申脈聯 。
補瀉浮沉分逆順，隨時呼吸不為難，
仙傳秘訣神針法，萬病如拈立便安 。

Qián (☰) belongs to Gōng Sūn 公孫 (SP 4), gèn (☶) to Nèi Guān 內關 (PC 6);
xùn (☴) to Lín Qì 臨泣 (GB 41),

---

89. From *Zhēn Jiǔ Dà Quán* 《針灸大全》(Great Completion of Acupuncture-Moxibustion), Volume 4.

90. From *Zhēn Jiǔ Dà Quán* 《針灸大全》(Great Completion of Acupuncture-Moxibustion), Volume 4.

and the zhèn (☳) position returns to Wài Guān 外關 (SJ 5),
Lí (☲) resides in Liè Quē 列缺 (LU 7), kūn (☷) in Zhào Hǎi 照海 (KI 6);
Hòu Xī 後谿 (SI 3) in duì (☱), and kǎn (☵) joins with Shēn Mài 申脈 (UB 62),
Supplementing or draining, floating or sinking: these divide counterflow or proper
flow; it is not difficult to exhale and inhale according to the hour,
Immortals passed down a secret rhyme about the spirit needle method;
it is as if the ten-thousand diseases are picked up and immediately pacified.

八穴配合歌
Eight Points Matching Song[91]

公孫偏與內關合，列缺能消照海疴，
臨泣外關分主客，後谿申脈正相和，
左針右病知高下，以意通經廣按摩，
補瀉迎隨分逆順，五門八法是真科 。

Gōng Sūn 公孫 (SP 4) leans toward uniting with Nèi Guān 內關 (PC 6);
Liè Quē 列缺 (LU 7) is able to disperse sickness with Zhào Hǎi 照海 (KI 6).
Lín Qì 臨泣 (GB 41) and Wài Guān 外關 (SJ 5)
are divided into host and guest;
Hòu Xī 後谿 (SI 3) and Shēn Mài 申脈 (UB 62)
are correct and harmonious with each other,
Needle the left for disease on the right, know the high and the low;
use intention to free the channels, expand with massage [àn mó 按摩],
Supplementing or draining, facing or following
are divided up according to counterflow or proper flow;
the five doors and eight methods, these are true branches of knowledge.

刺法啟玄歌 （五言）
Song to Explain the Mystery of Acupuncture[92]
([a poem of] five characters [per line])

---

91. From *Zhēn Jiǔ Dà Quán*《針灸大全》(Great Completion of Acupuncture-Moxibustion),
Volume 4.

92. *Zhēn Jiǔ Jù Yīng*《針灸聚英》(Gatherings from Eminent Acupuncturists) has a poem in
Volume 4 with the same title, but different words. This poem does not appear to be from any of
Yáng's usual sources.

八法神針紗，飛騰法最奇，
砭針行內外，水火就中推，
上下交經足，疾如應手驅，
往來依進退，補瀉逐迎隨，
用似般推舵，應如弩發機，
氣聚時間散，身疼指下移，
這般玄紗訣，料得少人知。

The eight methods of the spirit needle are wonderful;
the flying and soaring method is most extraordinary,
The healing stone and needle travel to the inner and outer;
water and fire are thereby pushed to the center,
When above and below communicate sufficiently[93] through the channels;
the disease is expelled as if responding to the hands,[94]
Going and coming depend on advance and retreat;
supplement and drain, in succession face and follow,
The function resembles pushing a rudder;
it responds like the trigger on a crossbow,
Dissipate at the time qì gathers;
the body's pains can be moved under your finger,
This type of mysterious formula;
few people know the materials it holds.

八法五虎建元日時歌
Eight Methods Song of the Five Tigers
or Establishing the First Hour of the Day[95]

甲己之辰起丙寅，乙庚之日戊寅行，
丙辛便起庚寅始，丁壬壬寅亦順尋，
戊癸甲寅定時候，五門得合是元因。

The time periods of jiǎ 甲 and jǐ 己 [days] start with bǐng yín 丙寅;

---

93. Some editions have *zǒu* 走 (running) rather than *zú* 足 (sufficiently).

94. 應手 "responding to the hands" is a phrase that means "easily."

95. From *Zhēn Jiǔ Dà Quán*《針灸大全》(Great Completion of Acupuncture-Moxibustion), Volume 4.

針灸大成・卷之五

yǐ 乙 and gēng 庚 days go to wù yín 戊寅,
Bǐng 丙 and xīn 辛 [days] arise with a gēng yín 庚寅 beginning;
dīng 丁 and rén 壬 [days] are rén yín 壬寅 and search forward as well,
On wù 戊 and guǐ 癸 [days], jiǎ yín 甲寅 establishes the time;
the five doors are able to unify with this original cause.

Translator's note:

The "five doors" refers to the five unities, the pairing of the stems: jiǎ 甲 and jǐ 己, yǐ 乙 and gēng 庚, etc. The hourly cycle of sixty stem-branch combinations repeats every five days, so day stems paired by the five unities have the same stem-branch combinations for their twelve time periods.

This poem starts each day with the yín 寅 branch hour (3 – 5 am). The yín branch is associated with the tiger among the twelve animals, hence the name of this poem refers to the "five tigers." Once you know the stem of the yín branch hour, you can easily calculate the stem and branch for the rest of the hours, as they always progress in the same order.

Here is a table that works out the stem and branch for each hour, with the yín (tiger) branch hour at the top of each column.

The Stems and Branches of the Double-Hours						
Double-Hour		Day Stem and Branch				
Time	Branch	Jiǎ 甲 or Jǐ 己	Yǐ 乙 or Gēng 庚	Bǐng 丙 or Xīn 辛	Dīng 丁 or Rén 壬	Wù 戊 or Guǐ 癸
3-5 am	Yín 寅	Bǐng Yín 丙寅	Wù Yín 戊寅	Gēng Yín 庚寅	Rén Yín 壬寅	Jiǎ Yín 甲寅
5-7 am	Mǎo 卯	Dīng Mǎo 丁卯	Jǐ Mǎo 己卯	Xīn Mǎo 辛卯	Guǐ Mǎo 癸卯	Yǐ Mǎo 乙卯
7-9 am	Chén 辰	Wù Chén 戊辰	Gēng Chén 庚辰	Rén Chén 壬辰	Jiǎ Chén 甲辰	Bǐng Chén 丙辰
9-11am	Sì 巳	Jǐ Sì 己巳	Xīn Sì 辛巳	Guǐ Sì 癸巳	Yǐ Sì 乙巳	Dīng Sì 丁巳
11 am-1 pm	Wǔ 午	Gēng Wǔ 庚午	Rén Wǔ 壬午	Jiǎ Wǔ 甲午	Bǐng Wǔ 丙午	Wù Wǔ 戊午
1-3 pm	Wèi 未	Xīn Wèi 辛未	Guǐ Wèi 癸未	Yǐ Wèi 乙未	Dīng Wèi 丁未	Jǐ Wèi 己未
3-5 pm	Shēn 申	Rén Shēn 壬申	Jiǎ Shēn 甲申	Bǐng Shēn 丙申	Wù Shēn 戊申	Gēng Shēn 庚申
5-7 pm	Yǒu 酉	Guǐ Yǒu 癸酉	Yǐ Yǒu 乙酉	Dīng Yǒu 丁酉	Jǐ Yǒu 己酉	Xīn Yǒu 辛酉
7-9 pm	Xū 戌	Jiǎ Xū 甲戌	Bǐng Xū 丙戌	Wù Xū 戊戌	Gēng Xū 庚戌	Rén Xū 壬戌
9-11pm	Hài 亥	Yǐ Hài 乙亥	Dīng Hài 丁亥	Jǐ Hài 己亥	Xīn Hài 辛亥	Guǐ Hài 癸亥
11 pm-1 am	Zǐ 子	Bǐng Zǐ 丙子	Wù Zǐ 戊子	Gēng Zǐ 庚子	Rén Zǐ 壬子	Jiǎ Zǐ 甲子
1-3 am	Chǒu 丑	Dīng Chǒu 丁丑	Jǐ Chǒu 己丑	Xīn Chǒu 辛丑	Guǐ Chǒu 癸丑	Yǐ Chǒu 乙丑

For the Mystical Tortoise Method, you need to know the stem and branch of the day and hour of treatment.

八法逐日干支歌
Eight Methods Song of the Stems and Branches, Day by Day[96]

甲己辰戌丑未十，乙庚申酉九為期，
丁壬寅卯八成數，戊癸巳午七相宜，
丙辛亥子亦七數，逐日支干即得知。

Jiǎ 甲, jǐ 己, chén 辰, xū 戌, chǒu 丑, and wèi 未 [each have a value of] ten;
yǐ 乙, gēng 庚, shēn 申, and yǒu 酉 take nine as their period of time,
For dīng 丁, rén 壬, yín 寅, and mǎo 卯, eight is the completion number;
wù 戊 [stem], guǐ 癸, sì 巳, and wǔ 午 [branch] are appropriate for seven,
Bǐng 丙, xīn 辛, hài 亥, and zǐ 子 are also the number seven;
you have now obtained knowledge of the branches and stems, day by day.

Translator's note:

The table below sums up the information in this poem. The stem and branch of the day have assigned values that will be used in the calculation to find the open point in the Mystical Tortoise Method.

Representative Number for the DAY Stem and Branch				
Representative Number	**10**	**9**	**8**	**7**
Stem	Jiǎ 甲 Jǐ 己	Yǐ 乙 Gēng 庚	Dīng 丁 Rén 壬	Bǐng 丙　Wù 戊 Xīn 辛　Guǐ 癸
Branch	Chén 辰　Chǒu 丑 Xū 戌　　Wèi 未	Shēn 申 Yǒu 酉	Yín 寅 Mǎo 卯	Sì 巳　　Wǔ 午 Hài 亥　Zǐ 子
Element	earth	metal	wood	water and fire

The representative number is determined by the element. The two stems that are placed in the same column are paired according to the five unities. While their individual elements may be different, when the two stems combine, they transform into the element given in the bottom row. The branches directly correspond to the element in the bottom row.

---

96. From *Zhēn Jiǔ Dà Quán* 《針灸大全》 (Great Completion of Acupuncture-Moxibustion), Volume 4.

According to the Hé Tú 河圖, certain numbers belong to the different elements. Five and ten belong to the center and so are associated with earth. Four and nine correspond to the west and metal. Three and eight go with east and wood. Two and seven belong to the south and fire. One and six are north and water, although in this calculation for the representative number of the day, water is put into the same column as fire.

八法臨時干支歌
Eight Methods Song of Approaching the Hour Stem and Branch[97]

甲己子午九宜用，乙庚丑未八無疑，
丙辛寅申七作數，丁壬卯酉六順知，
戊癸辰戌各有五，巳亥單加四共齊 。
陽日除九陰除六，不及零餘穴下推 。

**For jiǎ 甲, jǐ 己, zǐ 子, and wǔ 午 [branch], nine is suitable to use;
for yǐ 乙, gēng 庚, chǒu 丑, and wèi 未, it is eight without a doubt,
For bǐng 丙, xīn 辛, yín 寅, and shēn 申, seven makes the count;
for dīng 丁, rén 壬, mǎo 卯, and yǒu 酉, six is favorable to know,
Wù 戊 [stem], guǐ 癸, chén 辰, xū 戌: each has five;
for sì 巳 and hài 亥 alone, add four all together,
On yáng days eliminate by nines, on yīn [days] eliminate by sixes;
the remainder is the point chosen below.**

Translator's note:
The previous poem listed the values for the day stem and branch. This poem lists the values for the hour stem and branch. These numbers are listed in the following table:

Representative Number for the HOUR Stem and Branch						
Representative Number	**9**	**8**	**7**	**6**	**5**	**4**
Stem	Jiǎ 甲 Jǐ 己	Yǐ 乙 Gēng 庚	Bǐng 丙 Xīn 辛	Dīng 丁 Rén 壬	Wù 戊 Guǐ 癸	--
Branch	Zǐ 子 Wǔ 午	Chǒu 丑 Wèi 未	Yín 寅 Shēn 申	Mǎo 卯 Yǒu 酉	Chén 辰 Xū 戌	Sì 巳 Hài 亥

Here, the values are found using a different logic. The stems are still paired into the five unities, but the resulting element is not used. For the stems, take the lower number of the two stems. For ex-

---

97. From *Zhēn Jiŭ Dà Quán* 《 針灸大全 》 (Great Completion of Acupuncture-Moxibustion), Volume 4.

ample, jiǎ 甲 and jǐ 己 are paired with each other. Jiǎ is the first stem and jǐ is the sixth stem. Jiǎ (one) is the lower number. Subtract this from ten and the result is nine. So jiǎ and jǐ are in the column with nine on top. Yǐ 乙 is the second stem. Subtract two from ten and you get eight. So yǐ and its pair gēng 庚 are in the 'eight' column.

If the branches were put on a clock face, opposite branches are now paired with each other. We use the same calculation as for the stems. Zǐ 子 is the first branch. Subtract one from ten and we see zǐ and its pair wǔ 午 go in the 'nine' column.

There are ten stems, so they fill five columns. There are twelve branches so we need a sixth column for sì 巳 and hài 亥, which receive a value of four.

The last line of this poem tells us that we will add everything up (day stem, day branch, hour stem, and hour branch values). Then on yáng days divide the sum by nine and on yīn days divide by six.[98] The remainder of this calculation will tell you which point to use during that time-period. This process is described in more detail below.

其法如甲丙戊庚壬為陽日，乙丁己辛癸為陰日，以日時干支算計何數，陽日除九數，陰日除六數，陽日多，或一九二九三九四九，陰日多，或二六三六四六五六，剩下若干，同配卦數，日時得何卦，即知何穴開矣！

In this method, jiǎ 甲, bǐng 丙, wù 戊 [stem], gēng 庚 and rén 壬, are yáng days; yǐ 乙, dīng 丁, jǐ 己, xīn 辛, and guǐ 癸 are yīn days. Calculate the stem and branch of the day and hour to calculate which number [is the sum]. On yáng days subtract by nines. On yīn days subtract by sixes. On yáng days there may be too many; perhaps it is one times nine, two times nine, three times nine, or four times nine. On yīn days there may be too many; perhaps it is two times six, three times six, four times six, or five times six. The remainder amount is matched with the guà 卦 number. The day and time period get whichever guà 卦 and then you know what point is open.

假如甲子日戊辰時，以日上甲得十數，子得七數，以時上戊得五數，辰得五數，共成二十七數，此是陽日，以九除去二九一十八，餘有九數合離卦即列缺穴開也。

For example, on a jiǎ zǐ 甲子 day in a wù chén 戊辰 hour [7-9 am]: Take the jiǎ 甲 from the day to get 10. Zǐ 子 gives 7. Take the wù 戊 stem of the hour to get 5. Chén 辰 gives 5. Altogether this makes 27. This is a yáng day, so use 9. Remove two nines: 18. The remainder of 9 unites with lí guà (☲), meaning Liè Quē 列缺 (LU 7) is open.

---

98. Nine is yáng, being an odd number. Six is yīn because it is an even number. Sixes and nines are commonly used to represent yīn and yáng in calculations related to the *Book of Changes*.

假如乙丑日壬午時，以日上乙為九，丑為十，以時上壬為六，午為九，共成三十四數，此日陰日，以六除去五六三十數，零下四數，合巽四，即臨泣穴開也。餘倣此。

For example, on an yǐ chǒu 乙丑 day in a rén wǔ 壬午 hour [11 am – 1 pm]: Take the yǐ 乙 from the day as 9. Chǒu 丑 is 10. Take rén 壬 of the hour as 6. Wǔ 午 branch is 9. Altogether this is 34. This is a yīn day, so use 6. Remove five sixes: 30. A remainder of 4 unites with xùn 4 (☴), so Lín Qì 臨泣 (GB 41) is open. The rest are like this.

Translator's note:
To find the open point, add all the values for the day stem, day branch, hour stem, and hour branch. Remember that the day values come from a different table than the hour values.

Determine whether it is a yīn or yáng day. If the day stem is jiǎ 甲, bǐng 丙, wù 戊, gēng 庚 or rén 壬, it is a yáng day and you divide the sum by 9. If the day stem is yǐ 乙, dīng 丁, jǐ 己, xīn 辛, or guǐ 癸, it is a yīn day so you divide the sum by six. The remainder is the answer. Do not turn the number into a fraction. This number, the remainder, is then used to find the appropriate trigram and point according to the information Yáng gave at the beginning of this section. The diagram is repeated here for convenience. Find the palace (one of the nine cells in the diagram below) that contains the remainder number from the calculation. The acu-moxa point listed in the same palace is the open point for that time.

Xùn 4 Lín Qì 臨泣 (GB 41)	Lí 9 Liè Quē 列缺 (LU 7)	Kūn 2 Zhào Hǎi 照海 (KI 6)
Zhèn 3 Wài Guān 外關 (SJ 5)	Center 5 goes to Kūn Zhào Hǎi 照海 (KI 6)	Duì 7 Hòu Xī 後谿 (SI 3)
Gèn 8 Nèi Guān 內關 (PC 6)	Kǎn 1 Shēn Mài 申脈 (UB 62)	Qián 6 Gōng Sūn 公孫 (SP 4)

Yáng gave two examples. The first resulted in a remainder of 9. This is found in the top center of the above diagram. It belongs to lí guà (☲) and Liè Quē 列缺 (LU 7).

The second example had a final result of 4. You can see in the above diagram that 4 is in the upper left corner. It is associated with xùn guà (☴) and Zú Lín Qì 足臨泣 (GB 41).

Yáng never directly states how to deal with a remainder of zero, but it can be inferred from the first example. On a yáng day, a remainder of zero is equivalent to nine. On a yīn day, a remainder of zero is equivalent to six.

Below, Yáng provided a table that was meant to cover the calculation for business hours. It begins at the yín 寅 hour (3-5 am) and runs until the yǒu 酉 hour (5-7 pm).

There is a different pattern for each day of the sixty day cycle of stems and branches. Find the day in question and then read the open point for the time of treatment.

To save space, Yáng gave the stem and branch for the yáng time periods but only the branch for the yīn time periods. Since the stems always run in order, if you know the stem for one time period, it is easy to deduce the stem for the following hour.

推定六十甲子日時穴開圖例
Table to Deduce the Point Opening from the Sixty Jiǎ Zǐ 甲子 Days and Hours

甲子日	乙丑日	丙寅日	丁卯日	戊辰日	己巳日
丙寅臨卯照 戊辰列巳外 庚午後未照 壬申外酉申	戊寅申卯臨 庚辰照巳公 壬午臨未照 甲申照酉外	庚寅外卯申 壬辰內巳公 甲午公未臨 丙申照酉列	壬寅照卯外 甲辰公巳臨 丙午照未公 戊申臨酉申	甲寅公卯臨 丙辰照巳列 戊午臨未後 庚申照酉外	丙寅申卯照 戊辰外巳公 庚午臨未照 壬申公酉臨

庚午日	辛未日	壬申日	癸酉日	甲戌日	乙亥日
戊寅申卯臨 庚辰照巳列 壬午臨未照 甲申照酉外	庚寅照卯公 壬辰臨巳照 甲午照未外 丙申申酉照	壬寅外卯申 甲辰臨巳照 丙午公未臨 戊申照酉照	甲寅外卯申 丙辰臨巳照 戊午公未外 庚申申酉照	丙寅後卯照 戊辰外巳公 庚午申未內 壬申公酉臨	戊寅臨卯申 庚辰照巳外 壬午申未照 甲申照酉公

丙子日	丁丑日	戊寅日	己卯日	庚辰日	辛巳日
庚寅照卯列 壬辰後巳照 甲午照未外 丙申申酉內	壬寅申卯照 甲辰照巳公 丙午臨未照 戊申公酉外	甲寅臨卯照 丙辰列巳後 戊午照未照 庚申外酉申	丙寅照卯公 戊辰臨巳申 庚午照未外 壬申申酉照	戊寅臨卯後 庚辰照巳外 壬午後未照 甲申內酉公	庚寅照卯外 壬辰申巳照 甲午照未公 丙申臨酉照

壬午日	癸未日	甲申日	乙酉日	丙戌日	丁亥日
壬寅申卯內 甲辰照巳列 丙午臨未照 戊申列酉外	甲寅外卯申 丙辰照巳外 戊午申未臨 庚申照酉公	丙寅公卯臨 戊辰照巳照 庚午列未後 壬申照酉外	戊寅公卯外 庚辰申巳照 壬午外未申 甲申臨酉照	庚寅照卯外 壬辰申巳內 甲午內未公 丙申臨酉照	壬寅臨卯照 甲辰照巳外 丙午申未照 戊申外酉公

戊子日	己丑日	庚寅日	辛卯日	壬辰日	癸巳日
甲寅外卯申 丙辰內巳公 戊午申未臨 庚申照酉列	丙寅臨卯照 戊辰公巳外 庚午申未照 壬申外酉申	戊寅照卯照 庚辰外巳申 壬午照未外 甲申公酉臨	庚寅公卯臨 壬辰照巳公 甲午外未申 丙申照酉外	壬寅臨卯照 甲辰照巳外 丙午後未照 戊申外酉公	甲寅公卯臨 丙辰照巳公 戊午臨未申 庚申照酉外

甲午日	乙未日	丙申日	丁酉日	戊戌日	己亥日
丙寅臨卯照	戊寅申卯臨	庚寅臨卯照	壬寅公卯臨	甲寅公卯臨	丙寅申卯照
戊辰列巳外	庚辰照巳公	壬辰列巳後	甲辰申巳照	丙辰照巳列	戊辰外巳公
庚午後未照	壬午臨未照	甲午後未照	丙午外未申	戊午臨未後	庚午臨未照
壬申外酉申	甲申照酉外	丙申外酉申	戊申照酉照	庚申照酉外	壬申公酉臨
庚子日	辛丑日	壬寅日	癸卯日	甲辰日	乙巳日
戊寅申卯臨	庚寅照卯公	壬寅照卯列	甲寅申卯照	丙寅後卯照	戊寅臨卯申
庚辰照巳列	壬辰臨巳照	甲辰外巳申	丙辰外巳申	戊辰外巳公	庚辰照巳外
壬午臨未照	甲午照未外	丙午照未外	戊午照未照	庚午申未內	壬午申未照
甲申照酉外	丙申申酉照	戊申申酉臨	庚申公酉臨	壬申公酉臨	甲申照酉公
丙午日	丁未日	戊申日	己酉日	庚戌日	辛亥日
庚寅照卯列	壬寅申卯照	甲寅照卯外	丙寅外卯申	戊寅臨卯後	庚寅照卯外
壬辰後巳照	甲辰照巳公	丙辰申巳內	戊辰照巳照	庚辰照巳外	壬辰申巳照
甲午照未外	丙午臨未照	戊午外未公	庚午公未臨	壬午後未照	甲午照未外
丙申申酉內	戊申公酉外	庚申臨酉照	壬申照酉公	甲申內酉公	丙申臨酉照
壬子日	癸丑日	甲寅日	乙卯日	丙辰日	丁巳日
壬寅申卯內	甲寅外卯申	丙寅照卯外	戊寅照卯照	庚寅照卯外	壬寅臨卯照
甲辰照巳列	丙辰照巳外	戊辰申巳臨	庚辰公巳臨	壬辰申巳內	甲辰照巳外
丙午臨未照	戊午申未臨	庚午內未公	壬午照未公	甲午內未公	丙午申未照
戊申列酉外	庚申照酉公	壬申臨酉照	甲申外酉申	丙申臨酉照	戊申外酉公
戊午日	己未日	庚申日	辛酉日	壬戌日	癸亥日
甲寅外卯申	丙寅臨卯照	戊寅外卯公	庚寅申卯照	壬寅臨卯照	甲寅公卯臨
丙辰內巳公	戊辰公巳外	庚辰臨巳照	壬辰外巳照	甲辰照巳外	丙辰照巳公
戊午申未臨	庚午申未照	壬午公未臨	甲午臨未照	丙午後未照	戊午臨未申
庚申照酉列	壬申外酉申	甲申後酉照	丙申公酉臨	戊申外酉公	庚申照酉外

Stem										
jiǎ 甲	yǐ 乙	bǐng 丙	dīng 丁	wù 戊	jǐ 己	gēng 庚	xīn 辛	rén 壬	guǐ 癸	
Branch										
zǐ 子	chǒu 丑	yín 寅	mǎo 卯	chén 辰	sì 巳	wǔ 午	wèi 未	shēn 申	yǒu 酉	xū 戌	hài 亥

Jiǎ Zǐ 甲子 day		Yǐ Chǒu 乙丑 day		Bǐng Yín 丙寅 day		Dīng Mǎo 丁卯 day		Wù Chén 戊辰 day		Jǐ Sì 己巳 day	
丙寅	GB 41	戊寅	UB 62	庚寅	SJ 5	壬寅	KI 6	甲寅	SP 4	丙寅	UB 62
卯	KI 6	卯	GB 41	卯	UB 62	卯	SJ 5	卯	GB 41	卯	KI 6
戊辰	LU 7	庚辰	KI 6	壬辰	PC 6	甲辰	SP 4	丙辰	KI 6	戊辰	SJ 5
巳	SJ 5	巳	SP 4	巳	SP 4	巳	GB 41	巳	LU 7	巳	SP 4
庚午	SI 3	壬午	GB 41	甲午	SP 4	丙午	KI 6	戊午	GB 41	庚午	GB 41
未	KI 6	未	KI 6	未	GB 41	未	SP 4	未	SI 3	未	KI 6
壬申	SJ 5	甲申	KI 6	丙申	KI 6	戊申	GB 41	庚申	KI 6	壬申	SP 4
酉	UB 62	酉	SJ 5	酉	LU 7	酉	UB 62	酉	SJ 5	酉	GB 41

Gēng Wǔ 庚午 day

戊寅	UB 62
卯	GB 41
庚辰	KI 6
巳	LU 7
壬午	GB 41
未	KI 6
甲申	KI 6
酉	SJ 5

Xīn Wèi 辛未 day

庚寅	KI 6
卯	SP 4
壬辰	GB 41
巳	KI 6
甲午	KI 6
未	SJ 5
丙申	UB 62
酉	KI 6

Rén Shēn 壬申 day

壬寅	SJ 5
卯	UB 62
甲辰	GB 41
巳	KI 6
丙午	SP 4
未	GB 41
戊申	KI 6
酉	KI 6

Guǐ Yǒu 癸酉 day

甲寅	SJ 5
卯	UB 62
丙辰	GB 41
巳	KI 6
戊午	SP 4
未	SJ 5
庚申	UB 62
酉	KI 6

Jiǎ Xū 甲戌 day

丙寅	SI 3
卯	KI 6
戊辰	SJ 5
巳	SP 4
庚午	UB 62
未	PC 6
壬申	SP 4
酉	GB 41

Yǐ Hài 乙亥 day

戊寅	GB 41
卯	UB 62
庚辰	KI 6
巳	SJ 5
壬午	UB 62
未	KI 6
甲申	KI 6
酉	SP 4

Bǐng Zǐ 丙子 day

庚寅	KI 6
卯	LU 7
壬辰	SI 3
巳	KI 6
甲午	KI 6
未	SJ 5
丙申	UB 62
酉	PC 6

Dīng Chǒu 丁丑 day

壬寅	UB 62
卯	KI 6
甲辰	KI 6
巳	SP 4
丙午	GB 41
未	KI 6
戊申	SP 4
酉	SJ 5

Wù Yín 戊寅 day

甲寅	GB 41
卯	KI 6
丙辰	LU 7
巳	SI 3
戊午	KI 6
未	KI 6
庚申	SJ 5
酉	UB 62

Jǐ Mǎo 己卯 day

丙寅	KI 6
卯	SP 4
戊辰	GB 41
巳	UB 62
庚午	KI 6
未	SJ 5
壬申	UB 62
酉	KI 6

Gēng Chén 庚辰 day

戊寅	GB 41
卯	SI 3
庚辰	KI 6
巳	SJ 5
壬午	SI 3
未	KI 6
甲申	PC 6
酉	SP 4

Xīn Sì 辛巳 day

庚寅	KI 6
卯	SJ 5
壬辰	UB 62
巳	KI 6
甲午	KI 6
未	SP 4
丙申	GB 41
酉	KI 6

Rén Wǔ 壬午 day

壬寅	UB 62
卯	PC 6
甲辰	KI 6
巳	LU 7
丙午	GB 41
未	KI 6
戊申	LU 7
酉	SJ 5

Guǐ Wèi 癸未 day

甲寅	SJ 5
卯	UB 62
丙辰	KI 6
巳	SJ 5
戊午	UB 62
未	GB 41
庚申	KI 6
酉	SP 4

Jiǎ Shēn 甲申 day

丙寅	SP 4
卯	GB 41
戊辰	KI 6
巳	KI 6
庚午	LU 7
未	SI 3
壬申	KI 6
酉	SJ 5

Yǐ Yǒu 乙酉 day

戊寅	SP 4
卯	SJ 5
庚辰	UB 62
巳	KI 6
壬午	SJ 5
未	UB 62
甲申	GB 41
酉	KI 6

Bǐng Xū 丙戌 day

庚寅	KI 6
卯	SJ 5
壬辰	UB 62
巳	PC 6
甲午	PC 6
未	SP 4
丙申	GB 41
酉	KI 6

Dīng Hài 丁亥 day

壬寅	GB 41
卯	KI 6
甲辰	KI 6
巳	SJ 5
丙午	UB 62
未	KI 6
戊申	SJ 5
酉	SP 4

Wù Zǐ 戊子 day

甲寅	SJ 5
卯	UB 62
丙辰	PC 6
巳	SP 4
戊午	UB 62
未	GB 41
庚申	KI 6
酉	LU 7

Jǐ Chǒu 己丑 day

丙寅	GB 41
卯	KI 6
戊辰	SP 4
巳	SJ 5
庚午	UB 62
未	KI 6
壬申	SJ 5
酉	UB 62

Gēng Yín 庚寅 day

戊寅	KI 6
卯	KI 6
庚辰	SJ 5
巳	UB 62
壬午	KI 6
未	SJ 5
甲申	SP 4
酉	GB 41

Xīn Mǎo 辛卯 day

庚寅	SP 4
卯	GB 41
壬辰	KI 6
巳	SP 4
甲午	SJ 5
未	UB 62
丙申	KI 6
酉	SJ 5

Rén Chén 壬辰 day

壬寅	GB 41
卯	KI 6
甲辰	KI 6
巳	SJ 5
丙午	SI 3
未	KI 6
戊申	SJ 5
酉	SP 4

Guǐ Sì 癸巳 day

甲寅	SP 4
卯	GB 41
丙辰	KI 6
巳	SP 4
戊午	GB 41
未	UB 62
庚申	KI 6
酉	SJ 5

Jiǎ Wǔ 甲午 day

丙寅	GB 41
卯	KI 6
戊辰	LU 7
巳	SJ 5
庚午	SI 3
未	KI 6
壬申	SJ 5
酉	UB 62

Yǐ Wèi 乙未 day

戊寅	UB 62
卯	GB 41
庚辰	KI 6
巳	SP 4
壬午	GB 41
未	KI 6
甲申	KI 6
酉	SJ 5

Bǐng Shēn 丙申 day

庚寅	GB 41
卯	KI 6
壬辰	LU 7
巳	SI 3
甲午	SI 3
未	KI 6
丙申	SJ 5
酉	UB 62

Dīng Yǒu 丁酉 day

壬寅	SP 4
卯	GB 41
甲辰	UB 62
巳	KI 6
丙午	SJ 5
未	UB 62
戊申	KI 6
酉	KI 6

Wù Xū 戊戌 day

甲寅	SP 4
卯	GB 41
丙辰	KI 6
巳	LU 7
戊午	GB 41
未	SI 3
庚申	KI 6
酉	SJ 5

Jǐ Hài 己亥 day

丙寅	UB 62
卯	KI 6
戊辰	SJ 5
巳	SP 4
庚午	GB 41
未	KI 6
壬申	SP 4
酉	GB 41

Gēng Zǐ 庚子 day		Xīn Chǒu 辛丑 day		Rén Yín 壬寅 day		Guǐ Mǎo 癸卯 day		Jiǎ Chén 甲辰 day		Yǐ Sì 乙巳 day	
戊寅	UB 62	庚寅	KI 6	壬寅	KI 6	甲寅	UB 62	丙寅	SI 3	戊寅	GB 41
卯	GB 41	卯	SP 4	卯	LU 7	卯	KI 6	卯	KI 6	卯	UB 62
庚辰	KI 6	壬辰	GB 41	甲辰	SJ 5	丙辰	SJ 5	戊辰	SJ 5	庚辰	KI 6
巳	LU 7	巳	KI 6	巳	UB 62	巳	UB 62	巳	SP 4	巳	SJ 5
壬午	GB 41	甲午	KI 6	丙午	KI 6	戊午	KI 6	庚午	UB 62	壬午	UB 62
未	KI 6	未	SJ 5	未	SJ 5	未	KI 6	未	PC 6	未	KI 6
甲申	KI 6	丙申	UB 62	戊申	UB 62	庚申	SP 4	壬申	SP 4	甲申	KI 6
酉	SJ 5	酉	KI 6	酉	GB 41	酉	GB 41	酉	GB 41	酉	SP 4

Bǐng Wǔ 丙午 day		Dīng Wèi 丁未 day		Wù Shēn 戊申 day		Jǐ Yǒu 己酉 day		Gēng Xū 庚戌 day		Xīn Hài 辛亥 day	
庚寅	KI 6	壬寅	UB 62	甲寅	KI 6	丙寅	SJ 5	戊寅	GB 41	庚寅	KI 6
卯	LU 7	卯	KI 6	卯	SJ 5	卯	UB 62	卯	SI 3	卯	SJ 5
壬辰	SI 3	甲辰	KI 6	丙辰	UB 62	戊辰	KI 6	庚辰	KI 6	壬辰	UB 62
巳	KI 6	巳	SP 4	巳	PC 6	巳	KI 6	巳	SJ 5	巳	KI 6
甲午	KI 6	丙午	GB 41	戊午	SJ 5	庚午	SP 4	壬午	SI 3	甲午	KI 6
未	SJ 5	未	KI 6	未	SP 4	未	GB 41	未	KI 6	未	SP 4
丙申	UB 62	戊申	SP 4	庚申	GB 41	壬申	KI 6	甲申	PC 6	丙申	GB 41
酉	PC 6	酉	SJ 5	酉	KI 6	酉	SP 4	酉	SP 4	酉	KI 6

Rén Zǐ 壬子 day		Guǐ Chǒu 癸丑 day		Jiǎ Yín 甲寅 day		Yǐ Mǎo 乙卯 day		Bǐng Chén 丙辰 day		Dīng Sì 丁巳 day	
壬寅	UB 62	甲寅	SJ 5	丙寅	KI 6	戊寅	KI 6	庚寅	KI 6	壬寅	GB 41
卯	PC 6	卯	UB 62	卯	SJ 5	卯	KI 6	卯	SJ 5	卯	KI 6
甲辰	KI 6	丙辰	KI 6	戊辰	UB 62	庚辰	SP 4	壬辰	UB 62	甲辰	KI 6
巳	LU 7	巳	SJ 5	巳	GB 41	巳	GB 41	巳	PC 6	巳	SJ 5
丙午	GB 41	戊午	UB 62	庚午	PC 6	壬午	KI 6	甲午	PC 6	丙午	UB 62
未	KI 6	未	GB 41	未	SP 4	未	SP 4	未	SP 4	未	KI 6
戊申	LU 7	庚申	KI 6	壬申	GB 41	甲申	SJ 5	丙申	GB 41	戊申	SJ 5
酉	SJ 5	酉	SP 4	酉	KI 6	酉	UB 62	酉	KI 6	酉	SP 4

Wù Wǔ 戊午 day		Jǐ Wèi 己未 day		Gēng Shēn 庚申 day		Xīn Yǒu 辛酉 day		Rén Xū 壬戌 day		Guǐ Hài 癸亥 day	
甲寅	SJ 5	丙寅	GB 41	戊寅	SJ 5	庚寅	UB 62	壬寅	GB 41	甲寅	SP 4
卯	UB 62	卯	KI 6	卯	SP 4	卯	KI 6	卯	KI 6	卯	GB 41
丙辰	PC 6	戊辰	SP 4	庚辰	GB 41	壬辰	SJ 5	甲辰	KI 6	丙辰	KI 6
巳	SP 4	巳	SJ 5	巳	KI 6	巳	UB 62	巳	SJ 5	巳	SP 4
戊午	UB 62	庚午	UB 62	壬午	SP 4	甲午	GB 41	丙午	SI 3	戊午	GB 41
未	GB 41	未	KI 6	未	GB 41	未	KI 6	未	KI 6	未	UB 62
庚申	KI 6	壬申	SJ 5	甲申	SI 3	丙申	SP 4	戊申	SJ 5	庚申	KI 6
酉	LU 7	酉	UB 62	酉	KI 6	酉	GB 41	酉	SP 4	酉	SJ 5

右圖乃預先推定六十甲子，逐日逐時某穴所開以便用針，庶臨時倉卒之際，不致有差訛之失也。

The above table deduces in advance which point is open according to the sixty jiǎ zǐ 甲子, day by day and hour by hour, in order to make it convenient to use for acu-

puncture. This is so that when you are hurried during clinic hours, you do not arrive at an error [in the calculation].

Translator's note:

Because of space, the Pin Yin and characters for point names are not included in the above table. The times associated with the twelve branches are also left out. For clarity, they are repeated in the following tables:

Vessel	Point
Governing (Dū)	Hòu Xī 後谿 (SI 3)
Conception (Rèn)	Liè Quē 列缺 (LU 7)
Girdling (Dài)	Lín Qì 臨泣 (GB 41)
Thoroughfare (Chòng)	Gōng Sūn 公孫 (SP 4)
Yáng Springing (Yáng Qiāo)	Shēn Mài 申脈 (UB 62)
Yīn Springing (Yīn Qiāo)	Zhào Hǎi 照海 (KI 6)
Yáng Linking (Yáng Wéi)	Wài Guān 外關 (SJ 5)
Yīn Linking (Yīn Wéi)	Nèi Guān 內關 (PC 6)

Branch		Time Period
Zǐ 子	Not listed in Yáng's table	11 pm – 1 am
Chǒu 丑		1 – 3 am
Yín 寅		3 – 5 am
Mǎo 卯		5 – 7 am
Chén 辰		7 – 9 am
Sì 巳		9 – 11 am
Wǔ 午		11 am – 1 pm
Wèi 未		1 – 3 pm
Shēn 申		3 – 5 pm
Yǒu 酉		5 – 7 pm
Xū 戌	Not listed in Yáng's table	7 – 9 pm
Hài 亥		9 – 11 pm

Below is a table of the open points in a format more suitable for the modern acupuncturist. Correct for Daylight Savings Time if it is used in your location. To do this, generally you subtract one hour from the time given by your clock.

針灸大成 · 卷之五

Open Points for the Method of the Mystical Tortoise (Líng Guī Bā Fǎ 靈龜八法) – Correct for Daylight Savings Time, if necessary.

Time \ Day	Jiǎ Zǐ 甲子	Yǐ Chǒu 乙丑	Bǐng Yín 丙寅	Dīng Mǎo 丁卯	Wù Chén 戊辰	Jǐ Sì 己巳	Gēng Wǔ 庚午	Xīn Wèi 辛未	Rén Shēn 壬申	Guǐ Yǒu 癸酉	Jiǎ Xū 甲戌	Yǐ Hài 乙亥
11 pm–1am	PC 6	KI 6	KI 6	SJ 5	KI 6	KI 6	KI 6	UB 62	SI 3	UB 62	KI 6	KI 6
1 – 3 am	SP 4	SJ 5	KI 6	UB 62	SJ 5	SJ 5	SJ 5	GB 41	KI 6	KI 6	LU 7	SP 4
3 – 5 am	GB 41	UB 62	SJ 5	KI 6	SP 4	UB 62	UB 62	KI 6	SJ 5	KI 6	SI 3	GB 41
5 – 7am	KI 6	GB 41	UB 62	SJ 5	GB 41	KI 6	GB 41	SP 4	UB 62	SP 4	KI 6	UB 62
7 – 9am	LU 7	KI 6	PC 6	SP 4	KI 6	SJ 5	KI 6	GB 41	GB 41	GB 41	SJ 5	KI 6
9 – 11 am	SJ 5	SP 4	SP 4	GB 41	LU 7	SP 4	LU 7	KI 6	KI 6	KI 6	SP 4	SJ 5
11 am–1pm	SI 3	GB 41	SP 4	KI 6	GB 41	GB 41	GB 41	KI 6	SP 4	SP 4	UB 62	UB 62
1 – 3 pm	KI 6	KI 6	GB 41	SP 4	SI 3	KI 6	KI 6	SJ 5	GB 41	SJ 5	PC 6	KI 6
3 – 5 pm	SJ 5	KI 6	KI 6	GB 41	KI 6	SP 4	KI 6	UB 62	KI 6	UB 62	SP 4	KI 6
5 – 7 pm	UB 62	SJ 5	LU 7	UB 62	SJ 5	GB 41	SJ 5	KI 6	KI 6	KI 6	GB 41	SP 4
7 – 9 pm	GB 41	UB 62	SI 3	KI 6	UB 62	UB 62	UB 62	SJ 5	SJ 5	SJ 5	SI 3	GB 41
9 – 11 pm	KI 6	KI 6	UB 62	SJ 5	PC 6	KI 6	PC 6	SP 4	UB 62	UB 62	KI 6	KI 6

Open Points for the Method of the Mystical Tortoise (Líng Guī Bā Fǎ 靈龜八法) – Correct for Daylight Savings Time, if necessary.

Time \ Day	Bǐng Zǐ 丙子	Dīng Chǒu 丁丑	Wù Yín 戊寅	Jǐ Mǎo 己卯	Gēng Chén 庚辰	Xīn Sì 辛巳	Rén Wǔ 壬午	Guǐ Wèi 癸未	Jiǎ Shēn 甲申	Yǐ Yǒu 乙酉	Bǐng Xū 丙戌	Dīng Hài 丁亥
11 pm – 1 am	UB 62	KI 6	SJ 5	SP 4	PC 6	GB 41	KI 6	KI 6	UB 62	GB 41	GB 41	KI 6
1 – 3 am	GB 41	SJ 5	UB 62	GB 41	SP 4	UB 62	SJ 5	SP 4	PC 6	KI 6	SI 3	SP 4
3 – 5 am	KI 6	UB 62	GB 41	KI 6	GB 41	KI 6	UB 62	SJ 5	SP 4	SP 4	KI 6	GB 41
5 – 7 am	LU 7	KI 6	KI 6	SP 4	SI 3	SJ 5	PC 6	UB 62	GB 41	SJ 5	SJ 5	KI 6
7 – 9 am	SI 3	KI 6	LU 7	GB 41	KI 6	UB 62	KI 6	KI 6	KI 6	UB 62	UB 62	KI 6
9 – 11 am	KI 6	SP 4	SI 3	UB 62	SJ 5	KI 6	LU 7	SJ 5	KI 6	KI 6	PC 6	SJ 5
11 am – 1 pm	KI 6	GB 41	KI 6	KI 6	SI 3	KI 6	GB 41	UB 62	LU 7	SJ 5	PC 6	UB 62
1 – 3 pm	SJ 5	KI 6	KI 6	SJ 5	KI 6	SP 4	KI 6	GB 41	SI 3	UB 62	SP 4	KI 6
3 – 5 pm	PC 6	SP 4	SJ 5	UB 62	PC 6	GB 41	LU 7	KI 6	KI 6	GB 41	GB 41	SJ 5
5 – 7 pm	SP 4	SJ 5	UB 62	KI 6	SP 4	KI 6	SJ 5	SP 4	SJ 5	KI 6	KI 6	SP 4
7 – 9 pm	LU 7	UB 62	PC 6	KI 6	GB 41	SP 4	UB 62	GB 41	SP 4	SP 4	LU 7	GB 41
9 – 11 pm	KI 6	KI 6	SP 4	SP 4	KI 6	SJ 5	PC 6	KI 6	GB 41	GB 41	SJ 5	KI 6

Open Points for the Method of the Mystical Tortoise (Líng Guī Bā Fǎ 靈龜八法) – Correct for Daylight Savings Time, if necessary.

Day / Time	Wǔ Zǐ 戊子	Jǐ Chǒu 己丑	Gēng Yín 庚寅	Xīn Mǎo 辛卯	Rén Chén 壬辰	Guǐ Sì 癸巳	Jiǎ Wǔ 甲午	Yǐ Wèi 乙未	Bǐng Shēn 丙申	Dīng Yǒu 丁酉	Wù Xū 戊戌	Jǐ Hài 己亥
11 pm – 1 am	KI6	KI6	SP4	KI6	PC6	KI6	PC6	KI6	SJ5	GB41	KI6	KI6
1 – 3 am	LU7	SP4	GB41	KI6	SP4	SJ5	SP4	SJ5	SP4	KI6	SJ5	SJ5
3 – 5 am	SJ5	GB41	KI6	SP4	GB41	SP4	GB41	UB62	GB41	SP4	SP4	UB62
5 – 7 am	UB62	KI6	KI6	GB41	KI6	GB41	KI6	GB41	KI6	GB41	GB41	KI6
7 – 9 am	PC6	SP4	KI6	KI6	KI6	KI6	KI6	KI6	LU7	UB62	KI6	SJ5
9 – 11 am	SP4	SJ5	SJ5	SP4	SJ5	SP4	LU7	SP4	SI3	KI6	LU7	SP4
11 am – 1 pm	UB62	UB62	KI6	SJ5	SI3	GB41	SI3	GB41	SI3	SJ5	GB41	GB41
1 – 3 pm	GB41	KI6	SJ5	UB62	KI6	UB62	KI6	KI6	KI6	UB62	SI3	KI6
3 – 5 pm	KI6	SJ5	SP4	KI6	SJ5	KI6	SJ5	KI6	SJ5	KI6	KI6	SP4
5 – 7 pm	LU7	UB62	GB41	SJ5	SP4	SJ5	UB62	SJ5	UB62	KI6	SJ5	GB41
7 – 9 pm	SI3	GB41	KI6	UB62	GB41	UB62	GB41	UB62	PC6	SP4	UB62	UB62
9 – 11 pm	KI6	KI6	LU7	GB41	KI6	KI6	KI6	KI6	KI6	GB41	PC6	KI6

Open Points for the Method of the Mystical Tortoise (Líng Guī Bā Fǎ 靈龜八法) – Correct for Daylight Savings Time, if necessary.

Day / Time	Gēng Zǐ 庚子	Xīn Chǒu 辛丑	Rén Yín 壬寅	Guǐ Mǎo 癸卯	Jiǎ Chén 甲辰	Yǐ Sì 乙巳	Bǐng Wǔ 丙午	Dīng Wèi 丁未	Wù Shēn 戊申	Jǐ Yǒu 己酉	Gēng Xū 庚戌	Xīn Hài 辛亥
11 pm – 1 am	KI6	UB62	SP4	SP4	KI6	KI6	UB62	KI6	GB41	UB62	PC6	GB41
1 – 3 am	SJ5	GB41	GB41	GB41	LU7	SP4	GB41	SJ5	KI6	KI6	SP4	UB62
3 – 5 am	UB62	KI6	KI6	UB62	SI3	GB41	KI6	UB62	KI6	SJ5	GB41	KI6
5 – 7 am	GB41	SP4	LU7	KI6	KI6	UB62	LU7	KI6	SJ5	UB62	SI3	KI6
7 – 9 am	KI6	GB41	SJ5	SJ5	KI6	KI6	SI3	KI6	UB62	KI6	KI6	SJ5
9 – 11 am	LU7	KI6	UB62	UB62	SP4	SJ5	KI6	SP4	PC6	KI6	SJ5	UB62
11 am – 1 pm	GB41	KI6	KI6	KI6	UB62	UB62	KI6	GB41	SJ5	SP4	SI3	KI6
1 – 3 pm	KI6	SJ5	SJ5	KI6	PC6	KI6	SJ5	KI6	SP4	GB41	KI6	KI6
3 – 5 pm	KI6	UB62	UB62	SP4	SP4	KI6	UB62	SP4	GB41	KI6	PC6	GB41
5 – 7 pm	SJ5	KI6	GB41	GB41	GB41	SP4	PC6	SJ5	KI6	SP4	SP4	KI6
7 – 9 pm	UB62	GB41	KI6	KI6	SI3	GB41	SP4	UB62	LU7	SJ5	GB41	SP4
9 – 11 pm	PC6	SP4	LU7	SP4	KI6	KI6	LU7	KI6	SI3	UB62	KI6	SJ5

針灸大成 · 卷之五

Open Points for the Method of the Mystical Tortoise (Líng Guī Bā Fǎ 靈龜八法) – Correct for Daylight Savings Time, if necessary.

Time \ Day	Rén Zǐ 壬子	Guǐ Chǒu 癸丑	Jiǎ Yín 甲寅	Yǐ Mǎo 乙卯	Bǐng Chén 丙辰	Dīng Sì 丁巳	Wù Wǔ 戊午	Jǐ Wèi 己未	Gēng Shēn 庚申	Xīn Yǒu 辛酉	Rén Xū 壬戌	Guǐ Hài 癸亥
11 pm – 1 am	KI 6	KI 6	LU 7	SJ 5	GB 41	KI 6	KI 6	KI 6	SI 3	SP 4	PC 6	KI 6
1 – 3 am	SJ 5	SP 4	SI 3	UB 62	SI 3	SP 4	LU 7	SP 4	KI 6	SJ 5	SP 4	SJ 5
3 – 5 am	UB 62	SJ 5	KI 6	KI 6	KI 6	GB 41	SJ 5	GB 41	SJ 5	UB 62	GB 41	SP 4
5 – 7 am	PC 6	UB 62	SJ 5	KI 6	SJ 5	KI 6	UB 62	KI 6	SP 4	KI 6	KI 6	GB 41
7 – 9 am	KI 6	KI 6	UB 62	SP 4	UB 62	KI 6	PC 6	SP 4	GB 41	SJ 5	KI 6	KI 6
9 – 11 am	LU 7	SJ 5	GB 41	GB 41	PC 6	SJ 5	SP 4	SJ 5	KI 6	UB 62	SJ 5	SP 4
11 am – 1 pm	GB 41	UB 62	PC 6	KI 6	PC 6	UB 62	UB 62	UB 62	SP 4	GB 41	SI 3	GB 41
1 – 3 pm	KI 6	GB 41	SP 4	SP 4	SP 4	KI 6	GB 41	KI 6	GB 41	KI 6	KI 6	UB 62
3 – 5 pm	LU 7	KI 6	GB 41	SJ 5	GB 41	SJ 5	KI 6	SJ 5	SI 3	SP 4	SJ 5	KI 6
5 – 7 pm	SJ 5	SP 4	KI 6	UB 62	KI 6	SP 4	LU 7	UB 62	KI 6	GB 41	SP 4	SJ 5
7 – 9 pm	UB 62	GB 41	KI 6	KI 6	LU 7	GB 41	SI 3	GB 41	SJ 5	KI 6	GB 41	UB 62
9 – 11 pm	PC 6	KI 6	SJ 5	SJ 5	SJ 5	KI 6	KI 6	KI 6	UB 62	KI 6	KI 6	KI 6

129

八脈圖并治症穴（徐氏、楊氏）
Illustrations of the Eight Vessels, and Points for Treating Patterns (Master Xú, Master Yáng)[99]

衝脈
Chòng Mài

考穴：公孫二穴，脾經。足大指內側，本節後一寸陷中，舉足，兩足掌相對取之。針一寸，主心腹五臟病，與內關主客相應。

Examining the point: The two points of Gōng Sūn 公孫 (SP 4) are on the spleen channel. They are in the depression one *cùn* posterior to the base joint of the big toe on the medial aspect. To locate it, lift the feet so that the two soles oppose each other. Needle one *cùn* deep. It is indicated for diseases of the heart region, abdomen, and the five viscera. It responds to Nèi Guān 內關 (PC 6) as host and guest.

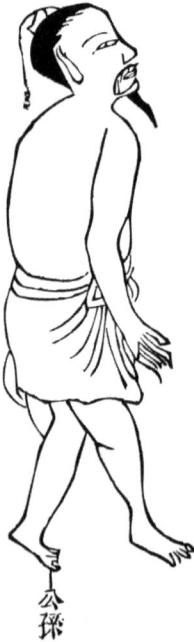

治病：〔西江月〕
　　　　九種心疼延悶，結胸翻胃難停。
　　　　酒食積聚胃腸鳴，水食氣疾膈病。
　　　　臍痛腹疼脅脹，腸風瘧疾心疼，
　　　　胎衣不下血迷心，泄瀉公孫立應。

Disease treatment: (West River Moon):[100]

The nine types of heart pain, drool oppression;[101]

---

99. Parts of this are taken from the *Zhēn Jiǔ Dà Quán*《針灸大全》(Great Completion of Acupuncture-Moxibustion), Volume 4. Yáng also added in his own point prescriptions and descriptions of the eight meeting points of the eight extraordinary vessels. The poem at the beginning of each entry was taken from Jù Yīng 聚英 *Gatherings of Eminent Acupuncturists*, Volume 4.

100. 〔西江月〕 "West River Moon" is the name of an old (non-medical) poem with a meter of *6-6-7-6*. Later, the term West River Moon was used for all poems with the same meter.

101. Here, the Chinese text says *yán mèn* 延悶 (prolonged oppression) but older books (including the *Great Completion*, which Yáng quotes correctly later) list *xián mèn* 涎悶 (drool oppression) and an indication for Gōng Sūn 公孫 (SP 4). Drool is the fluid of the spleen. In this context, the drool collects in the chest.

bound-up chest, stomach reflux that is difficult to stop;
Liquor and food accumulations and gatherings,
rumbling in the stomach and intestines;
water, food, and qì illness, and diseases of the diaphragm.
For pain in the umbilical region, abdominal pain, distention of the rib-sides;
intestinal wind, malaria, heart pain;
Retention of the placenta, blood confounding the heart;
and diarrhea, Gōng Sūn 公孫 (SP 4) immediately responds.

凡治後症，必先取公孫為主，次取各穴應之（徐氏）：

Generally to treat the following patterns, you must first select Gōng Sūn 公孫 (SP 4) as the host and next select each point that responds to it: (Master Xú)

九種心疼，一切冷氣：大陵、中脘、隱白

Nine types of heart pain, all from cold qì: Dà Líng 大陵 (PC 7), Zhōng Wǎn 中脘 (Ren 12), Yǐn Bái 隱白 (SP 1).

痰膈涎悶，胸中隱痛：勞宮、膻中、間使

Phlegm in the diaphragm, drool oppression, dull pain in the chest: Láo Gōng 勞宮 (PC 8), Dàn Zhōng 膻中 (Ren 17), Jiān Shǐ 間使 (PC 5).

氣膈五噎，飲食不下：膻中、三里、太白

Qì occlusion, the five [types of] dysphagia, inability to swallow food and drink: Dàn Zhōng 膻中 (Ren 17), Sān Lǐ 三里 (ST 36), Tài Bái 太白 (SP 3).

臍腹脹滿，食不消化：天樞、水分、內庭

Distention and fullness of the umbilicus and abdomen, non-transformation of food: Tiān Shū 天樞 (ST 25), Shuǐ Fēn 水分 (Ren 9), Nèi Tíng 內庭 (ST 44).

脅肋下痛，起止艱難：支溝、章門、陽陵泉

Pain below the rib-sides, difficulty getting up and lying down: Zhī Gōu 支溝 (SJ 6), Zhāng Mén 章門 (LV 13), Yáng Líng Quán 陽陵泉 (GB 34).

泄瀉不止，裏急後重：下脘、天樞、照海

Incessant diarrhea, tenesmus: Xià Wǎn 下脘 (Ren 10), Tiān Shū 天樞 (ST 25), Zhào Hǎi 照海 (KI 6).

胸中刺痛，隱隱不樂：內關、大陵、彧中

Pricking pain in the chest, dull discomfort: Nèi Guān 內關 (PC 6), Dà Líng 大陵 (PC 7), Yù Zhōng 彧中 (KI 26).

兩脅脹滿，氣攻疼痛：絕骨、章門、陽陵泉

Distention and fullness of the two rib-sides, pain due to attack of qì:[102] Jué Gǔ 絕骨 (GB 39), Zhāng Mén 章門 (LV 13), Yáng Líng Quán 陽陵泉 (GB 34).

中滿不快，翻胃吐食：中脘、太白、中魁

Center fullness and discomfort, stomach reflux, vomiting of food: Zhōng Wǎn 中脘 (Ren 12) Tài Bái 太白 (SP 3), Zhōng Kuí 中魁 (LI 5). [103]

胃脘停痰，口吐清水：巨闕、中脘、厲兌

Stomach duct collecting phlegm, clear water drooling from the mouth: Jù Què 巨闕 (Ren 14), Zhōng Wǎn 中脘 (Ren 12), Lì Duì 厲兌 (ST 45).

胃脘停食，疼刺不已：中脘、三里、解谿

Stomach duct collecting food, incessant pricking pain: Zhōng Wǎn 中脘 (Ren 12), Sān Lǐ 三里 (ST 36), Jiě Xī 解谿 (ST 41).

嘔吐痰涎，眩暈不已：膻中、中魁、豐隆

Vomiting phlegm drool, incessant dizziness: Dàn Zhōng 膻中 (Ren 17), Zhōng Kuí 中魁 (LI 5), Fēng Lóng 豐隆 (ST 40).

心瘧，令人心內怔忡：神門、心俞、百勞

Heart malaria making fearful throbbing inside the patient's heart: Shén Mén 神門 (HT 7), Xīn Shū 心俞 (UB 15), Bǎi Láo 百勞 (M-HN-30). [104]

---

102. "Attack of qì" meaning qì depression pressing horizontally onto the rib-sides.

103. There is a note in the *Great Completion* that says Zhōng Kuí 中魁 means Yáng Xī 陽溪 (LI 5). Zhōng Kuí is also a non-channel point (M-UE-16).

104. Bǎi Láo 百勞 (M-HN-30) is a non-channel point two cun above and one cun lateral to Dà Zhuī 大椎 (Du 14). However, Bǎi Láo is also an alternate name for Du 14. This question does not seem to be answered in Yáng's later sections on the points. He does not discuss Bǎi Láo among

脾瘧，令人怕寒腹痛：商丘、脾俞、三里

Spleen malaria making the patient fear cold and suffer abdominal pain: Shāng Qiū 商邱 (SP 5), Pí Shū 脾俞 (UB 20), Sān Lǐ 三里 (ST 36).

肝瘧，令人氣色蒼，惡寒發熱：中封、肝俞、絕骨

Liver malaria making the patient's qì color [complexion] dark green, aversion to cold, fever: Zhōng Fēng 中封 (LV 4), Gān Shū 肝俞 (UB 18), Jué Gǔ 絕骨 (GB 39).

肺瘧，令人心寒怕驚：列缺、肺俞、合谷

Lung malaria making the patient's heart cold, with fear and fright: Liè Quē 列缺 (LU 7), Fèi Shū 肺俞 (UB 13), Hé Gǔ 合谷 (LI 4).

腎瘧，令人洒熱，腰脊強痛：大鍾、腎俞、申脈

Kidney malaria making the patient [experience aversion to cold as if after] a soaking and fever,[105] stiffness and pain of the lumbar spine: Dà Zhōng 大鍾 (KI 4), Shèn Shū 腎俞 (UB 23), Shēn Mài 申脈 (UB 62).

瘧疾大熱不退：間使、百勞、絕骨

Malaria with great fever that does not abate: Jiān Shǐ 間使 (PC 5), Bǎi Láo 百勞 (M-HN-30), Jué Gǔ 絕骨 (GB 39).

瘧疾先寒後熱：後谿、曲池、勞宮

Malaria, first cold and later hot: Hòu Xī 後谿 (SI 3), Qū Chí 曲池 (LI 11), Láo Gōng 勞宮 (PC 8).

瘧疾先熱後寒：曲池、百勞、絕骨

Malaria, first hot and later cold: Qū Chí 曲池 (LI 11), Bǎi Láo 百勞 (M-HN-30), Jué Gǔ 絕骨 (GB 39).

---

the non-channel points and he does not mention it as an alternate name for Du 14. In this section of the *Great Completion* (Yáng's source here), Xú Fèng said Bǎi Láo is the same as Tiān Shū 天樞 (ST 25), but Yáng did not copy this note. I will label Bǎi Láo as the non-channel point, but the authors could have meant something else.

105. This statement is related to *Elementary Questions*, Chapter 36, but a few words are changed. The most important difference is that this chapter of the *Inner Classic* has (*sǎ sǎ rán* 洒洒然 or aversion to cold as if after a soaking) rather than (*sǎ rè* 洒熱, literally "sprinking fever"). It is quote possible that *rè* 熱 is a copying error for *rán* 然.

133

瘧疾心胸疼痛：內關、上脘、大陵

Malaria with heart and chest pain: Nèi Guān 內關 (PC 6), Shàng Wǎn 上脘 (Ren 13), Dà Líng 大陵 (PC 7).

瘧疾頭痛眩暈，吐痰不已：合谷、中脘、列缺

Malaria with headache, dizziness, and incessant vomiting of phlegm: Hé Gǔ 合谷 (LI 4), Zhōng Wǎn 中脘 (Ren 12), Liè Quē 列缺 (LU 7).

瘧疾骨節痠痛：魄戶、百勞、然谷

Malaria with soreness and pain of the bones and joints: Pò Hù 魄戶 (UB 42), Bǎi Láo 百勞 (M-HN-30), Rán Gǔ 然谷 (KI 2).

瘧疾口渴不已：關衝、人中、間使

Malaria with incessant thirst: Guān Chōng 關衝 (SJ 1), Rén Zhōng 人中 (Du 26), Jiān Shǐ 間使 (PC 5).

胃瘧，令人善飢，不能食：厲兌、胃俞、大都

Stomach malaria, making the patient frequently hungry but unable to eat: Lì Duì 厲兌 (ST 45), Wèi Shū 胃俞 (UB 21), Dà Dū 大都 (SP 2).

膽瘧，令人惡寒怕驚，睡臥不安：臨泣、膽俞、期門

Gall bladder malaria, making the patient averse to cold, with fear and fright, and unquiet sleep: Lín Qì 臨泣 (GB 41), Dǎn Shū 膽俞 (UB 19), Qī Mén 期門 (LV 14).

黃疸，四肢俱腫，汗出染衣：至陽、百勞、腕骨、中脘、三里

Jaundice, swelling of all four limbs, sweating that stains the clothes: Zhì Yáng 至陽 (Du 9), Bǎi Láo 百勞 (M-HN-30), Wàn Gǔ 腕骨 (SI 4), Zhōng Wǎn 中脘 (Ren 12), Sān Lǐ 三里 (ST 36).

黃疸，遍身皮膚面目小便俱黃：脾俞、隱白、百勞、至陽、三里、腕骨

Jaundice, the whole body's skin, face, eyes, and urine are all yellow: Pí Shū 脾俞 (UB 20), Yǐn Bái 隱白 (SP 1), Bǎi Láo 百勞 (M-HN-30), Zhì Yáng 至陽 (Du 9), Sān Lǐ 三里 (ST 36), Wàn Gǔ 腕骨 (SI 4).

穀疸，食畢則心眩，心中拂鬱，遍體發黃：胃俞、內庭、至陽、三里、腕骨、陰谷

Dietary irregularity jaundice, heart dizziness after eating, depression in the heart, yellowing of the entire body: Wèi Shū 胃俞 (ST 21), Nèi Tíng 內庭 (ST 44), Zhì Yáng 至陽 (Du 9), Sān Lǐ 三里 (ST 36), Wàn Gǔ 腕骨 (SI 4), Yīn Gǔ 陰谷 (KI 10).

酒疸，身目俱黃，心中痛，面發赤斑，小便赤黃：膽俞、至陽、委中、腕骨

Liquor jaundice, both the body and eyes are yellow, pain in the heart, eruptions of red macules on the face, reddish yellow urine: Dǎn Shū 膽俞 (UB 19), Zhì Yáng 至陽 (Du 9), Wěi Zhōng 委中 (UB 40), Wàn Gǔ 腕骨 (SI 4).

女癆疸，身目俱黃，發熱惡寒，小便不利：關元、腎俞、至陽、然谷

Sexual taxation jaundice, both the body and eyes are yellow, fever, aversion to cold, inhibited urination: Guān Yuán 關元 (Ren 4), Shèn Shū 腎俞 (UB 23), Zhì Yáng 至陽 (Du 9), Rán Gǔ 然谷 (KI 2).

楊氏治症：
Master Yáng's treatment of patterns:

月事不調：關元、氣海、天樞、三陰交

Irregular menstruation: Guān Yuán 關元 (Ren 4), Qì Hǎi 氣海 (Ren 6), Tiān Shū 天樞 (ST 25), Sān Yīn Jiāo 三陰交 (SP 6).

胸中滿痛：勞宮、通里、大陵、膻中

Fullness and pain in the chest: Láo Gōng 勞宮 (PC 8), Tōng Lǐ 通里 (HT 5), Dà Líng 大陵 (PC 7), Dàn Zhōng 膻中 (Ren 17).

痰熱結胸：列缺、大陵、湧泉

Phlegm-heat binding the chest: Liè Quē 列缺 (LU 7), Dà Líng 大陵 (PC 7), Yǒng Quán 湧泉 (KI 1).

四肢風痛：曲池、風市、外關、陽陵泉、三陰交、手三里

Wind pain in the four limbs: Qū Chí 曲池 (LI 11), Fēng Shì 風市 (GB 31), Wài Guān 外關 (SJ 5), Yáng Líng Quán 陽陵泉 (GB 34), Sān Yīn Jiāo 三陰交 (SP 6), Shǒu Sān Lǐ 手三里 (LI 10).

咽喉閉塞：少商、風池、照海、頰車。

Throat blockage: Shào Shāng 少商 (LU 11), Fēng Chí 風池 (GB 20), Zhào Hǎi 照海 (KI 6), Jiá Chē 頰車 (ST 6).

陰維脈
Yīn Wéi Mài

考穴：內關二穴，心包經。去掌二寸兩筋間，緊握拳取之。針一寸二分，主心膽脾胃之病，與公孫二穴，主客相應。

Examining the point: The two points of Nèi Guān 內關 (PC 6) are on the pericardium channel. They are two *cùn* proximal to the palm, between the two sinews. Make a tight fist to find it. Needle 1.2 *cùn* deep. It is indicated for diseases of the heart, gall bladder, spleen, and stomach. It responds to the two points of Gōng Sūn 公孫 (SP 4) as host and guest.

治病：〔西江月〕
中滿心胸痞脹，腸鳴泄瀉脫肛，
食難下膈酒來傷，積塊堅橫脅搶。
婦女脅疼心痛，結胸裏急難當，
傷寒不解結胸膛，瘧疾內關獨當。

Disease treatment: (West River Moon):

Fullness in the center, glomus and distention of the heart region and chest; intestinal rumbling, diarrhea, prolapse of the rectum;
Difficulty swallowing food through the diaphragm, damage brought about by liquor;
hard accumulations and lumps plundering the transverse rib-sides.
For rib-side pain in females, heart pain;
bound up chest, intolerable abdominal urgency;
Unresolved cold damage, bound up chest;
and malaria, only Nèi Guān 內關 (PC 6) is correct.

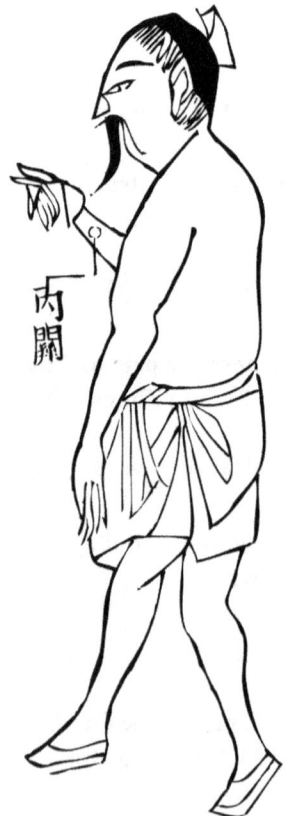

凡治後症，必先取內關為主，次取各穴應之（徐氏）：

Generally to treat the following patterns, you must first select Nèi Guān 內關 (PC 6) as the host and next select each point that responds to it:
(Master Xú)

中滿不快，胃脘傷寒：中脘、大陵、三里、膻中

Central fullness and discomfort, cold damage of the stomach duct: Zhōng Wǎn 中脘 (Ren 12), Dà Líng 大陵 (PC 7), Sān Lǐ 三里 (ST 36), Dàn Zhōng 膻中 (Ren 17).

中焦痞滿，兩脅刺痛：支溝、章門、膻中

Glomus and fullness of the central burner, pricking pain of both rib-sides: Zhī Gōu 支溝 (SJ 6), Zhāng Mén 章門 (LV 13), Dàn Zhōng 膻中 (Ren 17).

脾胃虛冷，嘔吐不已：內庭、中脘、氣海、公孫

Vacuity cold of the spleen-stomach, unceasing vomiting: Nèi Tíng 內庭 (ST 44), Zhōng Wǎn 中脘 (Ren 12), Qì Hǎi 氣海 (Ren 6), Gōng Sūn 公孫 (SP 4).

脾胃氣虛，心腹脹滿：太白、三里、氣海、水分

Qì vacuity of the spleen-stomach, distention and fullness of the heart region and abdomen: Tài Bái 太白 (SP 3), Sān Lǐ 三里 (ST 36), Qì Hǎi 氣海 (Ren 6), Shuǐ Fēn 水分 (Ren 9).

脅肋下疼，心脘刺痛：氣海、行間、陽陵泉

Pain below the rib-sides, pricking pain of the heart duct: Qì Hǎi 氣海 (Ren 6), Xíng Jiān 行間 (LV 2), Yáng Líng Quán 陽陵泉 (GB 34).

痞塊不散，心中悶痛：大陵、中脘、三陰交

Glomus lumps that do not disperse, oppression and pain in the heart: Dà Líng 大陵 (PC 7), Zhōng Wǎn 中脘 (Ren 12), Sān Yīn Jiāo 三陰交 (SP 6).

食癥不散，人漸羸瘦：腕骨、脾俞、公孫

Food concretions that do not disperse while the patient gradually becomes emaciated: Wàn Gǔ 腕骨 (SI 4), Pí Shū 脾俞 (UB 20), Gōng Sūn 公孫 (SP 4).

食積血瘕，腹中隱痛：胃俞、行間、氣海

Food accumulation, blood conglomeration, dull pain in the abdomen: Wèi Shū 胃俞 (UB 21), Xíng Jiān 行間 (LV 2), Qì Hǎi 氣海 (Ren 6).

五積氣塊，血積血癖：膈俞、肝俞、大敦、照海

The five accumulations, qì lumps, blood accumulations, blood aggregations: Gé Shū 膈俞 (UB 17), Gān Shū 肝俞 (UB 18), Dà Dūn 大敦 (LV 1), Zhào Hǎi 照海 (KI 6).

臟腑虛冷，兩脅痛疼：支溝、通里、章門、陽陵泉

Vacuity cold of the viscera and bowels, pain of both rib-sides: Zhī Gōu 支溝 (SJ 6), Tōng Lǐ 通里 (HT 5),[106] Zhāng Mén 章門 (LV 14), Yáng Líng Quán 陽陵泉 (GB 34).

風壅氣滯，心腹刺痛：風門、膻中、勞宮、三里

Wind congestion, qì stagnation, pricking pain in the heart region and abdomen: Fēng Mén 風門 (UB 12), Dàn Zhōng 膻中 (Ren 17), Láo Gōng 勞宮 (PC 8), Sān Lǐ 三里 (ST 36).

大腸虛冷，脫肛不收：百會、命門、長強、承山

Vacuity cold of the large intestine, unretractable prolapse of the rectum: Bǎi Huì 百會 (Du 20), Mìng Mén 命門 (Du 4), Cháng Qiáng 長強 (Du 1), Chéng Shān 承山 (UB 57).

大便艱難，用力脫肛：照海、百會、支溝

Difficult defecation, prolapse of the rectum when straining: Zhào Hǎi 照海 (KI 6), Bǎi Huì 百會 (Du 20), Zhī Gōu 支溝 (SJ 6).

臟毒腫痛，便血不止：承山、肝俞、膈俞、長強

Toxins, swelling, and pain of the viscera, unceasing bloody stool: Chéng Shān 承山 (UB 57), Gān Shū 肝俞 (UB 18), Gé Shū 膈俞 (UB 17), Cháng Qiáng 長強 (Du 1).

五種痔疾，攻痛不已：合陽、長強、承山

The five accumulations, hemorrhoidal diseases, unceasing attacks of pain: Hé Yáng 合陽 (UB 55), Cháng Qiáng 長強 (Du 1), Chéng Shān 承山 (UB 57).

五癇等病，口中吐沫：後谿、神門、心俞、鬼眼

The five epilepsies class of diseases, foaming at the mouth: Hòu Xī 後谿 (SI 3), Shén Mén 神

---

106. The *Great Completion* has Jiàn Lǐ 建里 (Ren 11) instead of Tōng Lǐ 通里 (HT 5).

門 (HT 7), Xīn Shū 心俞 (UB 15), Guǐ Yǎn 鬼眼 (Ghost Eye). [107]

心性呆痴，悲泣不已：通里、後谿、神門、大鍾

Feeble-minded nature of the heart [or mind], unceasing tears of sorrow: Tōng Lǐ 通里 (HT 5), Hòu Xī 後谿 (SI 3), Shén Mén 神門 (HT 7), Dà Zhōng 大鍾 (KI 4).

心驚發狂，不識親疏：少衝、心俞、中脘、十宣

Frightened heart triggering mania, doesn't recognize family: Shào Chōng 少衝 (HT 9), Xīn Shū 心俞 (UB 15), Zhōng Wǎn 中脘 (Ren 12), Shí Xuān 十宣 (M-UE-1).

健忘易失，言語不紀：心俞、通里、少衝

Forgetfulness, easily gets lost, disordered speech: Xīn Shū 心俞 (UB 15), Tōng Lǐ 通里 (HT 5), Shào Chōng 少衝 (HT 9).

心氣虛損，或歌或笑：靈道、心俞、通里

Heart qì vacuity detriment, sometimes singing, sometimes laughing: Líng Dào 靈道 (HT 4), Xīn Shū 心俞 (UB 15), Tōng Lǐ 通里 (HT 5).

心中驚悸，言語錯亂：少海、少府、心俞、後谿

Fright palpitations in the heart, deranged speech: Shào Hǎi 少海 (HT 3), Shào Fǔ 少府 (HT 8), Xīn Shū 心俞 (UB 15), Hòu Xī 後谿 (SI 3).

心中虛惕，神思不安：乳根、通里、膽俞、心俞

Vacuity and apprehension in the heart, disquieted spirit and thought: Rǔ Gēn 乳根 (ST 18), Tōng Lǐ 通里 (HT 5), Dǎn Shū 膽俞 (UB 19), Xīn Shū 心俞 (UB 15).

心驚中風，不省人事：中衝、百會、大敦

Frightened heart leading to wind stroke, loss of consciousness: Zhōng Chōng 中衝 (PC 9), Bǎi Huì 百會 (Du 20), Dà Dūn 大敦 (LV 1).

心膽諸虛，怔忡驚悸：陰郄、心俞、通里

---

107. Guǐ Yǎn 鬼眼 or Ghost Eye: Hand Ghost Eye is Shào Shāng 少商 (LU 11). Foot Ghost Eye is Yǐn Bái 隱白 (SP 1). These are also two of Sūn Sī Miǎo's 孫思邈 Thirteen Ghost Points. When called 'Ghost Eye,' they are treated with a special moxibustion technique. The two thumbs or big toes are tied together and large cones are placed so that one cone covers a bit of the flesh and the nail surrounding these points. One cone covers the area on both thumbs or big toes. Seven or fourteen cones are burned.

Dual vacuity of the heart and gall bladder, fearful throbbing, fright palpitations: Yīn Xī 陰郤 (HT 6), Xīn Shū 心俞 (UB 15), Tōng Lǐ 通里 (HT 5).

心虛膽寒，四體顫掉：膽俞 、通里 、臨泣

Heart vacuity, cold in the gall bladder, tremor and shaking of the four limbs: Dǎn Shū 膽俞 (UB 19), Tōng Lǐ 通里 (HT 5), Lín Qì 臨泣 (GB 41).

督脈
Dū Mài

考穴：後谿二穴，小腸經 。小指本節後外側骨縫中，緊握拳尖上 。針一寸，主頭面項頸病，與申脈主客相應 。

Examining the point: The two points of Hòu Xī 後谿 (SI 3) are on the small intestine channel. They are on the seam at the posterior lateral aspect of the bone at the base joint of the little finger. When you make a tight fist, it is at the tip [of the seam]. Needle one *cùn* deep. It is indicated for diseases of the head, face, nape, and neck. It responds to Shēn Mài 申脈 (UB 62) as host and guest.

治病：〔西江月〕
　　　手足拘攣戰掉，中風不語癇癲，
　　　頭疼眼腫淚漣漣，腿膝腰背痛遍 。
　　　項強傷寒不解，牙齒腮腫喉咽，
　　　手麻足麻破傷牽，盜汗後谿先砭 。

Disease treatment: (West River Moon):

Hypertonicity or trembling and
shaking of the hands and feet;
wind stroke with loss of speech, epilepsy and withdrawal;
Headache, swollen eyes with tears continually flowing; pain all
over the legs, knees, low back, and upper back.
For stiff nape, unresolved cold damage;
swelling of the teeth, cheeks, and throat;
Numb hands and feet,
tetany pulling [the face into a grimace];
and night sweating, first use the healing stone [*biān* 砭] on
Hòu Xī 後谿 (SI 3).

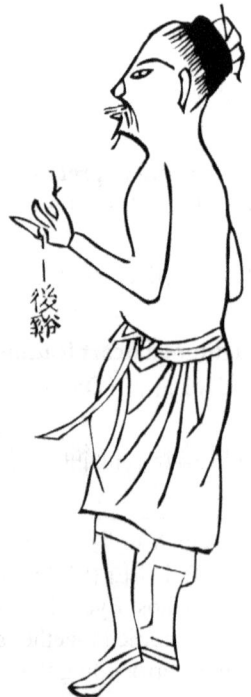

凡治後症，必先取後谿為主，次取各穴應之（ 徐氏 ）：

Generally to treat the following patterns, you must first select Hòu Xī 後谿 (SI 3) as the host and next select each point that responds to it: (Master Xú):

手足攣急，屈伸艱難：三里 、曲池 、尺澤 、合谷 、行間 、陽陵泉

Hypertonicity of hands and feet, difficulty bending and stretching: Sān Lǐ 三里 (ST 36), Qū Chí 曲池 (LI 11), Chǐ Zé 尺澤 (LU 5), Hé Gǔ 合谷 (LI 4), Xíng Jiān 行間 (LV 2), Yáng Líng Quán 陽陵泉 (GB 34).

手足俱顫，不能行步握物：陽谿 、曲池 、腕骨 、太衝 、絕骨 、公孫 、陽陵泉

Tremor of both the hands and feet, inability to walk or grasp things: Yáng Xī 陽谿 (LI 5), Qū Chí 曲池 (LI 11), Wàn Gǔ 腕骨 (SI 4), Tài Chōng 太衝 (LV 3), Jué Gǔ 絕骨 (GB 39), Gōng Sūn 公孫 (SP 4), Yáng Líng Quán 陽陵泉 (GB 34).

頸項強痛，不能回顧：承漿 、風池 、風府

Stiff painful neck, inability to turn the head: Chéng Jiāng 承漿 (Ren 24), Fēng Chí 風池 (GB 20), Fēng Fǔ 風府 (Du 16).

兩腮頰痛紅腫：大迎 、頰車 、合谷

Both cheeks painful, red, and swollen: Dà Yíng 大迎 (ST 5), Jiá Chē 頰車 (ST 6), Hé Gǔ 合谷 (LI 4).

咽喉閉塞，水粒不下：天突 、商陽 、照海 、十宣

Throat blockage, inability to swallow water and grain: Tiān Tú 天突 (Ren 22), Shāng Yáng 商陽 (LI 1), Zhào Hǎi 照海 (KI 6), Shí Xuān 十宣 (M-UE-1).

雙蛾風，喉閉不通：少商 、金津 、玉液 、十宣

Double moth wind, throat blocked and lacking passage: Shào Shāng 少商 (LU 11), Jīn Jīn Yù Yè 金津玉液 (M-HN-20), Shí Xuān 十宣 (M-UE-1).

單蛾風，喉中腫痛：關衝 、天突 、合谷

Single moth wind, swelling and pain in the throat: Guān Chōng 關衝 (SJ 1), Tiān Tú 天突 (Ren 22), Hé Gǔ 合谷 (LI 4).

偏正頭風，及兩額角痛：列缺 、合谷 、太陽紫脈 、頭臨泣 、絲竹空

Hemilateral or bilateral head wind, as well as pain in both corners of the forehead: Liè Quē 列缺 (LU 7), Hé Gǔ 合谷 (LI 4), the purple vessels at Tài Yáng 太陽 (M-HN-9), Tóu Lín Qì 頭臨泣 (GB 15), Sī Zhú Kōng 絲竹空 (SJ 23).

兩眉角痛不已：攢竹 、陽白 、印堂 、合谷 、頭維

Incessant pain at both corners of the eyebrows: Zǎn Zhú 攢竹 (UB 2), Yáng Bái 陽白 (GB 14), Yìn Táng 印堂 (M-HN-3), Hé Gǔ 合谷 (LI 4), Tóu Wéi 頭維 (ST 8).

頭目昏沉，太陽痛：合谷 、太陽紫脈 、頭縫

Head and eyes dazed, pain at Tài Yáng 太陽 (M-HN-9): Hé Gǔ 合谷 (LI 4), the purple vessels at Tài Yáng 太陽 (M-HN-9), Tóu Fèng 頭縫 (Fontanel).[108]

頭項拘急，引肩背痛：承漿 、百會 、肩井 、中渚

Hypertonicity of the head and neck, upper back pain radiating to the shoulders: Chéng Jiāng 承漿 (Ren 24), Bǎi Huì 百會 (Du 20), Jiān Jǐng 肩井 (GB 21), Zhōng Zhǔ 中渚 (SJ 3).

醉頭風，嘔吐不止，惡聞人言：湧泉 、列缺 、百勞 、合谷

Head wind from drunkenness, incessant vomiting, aversion to sounds and human speech: Yǒng Quán 湧泉 (KI 1), Liè Quē 列缺 (LU 7), Bǎi Láo 百勞 (M-HN-30), Hé Gǔ 合谷 (LI 4).

眼赤腫，衝風淚下不已：攢竹 、合谷 、小骨空 、臨泣

Eyes red and swollen, tears fall incessantly when hit by wind: Zǎn Zhú 攢竹 (UB 2), Hé Gǔ 合谷 (LI 4), Xiǎo Gǔ Kōng 小骨空 (Small Bone Hollow),[109] Lín Qì 臨泣 (GB 41).

破傷風，因他事搐發，渾身發熱顛強：大敦 、合谷 、行間 、十宣 、太陽紫脈（ 宜鋒針出血 ）

Lockjaw caused by other convulsions, the whole body is feverish, stiffness at the vertex:[110] Dà Dūn 大敦 (LV 1), Hé Gǔ 合谷 (LI 4), Xíng Jiān 行間 (LV 2), Shí Xuān 十宣 (M-UE-

---

108. Tóu Fèng 頭縫 (Fontanel) is in the corner of the forehead at the "point" of the hair, according to the *Zhēn Jiǔ Dà Quán*《 針灸大全 》(Great Completion of Acupuncture-Moxibustion).

109. Xiǎo Gǔ Kōng 小骨空 (Small Bone Hollow) is on the proximal interphalangeal joint of the little finger, on the dorsal side. Apply seven cones of moxibustion. This point treats pain in the eyes and the joints of the hands.

110. "Stiffness at the vertex" probably means a distended pulling sensation at the vertex.

1), the purple vessels at Tài Yáng 太陽 (M-HN-9) (it is appropriate to use the sharp-edged needle to let blood).

楊氏治症：
Master Yáng's treatment of patterns:

咳嗽寒痰：列缺、湧泉、申脈、肺俞、天突、絲竹空

Cough with cold phlegm: Liè Quē 列缺 (LU 7), Yǒng Quán 湧泉 (KI 1), Shēn Mài 申脈 (UB 62), Fèi Shū 肺俞 (UB 13), Tiān Tú 天突 (Ren 22), Sī Zhú Kōng 絲竹空 (SJ 23).

頭目眩暈：風池、命門、合谷

Dizziness in the head and eyes: Fēng Chí 風池 (GB 20), Mìng Mén 命門 (Du 4), Hé Gǔ 合谷 (LI 4).

頭項強硬：承漿、風府、風池、合谷

Stiffness and hardness of the head and neck: Chéng Jiāng 承漿 (Ren 24), Fēng Fǔ 風府 (Du 16), Fēng Chí 風池 (GB 20), Hé Gǔ 合谷 (LI 4).

牙齒疼痛：列缺、人中、頰車、呂細、太淵、合谷

Toothache: Liè Quē 列缺 (LU 7), Rén Zhōng 人中 (Du 26), Jiá Chē 頰車 (ST 6), Lǚ Xì 呂 細 (Small Lǚ),[111] Tài Yuān 太淵 (LU 9), Hé Gǔ 合谷 (LI 4).

耳不聞聲：聽會、商陽、少衝、中衝

Deafness: Tīng Huì 聽會 (GB 2), Shāng Yáng 商陽 (LI 1), Shào Chōng 少衝 (HT 9), Zhōng Chōng 中衝 (PC 9).

破傷風症：承漿、合谷、八邪、後谿、外關、四關

Lockjaw patterns: Chéng Jiāng 承漿 (Ren 24), Hé Gǔ 合谷 (LI 4), Bā Xié 八邪 (M-UE-22), Hòu Xī 後谿 (SI 3), Wài Guān 外關 (SJ 5), Sì Guān 四關 (Four Gates, Hé Gǔ 合谷 - LI 4 and Tài Chōng 太衝 - LV 3).

---

111. Lǚ Xì 呂細 (Small Lǚ) is an alternate name for Tài Xī 太谿 (KI 3) according to the *Great Completion*. The word Lǚ in the name of this point refers to the fifth note of the Chinese musical scale, the note corresponding to water element and the kidneys.

陽蹻脈
Yáng Qiāo Mài

考穴：申脈二穴，膀胱經 。足外踝下陷中，赤白肉際，直立取之 。針一寸，主四肢風邪，及癰毒病，與後溪主客相應 。

Examining the point: The two points of Shēn Mài 申脈 (UB 62) are on the urinary bladder channel. They are in the depression below the lateral malleolus, at the border of the red and white flesh. Stand straight to locate it. Needle it one *cùn* deep. It is indicated for diseases of the four limbs, wind evils, and abscess toxins. It responds to Hòu Xī 後谿 (SI 3) as host and guest.

治病：〔西江月〕
　　　腰背屈強腿腫，惡風自汗頭疼，
　　　雷頭赤目痛眉稜，手足麻攣臂冷 。
　　　吹乳耳聾鼻衄，癲癇肢節煩憎，
　　　遍身腫滿汗頭淋，申脈先針有應 。

Disease treatment: (West River Moon):

Back bent and stiff, swollen legs;
aversion to wind, spontaneous sweating, headache;
Thunder head, red eyes, pain on the ridge of the eyebrows;
numbness and hypertonicity of the hands and feet, cold arms.
Breast blowing,[112] deafness, nosebleeds;
epilepsy and withdrawal, vexation in the joints of the limbs;
For swelling and fullness of the entire body
and sweat dripping from the head;
first needle Shēn Mài 申脈 (UB 62) to have a [good] response.

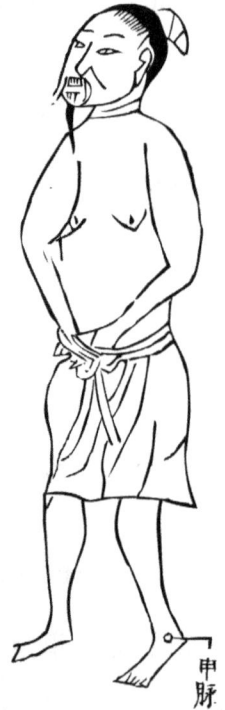

Fig. 5.28

凡治後症，必先取申脈為主，次取各穴應之（徐氏）：

Generally to treat the following patterns, you must first select Shēn Mài 申脈 (UB 62) as the host and next select each point that responds to it: (Master Xú)

---

112. Breast blowing: A type of breast abscess that occurs during the period of breast feeding.

腰背強，不可俛仰：腰俞、膏肓、委中（ 刺紫脈出血 ）

Stiff back, cannot bend forward and backward: Yāo Shū 腰俞 **(Du 2), Gāo Huāng** 膏肓 **(UB 43), Wěi Zhōng** 委中 **(UB 40) (pierce the purple vessels to let blood).**

肢節煩痛，牽引腰腳疼：肩髃、曲池、崑崙、陽陵

Vexing pain of the joints of the limbs, pulling pain that radiates through the low back and legs: Jiān Yú 肩髃 **(LI 15), Qū Chí** 曲池 **(LI 11), Kūn Lún** 崑崙 **(UB 60), Yáng Líng** 陽陵 **(GB 34).**

中風不省人事：中衝、百會、大敦、印堂、合谷

Wind stroke with unconsciousness: Zhōng Chōng 中衝 **(PC 9), Bǎi Huì** 百會 **(Du 20), Dà Dūn** 大敦 **(LV 1), Yìn Táng** 印堂 **(M-HN-3), Hé Gǔ** 合谷 **(LI 4).**

中風不語：少商、前頂、人中、膻中、合谷、啞門

Wind stroke, loss of speech: Shào Shāng 少商 **(LU 11), Qián Dǐng** 前頂 **(Du 21), Rén Zhōng** 人中 **(Du 26), Dàn Zhōng** 膻中 **(Ren 17), Hé Gǔ** 合谷 **(LI 4), Yǎ Mén** 啞門 **(Du 15).**

中風半身癱瘓：手三里、腕骨、合谷、絕骨、行間、風市、三陰交

Wind stroke with hemiplegia: Shǒu Sān Lǐ 手三里 **(LI 10), Wàn Gǔ** 腕骨 **(SI 4), Hé Gǔ** 合谷 **(LI 4), Jué Gǔ** 絕骨 **(GB 39), Xíng Jiān** 行間 **(LV 2), Fēng Shì** 風市 **(GB 31), Sān Yīn Jiāo** 三陰交 **(SP 6).**

中風偏枯，疼痛無時：絕骨、太淵、曲池、肩髃、三里、崑崙

Wind stroke with hemilateral withering, sporadic pain: Jué Gǔ 絕骨 **(GB 39), Tài Yuān** 太淵 **(LU 9), Qū Chí** 曲池 **(LI 11), Jiān Yú** 肩髃 **(LI 15), Sān Lǐ** 三里 **(ST 36), Kūn Lún** 崑崙 **(UB 60).**

中風四肢麻痹不仁：肘髎、上廉、魚際、風市、膝關、三陰交

Wind stroke with numbness of the four limbs: Zhǒu Liáo 肘髎 **(LI 12), Shàng Lián** 上廉 **(LI 9), Yú Jì** 魚際 **(LU 10), Fēng Shì** 風市 **(GB 31), Xī Guān** 膝關 **(LV 7), Sān Yīn Jiāo** 三陰交 **(SP 6).**

中風手足搔癢，不能握物：臑會、腕骨、合谷、行間、風市、陽陵泉

Wind stroke, scratching and itching on the hands and feet, inability to grasp things: Nào Huì 臑會 **(SJ 13), Wàn Gǔ** 腕骨 **(SI 4), Hé Gǔ** 合谷 **(LI 4), Xíng Jiān** 行間 **(LV 2), Fēng Shì** 風市 **(GB 31), Yáng Líng Quán** 陽陵泉 **(GB 34).**

針灸大成・卷之五

中風口眼喎斜，牽連不已：人中、合谷、太淵、十宣、瞳子髎、頰車（ 此穴
針入一分，沿皮向下透地倉穴 。喎左瀉右，喎右瀉左，可灸二七壯 ）

Wind stroke with deviation of the eyes and mouth, incessant pulling [of the eyes and mouth]: Rén Zhōng 人中 (Du 26), Hé Gǔ 合谷 (LI 4), Tài Yuān 太淵 (LU 9), Shí Xuān 十宣 (M-UE-1), Tóng Zǐ Liáo 瞳子髎 (GB 1), Jiá Chē 頰車 (ST 6) (needle this point one *fēn* deep, [then make the needle] follow down along the skin to join it to Dì Cāng 地倉 (ST 4). If the deviation is on the left, drain the right; if the deviation is on the right, drain the left. You can apply two times seven cones of moxibustion).

中風角弓反張，眼目盲視：百會、百勞、合谷、行間、曲池、十宣、陽陵泉

Wind stroke with arched-back rigidity and blindness: Bǎi Huì 百會 (Du 20), Bǎi Láo 百勞 (M-HN-30), Hé Gǔ 合谷 (LI 4), Xíng Jiān 行間 (LV 2), Qū Chí 曲池 (LI 11), Shí Xuān 十宣 (M-UE-1), Yáng Líng Quán 陽陵泉 (GB 34).

中風口噤不開，言語蹇澀：地倉（ 宜針透 ）頰車、人中、合谷

Wind stroke with clenched jaw that cannot open and sluggish speech: Dì Cāng 地倉 (ST 4) (it is appropriate to join the needle to) Jiá Chē 頰車 (ST 6), Rén Zhōng 人中 (Du 26), Hé Gǔ 合谷 (LI 4).

腰脊項背疼痛：腎俞、人中、肩井、委中

Pain of the low back, spine, nape, or upper back: Shèn Shū 腎俞 (UB 23), Rén Zhōng 人中 (Du 26), Jiān Jǐng 肩井 (GB 21), Wěi Zhōng 委中 (UB 40).

腰痛，起止艱難：然谷、膏肓、委中、腎俞

Low back pain, difficulty getting up and lying down: Rán Gǔ 然谷 (KI 2), Gāo Huāng 膏肓 (UB 43), Wěi Zhōng 委中 (UB 40), Shèn Shū 腎俞 (UB 23).

足背生毒，名曰發背：內庭、俠谿、行間、委中

Toxins erupting on the dorsum of the feet. This is called effusion of the back: Nèi Tíng 內庭 (ST 44), Xiá Xī 俠谿 (GB 43), Xíng Jiān 行間 (LV 2), Wěi Zhōng 委中 (UB 40).

手背生毒，名附筋發背：液門、中渚、合谷、外關

Toxins erupting on the dorsum of the hands. This is called sinew effusion of the back: Yè Mén 液門 (SJ 2), Zhōng Zhǔ 中渚 (SJ 3), Hé Gǔ 合谷 (LI 4), Wài Guān 外關 (SJ 5).

手臂背生毒，名曰附骨疽：天府、曲池、委中

Toxins erupting on the hands, arms, and back. This is called abscess attached to the bone: Tiān Fǔ 天府 (LU 3), Qū Chí 曲池 (LI 11), Wěi Zhōng 委中 (UB 40).

楊氏治症：
Master Yáng's treatment of patterns:

背腰生癰：委中、俠谿、十宣、曲池、液門、內關、外關

Abscesses erupting on the back: Wěi Zhōng 委中 (UB 40), Xiá Xī 俠谿 (GB 43), Shí Xuān 十宣 (M-UE-1), Qū Chí 曲池 (LI 11), Yè Mén 液門 (SJ 2), Nèi Guān 內關 (PC 6), Wài Guān 外關 (SJ 5).

遍體疼痛：太淵、三里、曲池

Pain all over the body: Tài Yuān 太淵 (LU 9), Sān Lǐ 三里 (ST 36), Qū Chí 曲池 (LI 11).

鬢髭發毒：太陽、申脈、太谿、合谷、外關

Toxins erupting in the hair on the temples and in the mustache: Tài Yáng 太陽 (M-HN-9), Shēn Mài 申脈 (UB 62), Tài Xī 太谿 (KI 3), Hé Gǔ 合谷 (LI 4), Wài Guān 外關 (SJ 5).

頭腦攻瘡：百勞、合谷、申脈、強間、委中

Sores attacking the head and brain: Bǎi Láo 百勞 (M-HN-30), Hé Gǔ 合谷 (LI 4), Shēn Mài 申脈 (UB 62), Qiáng Jiān 強間 (Du 18), Wěi Zhōng 委中 (UB 40).

頭痛難低：申脈、金門、承漿

Headache, difficulty bowing the head: Shēn Mài 申脈 (UB 62), Jīn Mén 金門 (UB 63), Chéng Jiāng 承漿 (Ren 24).

頸項難轉：後谿、合谷、承漿

Difficulty rotating the neck: Hòu Xī 後谿 (SI 3), Hé Gǔ 合谷 (LI 4), Chéng Jiāng 承漿 (Ren 24).

帶脈
Dài Mài

考穴：臨泣二穴，膽經 。足小指次指外側，本節中筋骨縫內，去一寸是 。針五分，放水隨皮過一寸 。主四肢病，與外關主客相應 。

Examining the point: The two points of Lín Qì 臨泣 (GB 41) are on the gall bladder channel. They are on the lateral aspect of the fourth toe, one *cùn* proximal to the base joint inside the seam between the sinew and the bone. Needle it five *fēn* deep. To let out water, follow the skin more than one *cùn*.[113] It is indicated for diseases of the four limbs. It responds to Wài Guān 外關 (SJ 5) as host and guest.

治病：〔西江月〕
手足中風不舉，痛麻發熱拘攣，
頭風痛腫項腮連，眼腫赤疼頭旋 。
齒痛耳聾咽腫，浮風搔痒筋牽，
腿疼脅脹肋肢偏，臨泣針時有驗 。

Disease treatment: (West River Moon):

Inability to raise the limbs due to windstroke;
pain, numbness, fever, hypertonicity;
Head wind pain and swelling radiating to the
nape and cheeks;
swollen red painful eyes, spinning head.
Toothache, deafness, swollen throat;
scratching and itching due to superficial wind,
pulling of sinews;
Leg pain, one-sided distention of the rib-sides and limbs;
at the time you needle Lín Qì 臨泣 (GB 41),
you will have results.

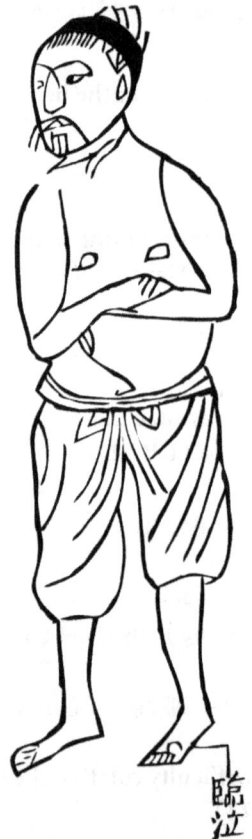

臨泣

Fig. 5.29

113. "To let out water" This means to let fluids out of a point, similar to blood-letting. In Volume 3 of the *Great Compendium*, Yáng discussed letting water in a little more detail. He wrote that to drain Shuǐ Fēn 水分 (Ren 9), first needle it with a small needle, then with a large needle. After that, insert the quill from a feather into the hole. If clear water comes out, the patient will live. If turbid water comes out, the patient will die. He also recommended this procedure on Fù Liū 復溜 (KI 7) if there is a lot of swelling in the legs.

凡治後症，必先取臨泣為主，次取各穴應之（ 徐氏 ）：

Generally to treat the following patterns, you must first select Lín Qì 臨泣 (GB 41) as the host and next select each point that responds to it:
(Master Xú)

足跗腫痛，久不能消：行間 、申脈

Enduring swelling and pain of the dorsum of the feet which cannot be dispersed: Xíng Jiān 行間 (LV 2), Shēn Mài 申脈 (UB 62).

手足麻痺，不知痒痛：太衝 、曲池 、大陵 、合谷 、三里 、中渚

Paralysis of the limbs, inability to perceive itching or pain: Tài Chōng 太衝 (LV 3), Qū Chí 曲池 (LI 11), Dà Líng 大陵 (PC 7), Hé Gǔ 合谷 (LI 4), Sān Lǐ 三里 (ST 36), Zhōng Zhǔ 中渚 (SJ 3).

兩足顫掉，不能移步：太衝 、崑崙 、陽陵泉

Tremor and shaking of both feet, inability to walk: Tài Chōng 太衝 (LV 3), Kūn Lún 崑崙 (UB 60), Yáng Líng Quán 陽陵泉 (GB 34).

兩手顫掉，不能握物：曲澤 、腕骨 、合谷 、中渚

Tremor and shaking of both hands, inability to grasp things: Qū Zé 曲澤 (PC 3), Wàn Gǔ 腕骨 (SI 4), Hé Gǔ 合谷 (LI 4), Zhōng Zhǔ 中渚 (SJ 3).

足指拘攣，筋緊不開：足十指節（ 握拳指尖，小麥炷，灸五壯 ）、邱墟 、公孫 、陽陵泉

Hypertonicity of the toes, hard sinews that will not open up: the joints of the ten toes (make a 'fist' [by curling the toes], apply moxibustion with five small grain-of-wheat size cones at the tips [of each joint] on the toes), Qiū Xū 邱墟 (GB 40), Gōng Sūn 公孫 (SP 4), Yáng Líng Quán 陽陵泉 (GB 34).

手指拘攣，伸縮疼痛：手十指節（ 握拳指尖，小麥炷，灸五壯 ）、尺澤 、陽谿 、中渚 、五虎

Hypertonicity of the fingers, pain when stretching out the contraction: the joints of the ten fingers (make a fist, apply moxibustion with five small grain-of-wheat size cones at the tips [of each joint] on the fingers), Chǐ Zé 尺澤 (LU 5), Yáng Xī 陽谿 (LI 5), Zhōng Zhǔ 中渚 (SJ 3), Wǔ Hǔ 五虎 (Five Tigers, M-UE-45).

足底發熱，名曰濕熱：湧泉、京骨、合谷

Feverish soles of the feet. This is called damp-heat: Yǒng Quán 湧泉 (KI 1), Jīng Gǔ 京骨 (UB 64), Hé Gǔ 合谷 (LI 4).

足外踝紅腫，名曰穿踝風：崑崙、邱墟、照海

Redness and swelling of the lateral malleolus. This is called ankle-boring wind: Kūn Lún 崑崙 (UB 60), Qiū Xū 邱墟 (GB 40), Zhào Hǎi 照海 (KI 6).

足跗發熱，五指節痛：衝陽、俠谿、足十宣

Feverish dorsum of the feet, pain in the joints of the five toes: Chōng Yáng 衝陽 (ST 42), Xiá Xī 俠谿 (GB 43), Shí Xuān 十宣 (M-UE-1) of the feet.

兩手發熱，五指疼痛：陽池、液門、合谷

Both hands feverish, pain in the five fingers: Yáng Chí 陽池 (SJ 4), Yè Mén 液門 (SJ 2), Hé Gǔ 合谷 (LI 4).

兩膝紅腫疼痛，名曰鶴膝風：膝關、行間、風市、陽陵泉

Redness, swelling, and pain of both knees. This is called crane's knee wind: Xī Guān 膝關 (LV 7), Xíng Jiān 行間 (LV 2), Fēng Shì 風市 (GB 31), Yáng Líng Quán 陽陵泉 (GB 34).

手腕起骨痛，名曰遶踝風：太淵、腕骨、大陵

Pain in the raised bones of the wrist. This is called wind around the styloid processes: Tài Yuān 太淵 (LU 9), Wàn Gǔ 腕骨 (SI 4), Dà Líng 大陵 (PC 7).

腰胯疼痛，名曰寒疝：五樞、委中、三陰交

Low back and hip pain. This is called cold shàn 疝 (mounting): Wǔ Shū 五樞 (GB 27), Wěi Zhōng 委中 (UB 40), Sān Yīn Jiāo 三陰交 (SP 6).

臂膊痛連肩背：肩井、曲池、中渚

Pain of the arms radiating to the shoulders and upper back: Jiān Jǐng 肩井 (GB 21), Qū Chí 曲池 (LI 11), Zhōng Zhǔ 中渚 (SJ 3).

腿胯疼痛，名腿叉風：環跳、委中、陽陵泉

Leg and hip pain. This is called leg fork wind: Huán Tiào 環跳 (GB 30), Wěi Zhōng 委中 (UB 40), Yáng Líng Quán 陽陵泉 (GB 34).

白虎歷節風疼痛：肩井、三里、曲池、委中、合谷、行間、天應（遇痛處針，強針出血）

White tiger running joint wind pain: Jiān Jǐng 肩井 (GB 21), Sān Lǐ 三里 (ST 36), Qū Chí 曲池 (LI 11), Wěi Zhōng 委中 (UB 40), Hé Gǔ 合谷 (LI 4), Xíng Jiān 行間 (LV 2), Tiān Yìng 天應[114] (when you meet a painful site, needle it, needle forcefully to let blood).

走注風，遊走，四肢疼痛：天應、曲池、三里、委中

Travelling influx[115] wind, wandering pain in the four limbs: Tiān Yìng 天應 (Natural Response), Qū Chí 曲池 (LI 11), Sān Lǐ 三里 (ST 36), Wěi Zhōng 委中 (UB 40).

浮風，渾身搔痒：百會、百勞、命門、太陽紫脈、風市、絕骨、水分、氣海、血海、委中、曲池

Superficial wind, scratching and itching over the whole body: Bǎi Huì 百會 (Du 20), Bǎi Láo 百勞 (M-HN-30), Mìng Mén 命門 (Du 4), the purple vessels at Tài Yáng 太陽 (M-HN-9), Fēng Shì 風市 (GB 31), Jué Gǔ 絕骨 (GB 39), Shuǐ Fēn 水分 (Ren 9), Qì Hǎi 氣海 (Ren 6), Xuè Hǎi 血海 (SP 10), Wěi Zhōng 委中 (UB 40), Qū Chí 曲池 (LI 11).

頭項紅腫強痛：承漿、風池、肩井、風府

Redness, swelling, stiffness, and pain in the head and nape: Chéng Jiāng 承漿 (Ren 24), Fēng Chí 風池 (GB 20), Jiān Jǐng 肩井 (GB 21), Fēng Fǔ 風府 (Du 16).

腎虛腰痛，舉動艱難：腎俞、脊中、委中

Kidney vacuity low back pain, difficulty moving around: Shèn Shū 腎俞 (UB 23), Jǐ Zhōng 脊中 (Du 6), Wěi Zhōng 委中 (UB 40).

閃挫腰痛，起止艱難：脊中、腰俞、腎俞、委中

Low back pain from wrenching and contusion, difficulty getting up and lying down: Jǐ Zhōng 脊中 (Du 6), Yāo Shū 腰俞 (Du 2), Shèn Shū 腎俞 (UB 23), Wěi Zhōng 委中 (UB 40).

虛損濕滯，腰痛行動無力：脊中、腰俞、腎俞、委中

Vacuity detriment damp stagnation, low back pain, feebly moving around: Jǐ Zhōng 脊中 (Du 6), Yāo Shū 腰俞 (Du 2), Shèn Shū 腎俞 (UB 23), Wěi Zhōng 委中 (UB 40).

---

114. Tiān Yìng 天應 can be translated as "Natural Response." Yang means an ouch (*a shi*) point.

115. Wiseman defines *zǒu zhù* 走注 travelling influx as moving impediment (*bì* 痹).

諸虛百損，四肢無力：百勞、心俞、三里、關元、膏肓

All types of vacuity, the hundred detriments, the four limbs lack strength: Bǎi Láo 百勞 (M-HN-30), Xīn Shū 心俞 (UB 15), Sān Lǐ 三里 (ST 36), Guān Yuán 關元 (Ren 4), Gāo Huāng 膏肓 (UB 43).

脅下肝積，氣塊刺痛：章門、支溝、中脘、大陵、陽陵泉，

Liver accumulation below the rib-sides, qì lumps, pricking pain: Zhāng Mén 章門 (LV 13), Zhī Gōu 支溝 (SJ 6), Zhōng Wǎn 中脘 (Ren 12), Dà Líng 大陵 (PC 7), Yáng Líng Quán 陽陵泉 (GB 34).

楊氏治症：
Master Yáng's treatment of patterns:

手足拘攣：中渚、尺澤、絕骨、八邪、陽谿、陽陵泉

Hypertonicity of the limbs: Zhōng Zhǔ 中渚 (SJ 3), Chǐ Zé 尺澤 (LU 5), Jué Gǔ 絕骨 (GB 39), Bā Xié 八邪 (M-UE-2), Yáng Xī 陽谿 (LI 5), Yáng Líng Quán 陽陵泉 (GB 34).

四肢走注：三里、委中、命門、天應、曲池、外關

Travelling influx of the four limbs: Sān Lǐ 三里 (ST 36), Wěi Zhōng 委中 (UB 40), Mìng Mén 命門 (Du 4), Tiān Yìng 天應 (Natural Response), Qū Chí 曲池 (LI 11), Wài Guān 外關 (SJ 5).

膝脛痠痛：行間、絕骨、太衝、膝眼、三里、陽陵泉

Aching pain of the knees and shins: Xíng Jiān 行間 (LV 2), Jué Gǔ 絕骨 (GB 39), Tài Chōng 太衝 (LV 3), Xī Yǎn 膝眼 (MN-LE-16), Sān Lǐ 三里 (ST 36), Yáng Líng Quán 陽陵泉 (GB 34).

腿寒痹痛：四關、絕骨、風市、環跳、三陰交

Cold legs with impediment (*bì* 痹) and pain: Sì Guān 四關 (Four Gates: Hé Gǔ 合谷 LI 4 and Tài Chōng 太衝 LV 3), Jué Gǔ 絕骨 (GB 39), Fēng Shì 風市 (GB 31), Huán Tiào 環跳 (GB 30), Sān Yīn Jiāo 三陰交 (SP 6).

臂冷痹痛：肩井、曲池、外關、三里

Cold arms with impediment (*bì* 痹) and pain: Jiān Jǐng 肩井 (GB 21), Qū Chí 曲池 (LI 11),

Wài Guān 外關 (SJ 5), Sān Lǐ 三里 (ST 36).

百節痰痛：魂門、絕骨、命門、外關

Aching pain of the hundred joints: Hún Mén 魂門 (UB 47), Jué Gǔ 絕骨 (GB 39), Mìng Mén 命門 (Du 4), Wài Guān 外關 (SJ 5).

陽維脈
Yáng Wéi Mài

考穴：外關二穴，三焦經。掌背去腕二寸，骨縫兩筋陷中，伏手取之。針一寸二分，主風寒經絡皮膚病，與臨泣主客相應。

Examining the point: The two points of Wài Guān 外關 (SJ 5) are on the triple burner channel. They are two *cùn* proximal to the wrist on the dorsal side, in the depression of the bone seam and the two sinews. Pronate the hand to locate it. Needle 1.2 *cùn* deep. It is indicated for diseases of wind-cold in the channels,[116] network vessels, and skin. It responds to Lín Qì 臨泣 (GB 41) as host and guest.

治病：〔西江月〕
　　肢節腫疼膝冷，四肢不遂頭風，
　　背胯內外骨筋攻，頭項眉稜皆痛。
　　手足熱麻盜汗，破傷眼腫睛紅，
　　傷寒自汗表烘烘，獨會外關為重。

Disease treatment: (West River Moon):

Swelling and pain of the joints of the limbs, cold knees;
paralysis of the four limbs, head wind;
Attacks in the bones and sinews
of the medial and lateral back and hips;
pain all over the head, nape, and ridge of the eyebrows.
Hot numb limbs, night sweating;
tetany, swollen red eyes;
Cold damage, spontaneous sweating,
the exterior feels as if it is roasting in a fire;
the only thing of value is to meet Wài Guān 外關 (SJ 5).

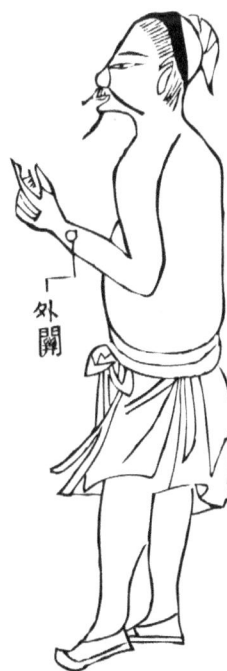

外關

---

116. Some editions have *jīng* 經 (channels) and others have *jīn* 筋 (sinews).

凡治後症，必先取外關為主，次取各穴應之（ 徐氏 ）：

Generally to treat the following patterns, you must first select Wài Guān 外關 (SJ 5) as the host and next select each point that responds to it:
(Master Xú)

臂膊紅腫，肢節疼痛：肘髎 、肩髃 、腕骨（ 髎音僚，髃音魚 ）

Red swollen arms, pain in the joints of the limbs: Zhǒu Liáo 肘髎 (LI 12), Jiān Yú 肩髃 (LI 15), Wàn Gǔ 腕骨 (SI 4). (A note on the pronunciation of *liáo* 髎 and *yú* 髃)

足內踝紅腫痛，名曰遶踝風：太谿 、邱墟 、臨泣 、崑崙

Red swollen painful medial malleolus. This is called wind around the ankles: Tài Xī 太谿 (KI 3), Qiū Xū 邱墟 (GB 40), Lín Qì 臨泣 (GB 41), Kūn Lún 崑崙 (UB 60).

手指節痛，不能伸屈：陽谷 、五虎 、腕骨 、合谷

Pain in the finger joints, inability to bend and stretch them: Yáng Gǔ 陽谷 (SI 5), Wǔ Hǔ 五虎 (Five Tigers, M-UE-45), Wàn Gǔ 腕骨 (SI 4), Hé Gǔ 合谷 (LI 4).

足指節痛，不能行步：內庭 、太衝 、崑崙

Pain in the toe joints, inability to walk: Nèi Tíng 內庭 (ST 44), Tài Chōng 太衝 (LV 3), Kūn Lún 崑崙 (UB 60).

五臟結熱，吐血不已，取五臟俞穴，並血會治之：心俞 、肺俞 、脾俞 、肝俞 、腎俞 、膈俞

Binding heat of the five viscera, incessant vomiting of blood. Apply treatment to the [back] transport points of the five viscera and the meeting point for blood: Xīn Shū 心俞 (UB 15), Fèi Shū 肺俞 (UB 13), Pí Shū 脾俞 (UB 20), Gān Shū 肝俞 (UB 18), Shèn Shū 腎俞 (UB 23), Gé Shū 膈俞 (UB 17).

六腑結熱，血妄行不已，取六腑俞穴，並血會治之：膽俞 、胃俞 、小腸俞 、大腸俞 、膀胱俞 、三焦俞 、膈俞

Binding heat of the six bowels, incessant frenetic movement of blood. Apply treatment to the [back] transport points of the six bowels and the meeting point for blood: Dǎn Shū 膽俞 (UB 19), Wèi Shū 胃俞 (UB 21), Xiǎo Cháng Shū 小腸俞 (UB 27), Dà Cháng Shū 大腸俞 (UB 25), Páng Guāng Shū 膀胱俞 (UB 28), Sān Jiāo Shū 三焦俞 (UB 22), Gé Shū 膈俞 (UB 17).

鼻衄不止，名血妄行：少澤、心俞、膈俞、湧泉

Incessant nosebleed. This is called frenetic movement of blood: Shào Zé 少澤 (SI 1), Xīn Shū 心俞 (UB 15), Gé Shū 膈俞 (UB 17), Yǒng Quán 湧泉 (KI 1).

吐血昏暈，不省人事：肝俞、膈俞、通里、大敦

Vomiting blood with clouding dizziness, loss of consciousness: Gān Shū 肝俞 (UB 18), Gé Shū 膈俞 (UB 17), Tōng Lǐ 通里 (HT 5), Dà Dūn 大敦 (LV 1).

虛損氣逆，吐血不已：膏肓、膈俞、丹田、肝俞

Vacuity detriment, qì counterflow, unceasing vomiting of blood: Gāo Huāng 膏肓 (UB 43), Gé Shū 膈俞 (UB 17), Dān Tián 丹田 (Ren 4),[117] Gān Shū 肝俞 (UB 18).

吐血衄血，陽乘於陰，血熱妄行：中衝、肝俞、膈俞、三里、三陰交

Vomiting blood, nosebleed, yáng overwhelms yin, frenetic movement of hot blood: Zhōng Zhǔ 中渚 (SJ 3), Gān Shū 肝俞 (UB 18), Gé Shū 膈俞 (UB 17), Sān Lǐ 三里 (ST 36), Sān Yīn Jiāo 三陰交 (SP 6).

血寒亦吐，陰乘於陽，名心肺二經嘔血：少商、心俞、神門、肺俞、膈俞、三陰交

Cold blood, also causing vomiting, yīn overwhelms yáng. This is called dual heart and lung channel vomiting of blood: Shào Shāng 少商 (LU 11), Xīn Shū 心俞 (UB 15), Shén Mén 神門 (HT 7), Fèi Shū 肺俞 (UB 13), Gé Shū 膈俞 (UB 17), Sān Yīn Jiāo 三陰交 (SP 6).

舌強難言，及生白胎：關衝、中衝、承漿、聚泉

Stiff tongue, difficulty speaking, and the growth of a white tongue coat:[118] Guān Chōng 關衝 (SJ 1), Zhōng Zhǔ 中渚 (SJ 3), Chéng Jiāng 承漿 (Ren 24), Jù Quán 聚泉 (M-HN-36).

重舌腫脹，熱極難言：十宣、海泉、金津、玉液

Double tongue with swelling and and distention, extreme heat, difficulty speaking: Shí Xuān 十宣 (M-UE-1), Hǎi Quán 海泉 (M-HN-37), Jīn Jīn Yù Yè 金津玉液 (M-HN-20).

---

117. In Volume 7 Yáng tells us that Dān Tián 丹田 (Elixir Field) is another name for both Guān Yuán 關元 (Ren 4) and for Shí Mén 石門 (Ren 5). Most of this section came from the *Great Completion*, which also lists Dān Tián as an alternate name for both points. We cannot know which point was intended; however in two out of the three times Dān Tián is listed, it seems that Guān Yuán (Ren 4) is a better choice. Therefore, Dān Tián will be translated as "Ren 4."

118. This was written before tongue diagnosis was commonly used.

口內生瘡，名枯曹風：兌端、支溝、承漿、十宣

Sores erupting inside the mouth. This is called desiccated trough wind [*kū cáo fēng* 枯曹風]:[119] Duì Duān 兌端 (Du 27), Zhī Gōu 支溝 (SJ 6), Chéng Jiāng 承漿 (Ren 24), Shí Xuān 十宣 (M-UE-1).

舌吐不收，名曰陽強：湧泉、兌端、少衝、神門

Protruding tongue that does not retract. This is called yáng overly strong: Yǒng Quán 湧泉 (KI 1), Duì Duān 兌端 (Du 27), Shào Chōng 少衝 (HT 9), Shén Mén 神門 (HT 7).

舌縮難言，名曰陰強：心俞、膻中、海泉

Contracted tongue, difficulty speaking. This is called yīn overly strong: Xīn Shū 心俞 (UB 15), Dàn Zhōng 膻中 (Ren 17), Hǎi Quán 海泉 (M-HN-37).

唇裂破，血出乾痛：承漿、少商、關衝

Lips cracked and broken, bleeding, dryness, pain: Chéng Jiāng 承漿 (Ren 24), Shào Shāng 少商 (LU 11), Guān Chōng 關衝 (SJ 1).

項生瘰癧，繞項起核，名曰蟠蛇癧：天井、風池、肘尖、缺盆、十宣

Scrofula erupting on the nape, winding around the nape, nodes rising up. This is called coiled snake scrofula: Tiān Jǐng 天井 (SJ 10), Fēng Chí 風池 (GB 20), Zhǒu Jiān 肘尖 (M-UE-46), Quē Pén 缺盆 (ST 12), Shí Xuān 十宣 (M-UE-1).

瘰癧延生胸前，連腋下者，名曰瓜藤癧：肩井、膻中、大陵、支溝、陽陵泉

Scrofula spreading from the anterior chest extending to the sub-axillary region. This is called melon vine scrofula: Jiān Jǐng 肩井 (GB 21), Dàn Zhōng 膻中 (Ren 17), Dà Líng 大陵 (PC 7), Zhī Gōu 支溝 (SJ 6), Yáng Líng Quán 陽陵泉 (GB 34).

---

119. *kū cáo fēng* 枯曹風 (desiccated trough wind): *Cáo* 曹 is a family name, and also is a kind of official. Unless this pattern was named after a person, this character is probably an abbreviation for *cáo* 槽 or *cáo* 蠐. The former means a trough, for example a water trough. This fits the image of a sore that has eaten a hole in the flesh. It can also be used in phrases meaning the molars, which fits with mouth sores. The latter character means grubs in fruit, which spoil it and make holes. Various types of worms were thought to cause diseases including toothache and sores, so this is also possible. This desiccated trough wind [*kū cáo fēng*] is also described in Volume 9 of the *Great Compendium*. There, it says that in this condition, the cheeks are red and swollen, with sores erupting. It is also called Pig Cheek Wind. This is due to obstructing by hot qì above, phlegm stagnating in the triple burner channel, and swelling that doesn't disperse, so the cheeks erupt in sores.

左耳根腫核者，名曰惠袋癧：翳風、後谿、肘尖

Swollen nodes at the root of the left ear. This is called alms bag scrofula:[120] Yì Fēng 翳風 (SJ 17), Hòu Xī 後谿 (SI 3), Zhǒu Jiān 肘尖 (M-UE-46).

右耳根腫核者，名曰蜂窩癧：翳風、頰車、後谿、合谷

Swollen nodes at the root of the right ear. This is called hornet's nest scrofula: Yì Fēng 翳風 (SJ 17), Jiá Chē 頰車 (ST 6), Hòu Xī 後谿 (SI 3), Hé Gǔ 合谷 (LI 4).

耳根紅腫痛：合谷、翳風、頰車

Redness, swelling, and pain at the root of the ear: Hé Gǔ 合谷 (LI 4), Yì Fēng 翳風 (SJ 17), Jiá Chē 頰車 (ST 6).

頸項紅腫不消，名曰項疽：風府、肩井、承漿

Redness and swelling of the neck that doesn't disperse. This is called nape abscess: Fēng Fǔ 風府 (Du 16), Jiān Jǐng 肩井 (GB 21), Chéng Jiāng 承漿 (Ren 24).

目生翳膜，隱澀難開：晴明、合谷、肝俞、魚尾

Screen membrane engendered in the eyes, dull and dry, difficult to open: Jīng Míng 晴明 (UB 1), Hé Gǔ 合谷 (LI 4), Gān Shū 肝俞 (UB 18), Yú Wěi 魚尾 (M-HN-7).

風沿爛眼，迎風冷淚：攢竹、絲竹、二間、小骨空

Wind ulceration of the eyelid rim, tearing on exposure to wind and cold: Zǎn Zhú 攢竹 (UB 2), Sī Zhú 絲竹 (SJ 23), Èr Jiān 二間 (LI 2), Xiǎo Gǔ Kōng 小骨空 (Small Bone Hollow).[121]

目風腫痛，努肉攀睛：和髎、晴明、攢竹、肝俞、委中、合谷、肘尖、照海、列缺、十宣

Eye wind swelling and pain, outcrop creeping over the eye: Hé Liáo 和髎 (SJ 22), Jīng Míng 晴明 (UB 1), Zǎn Zhú 攢竹 (UB 2), Gān Shū 肝俞 (UB 18), Wěi Zhōng 委中 (UB 40), Hé Gǔ 合谷 (LI 4), Zhǒu Jiān 肘尖 (M-UE-46), Zhào Hǎi 照海 (KI 6), Liè Quē 列缺 (LU 7),

---

120. *huì dài lì* 惠袋癧 (alms bag scrofula): This is not a common medical term. The second and third characters are easy to translate. *Dài* is a sack or a bag. *Lì* is one type of scrofula. *Huì* means benefit, favor, or kindness. Therefore, I speculate that this may mean an alms bag, where a monk or a begger puts the money that people donate. In any case, the image is clear. This is a swelling below the left ear that is big and shaped like a sack or bag.

121. Xiǎo Gǔ Kōng 小骨空 (Small Bone Hollow) is on the dorsum of the proximal interphalangeal joint of the little finger. Apply seven cones of moxibustion. This point treats pain in the eyes and the joints of the hands.

Shí Xuān 十宣 (M-UE-1).

牙齒兩頷腫痛：人中、合谷、呂細

Swelling and pain of the teeth and both cheeks: Rén Zhōng 人中 (Du 26), Hé Gǔ 合谷 (LI 4), Lǚ Xì 呂細 (Small Lǚ).[122]

上丬牙痛，及牙關不開：太淵、頰車、合谷、呂細

Pain of the upper teeth, with inability to open the jaw: Tài Yuān 太淵 (LU 9), Jiá Chē 頰車 (ST 6), Hé Gǔ 合谷 (LI 4), Lǚ Xì 呂細 (Small Lǚ).

下丬牙痛，頰項紅腫痛：陽谿、承漿、頰車、太谿

Pain of the lower teeth, redness, swelling, and pain of the jaw and nape: Yáng Xī 陽谿 (LI 5), Chéng Jiāng 承漿 (Ren 24), Jiá Chē 頰車 (ST 6), Tài Xī 太谿 (KI 3).

耳聾，氣痞疼痛：聽會、腎俞、三里、翳風

Deafness, qì glomus pain: Tīng Huì 聽會 (GB 2), Shèn Shū 腎俞 (UB 23), Sān Lǐ 三里 (ST 36), Yì Fēng 翳風 (SJ 17).

耳內或鳴，或痒，或痛：客主人、合谷、聽會

Tinnitus or itching or pain inside the ear: Kè Zhǔ Rén 客主人 (GB 3), Hé Gǔ 合谷 (LI 4), Tīng Huì 聽會 (GB 2).

雷頭風暈，嘔吐痰涎：百會、中腕、太淵、風門

Thunder head wind dizziness, vomiting phlegm drool: Bǎi Huì 百會 (Du 20), Zhōng Wǎn 中脘 (Ren 12), Tài Yuān 太淵 (LU 9), Fēng Mén 風門 (UB 12).

腎虛頭痛，頭重不舉：腎俞、百會、太谿、列缺

Headache due to kidney vacuity, heavy head that cannot be raised: Shèn Shū 腎俞 (UB 23), Bǎi Huì 百會 (Du 20), Tài Xī 太谿 (KI 3), Liè Quē 列缺 (LU 7).

---

122. Lǚ Xì 呂細 (Small Lǚ) is an alternate name for Tài Xī 太谿 (KI 3) according to the *Great Completion*. The word Lǚ in the name of this point refers to the fifth note of the Chinese musical scale, the note corresponding to water element and the kidneys.

痰厥頭暈，頭目昏沉：大敦、肝俞、百會

Phlegm reversal dizzy head, dazed head and eyes: Dà Dūn 大敦 (LV 1), Gān Shū 肝俞 (UB 18), Bǎi Huì 百會 (Du 20).

頭頂痛，名曰正頭風：上星、百會、腦空、湧泉、合谷

Pain at the vertex of the head. This is called medial head wind: Shàng Xīng 上星 (Du 23), Bǎi Huì 百會 (Du 20), Nǎo Kōng 腦空 (GB 19), Yǒng Quán 湧泉 (KI 1), Hé Gǔ 合谷 (LI 4).

目暴赤腫疼痛：攢竹、合谷、迎香

Sudden redness, swelling, and pain of the eyes: Zǎn Zhú 攢竹 (UB 2), Hé Gǔ 合谷 (LI 4), Yíng Xiāng 迎香 (LI 20).

楊氏治症：
Master Yáng's treatment of patterns:

中風拘攣：中渚、陽池、曲池、八邪

Wind stroke with hypertonicity: Zhōng Zhǔ 中渚 (SJ 3), Yáng Chí 陽池 (SJ 4), Qū Chí 曲池 (LI 11), Bā Xié 八邪 (M-UE-22).

任脈
Rèn Mài

考穴：列缺二穴，肺經。手腕內側一寸五分，手交叉食指盡處骨間是。針八分，主心腹脅肋五臟病，與照海主客相應。

Examining the point: The two points of Liè Quē 列缺 (LU 7) are on the lung channel. They are 1.5 *cùn* from the inner aspect of the wrist. Make the forks of the hand intersect with each other. It is located on the bone at the end of the index finger. Needle eight *fèn* deep. It is indicated for diseases of the heart region, abdomen, rib-sides, and the five viscera. It responds to Zhào Hǎi 照海 (KI 6) as host and guest.

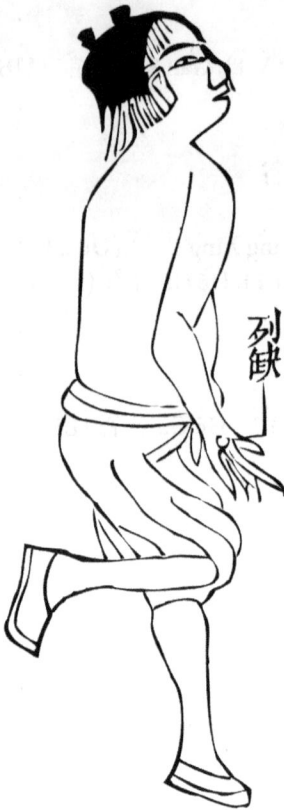

治病：〔西江月〕
　　痔瘻便腫泄痢，唾紅溺血咳痰，
　　牙疼喉腫小便難，心胸腹疼噎嗝。
　　產後發強不語，腰痛血疾臍寒，
　　死胎不下膈中寒，列缺乳癰多散。

Disease treatment: (West River Moon):

Hemorrhoids, malaria,
swelling after a bowel movement, diarrhea;
spitting red [-tinged saliva], blood in the urine,
coughing up phlegm;
Toothache, swollen throat, difficult urination;
pain in the heart, chest, and abdomen, dysphagia.
Postpartum stiffening and inability to speak;
low back pain, blood [or bleeding] diseases,
cold umbilicus;
Retention of dead fetus, cold in the diaphragm;
Liè Quē 列缺 (LU 7) often scatters breast abscesses.

Fig. 5.31

凡治後症，必先取列缺為主，次取各穴應之（徐氏）：

Generally to treat the following patterns, you must first select Liè Quē 列缺 (LU 7) as the host and next select each point that responds to it: (Master Xú)

鼻流涕臭，名曰鼻淵：曲差、上星、百會、風門、迎香

Running nose with malodorous snivel. This is called deep-source nasal congestion: Qū Chā 曲差 (UB 4), Shàng Xīng 上星 (Du 23), Bǎi Huì 百會 (Du 20), Fēng Mén 風門 (UB 12), Yíng Xiāng 迎香 (LI 20).

鼻生瘜肉，閉塞不通：印堂、迎香、上星、風門

Nasal polyps, blockage with flow stoppage: Yìn Táng 印堂 (M-HN-3), Yíng Xiāng 迎香 (LI 20), Shàng Xīng 上星 (Du 23), Fēng Mén 風門 (UB 12).

傷風面赤，發熱頭痛：通里、曲池、絕骨、合谷

Wind damage with red face, fever, headache: **Tōng Lǐ** 通里 (HT 5), **Qū Chí** 曲池 (LI 11), **Jué Gǔ** 絕骨 (GB 39), **Hé Gǔ** 合谷 (LI 4).

傷風感寒，咳嗽脹滿：膻中、風門、合谷、風府

Wind damage, cold contraction, cough with distention and fullness: **Dàn Zhōng** 膻中 (Ren 17), **Fēng Mén** 風門 (UB 12), **Hé Gǔ** 合谷 (LI 4), **Fēng Fǔ** 風府 (Du 16).

傷風，四肢煩熱，頭痛：經渠、曲池、合谷、委中

Wind damage, vexing heat of the four limbs, headache: **Jīng Qú** 經渠 (LU 8), **Qū Chí** 曲池 (LI 11), **Hé Gǔ** 合谷 (LI 4), **Wěi Zhōng** 委中 (UB 40).

腹中脹痛，下利不已：內庭、天樞、三陰交

Distending pain in the abdomen, incessant diarrhea: **Nèi Tíng** 內庭 (ST 44), **Tiān Shū** 天樞 (ST 25), **Sān Yīn Jiāo** 三陰交 (SP 6).

赤白痢疾，腹中冷痛：水道、氣海、外陵、天樞、三陰交、三里

Red and white dysentery, cold pain in the abdomen: **Shuǐ Dào** 水道 (ST 28), **Qì Hǎi** 氣海 (Ren 6), **Wài Líng** 外陵 (ST 26), **Tiān Shū** 天樞 (ST 25), **Sān Yīn Jiāo** 三陰交 (SP 6), **Sān Lǐ** 三里 (ST 36).

胸前兩乳紅腫痛：少澤、大陵、膻中

Redness, swelling, and pain of the anterior chest and two breasts: **Shào Zé** 少澤 (SI 1), **Dà Líng** 大陵 (PC 7), **Dàn Zhōng** 膻中 (Ren 17).

乳癰腫痛，小兒吹乳：中府、膻中、少澤、大敦

Breast abscess with swelling and pain, infantile breast blowing:[123] **Zhōng Fǔ** 中府 (LU 1), **Dàn Zhōng** 膻中 (Ren 17), **Shào Zé** 少澤 (SI 1), **Dà Dūn** 大敦 (LV 1).

腹中寒痛，泄瀉不止：天樞、中脘、關元、三陰交

Cold pain in the abdomen, incessant diarrhea: **Tiān Shū** 天樞 (ST 25), **Zhōng Wǎn** 中脘 (Ren 12), **Guān Yuán** 關元 (Ren 4), **Sān Yīn Jiāo** 三陰交 (SP 6).

---

123. Infantile breast blowing: A type of breast abscess that occurs during the period of breast feeding.

婦人血積痛，敗血不止：肝俞、腎俞、膈俞、三陰交

Painful blood accumulations in females, incessant vanquished blood: Gān Shū 肝俞 (UB 18), Shèn Shū 腎俞 (UB 23), Gé Shū 膈俞 (UB 17), Sān Yīn Jiāo 三陰交 (SP 6).

咳嗽寒痰，胸膈閉痛：肺俞、膻中、三里

Cough with cold phlegm, blockage and pain in the chest and diaphragm: Fèi Shū 肺俞 (UB 13), Dàn Zhōng 膻中 (Ren 17), Sān Lǐ 三里 (ST 36).

久咳不愈，咳唾血痰：風門、太淵、膻中

Enduring cough without recovery, coughing up spittle, blood, and phlegm: Fēng Mén 風門 (UB 12), Tài Yuān 太淵 (LU 9), Dàn Zhōng 膻中 (Ren 17).

哮喘氣促，痰氣壅盛：豐隆、俞府、膻中、三里

Wheezing and panting, hasty breathing, phlegm congestion and exuberance of qì: Fēng Lóng 豐隆 (ST 40), Shū Fǔ 俞府 (KI 27), Dàn Zhōng 膻中 (Ren 17), Sān Lǐ 三里 (ST 36).

吼喘胸膈急痛：彧中、天突、肺俞、三里

Rough panting, acute pain in the chest and diaphragm: Yù Zhōng 彧中 (KI 26), Tiān Tú 天突 (Ren 22), Fèi Shū 肺俞 (UB 13), Sān Lǐ 三里 (ST 36).

吼喘氣滿，肺脹不得臥：俞府、風門、太淵、中府、三里、膻中

Rough panting with qì fullness, lung distention, inability to lie down: Shū Fǔ 俞府 (KI 27), Fēng Mén 風門 (UB 12), Tài Yuān 太淵 (LU 9), Zhōng Fǔ 中府 (LU 1), Sān Lǐ 三里 (ST 36), Dàn Zhōng 膻中 (Ren 17).

鼻塞不知香臭：迎香、上星、風門

Nasal blockage, cannot tell the fragrant from the malodorous: Yíng Xiāng 迎香 (LI 20), Shàng Xīng 上星 (Du 23), Fēng Mén 風門 (UB 12).

鼻流清涕，腠理不密，噴嚏不止：神庭、肺俞、太淵、三里

Running nose with clear snivel, insecurity of the interstices, unceasing sneezing: Shén Tíng 神庭 (Du 24), Fèi Shū 肺俞 (UB 13), Tài Yuān 太淵 (LU 9), Sān Lǐ 三里 (ST 36).

婦人血瀝，乳汁不通：少澤、大陵、膻中、關衝

Female spotting of blood, breast milk doesn't flow: Shào Zé 少澤 (SI 1), Dà Líng 大陵 (PC

7), Dàn Zhōng 膻中 (Ren 17), Guān Chōng 關衝 (SJ 1).

乳頭生瘡，名曰妬乳：乳根、少澤、肩井、膻中

Sores erupting on the nipples. This is called jealous breasts: Rǔ Gēn 乳根 (ST 18), Shào Zé 少澤 (SI 1), Jiān Jǐng 肩井 (GB 21), Dàn Zhōng 膻中 (Ren 17).

胸中噎塞痛：大陵、內關、膻中、三里

Dysphagia obstruction and pain in the chest: Dà Líng 大陵 (PC 7), Nèi Guān 內關 (PC 6), Dàn Zhōng 膻中 (Ren 17), Sān Lǐ 三里 (ST 36).

五癭等症，項癭之症有五：一曰石癭，如石之硬；二曰氣癭，如綿之軟；三曰血癭，如赤脈細絲；四曰筋癭，乃無骨；五曰肉癭；如袋之狀；此乃五癭之形也：扶突、天突、天窗、缺盆、俞府、膺俞（喉上）、膻中、合谷、十宣（出血）

The five goiters and similar patterns. There are five goiter patterns of the neck:
- The first is called stone goiter, having the hardness of a stone.
- The second is called qì goiter, having the softness of silk floss.
- The third is called blood goiter, having red vessels like fine silk threads.
- The fourth is called sinew goiter, as it does not have a bone.
- The fifth is called flesh goiter, having the shape of a sack.

These are the forms of the five goiters. Fú Tú 扶突 (LI 18), Tiān Tú 天突 (Ren 22), Tiān Chuāng 天窗 (SI 16), Quē Pén 缺盆 (ST 12), Shū Fǔ 俞府 (KI 27), Yīng Shū 膺俞 (Chest Transport) (on the throat),[124] Dàn Zhōng 膻中 (Ren 17), Hé Gǔ 合谷 (LI 4), Shí Xuān 十宣 (M-UE-1) (let blood).

口內生瘡，臭穢不可近：十宣、人中、金津、玉液、承漿、合谷

Sores erupting inside the mouth, the odor is so foul that you cannot get near: Shí Xuān 十宣 (M-UE-1), Rén Zhōng 人中 (Du 26), Jīn Jīn Yù Yè 金津玉液 (M-HN-20), Chéng Jiāng 承漿 (Ren 24), Hé Gǔ 合谷 (LI 4).

三焦極熱，口內生瘡：關衝、外關、人中、迎香、金津、玉液、地倉

Extreme heat in the triple burner, sores erupting inside the mouth: Guān Chōng 關衝 (SJ 1), Wài Guān 外關 (SJ 5), Rén Zhōng 人中 (Du 26), Yíng Xiāng 迎香 (LI 20), Jīn Jīn Yù Yè 金津玉液 (M-HN-20), Dì Cāng 地倉 (ST 4).

---

124. This point is a bit of a mystery. Yīng Shū 膺俞 is another name for Zhōng Fǔ 中府 (LU 1), but the point in this passage is said to be on the throat. It is not described in Volume 7, where other points are discussed.

口氣衝人，臭不可近：少衝、通里、人中、十宣、金津、玉液

Smell of the breath knocks people over, so malodorous that you cannot get near: Shào Chōng 少衝 (HT 9), Tōng Lǐ 通里 (HT 5), Rén Zhōng 人中 (Du 26), Shí Xuān 十宣 (M-UE-1), Jīn Jīn Yù Yè 金津玉液 (M-HN-20).

冒暑大熱，霍亂吐瀉：委中、百勞、中脘、曲池、十宣、三里、合谷

Contraction of summerheat with great fever, sudden turmoil (cholera) with vomiting and diarrhea: Wěi Zhōng 委中 (UB 40), Bǎi Láo 百勞 (M-HN-30), Zhōng Wǎn 中脘 (Ren 12), Qū Chí 曲池 (LI 11), Shí Xuān 十宣 (M-UE-1), Sān Lǐ 三里 (ST 36), Hé Gǔ 合谷 (LI 4).

中暑自熱，小便不利：陰谷、百勞、中脘、委中、氣海、陰陵泉

Summerheat stroke with spontaneous fever, inhibited urination: Yīn Gǔ 陰谷 (KI 10), Bǎi Láo 百勞 (M-HN-30), Zhōng Wǎn 中脘 (Ren 12), Wěi Zhōng 委中 (UB 40), Qì Hǎi 氣海 (Ren 6), Yīn Líng Quán 陰陵泉 (SP 9).

小兒急驚風，手足搐搦：印堂、百會、人中、中衝、大敦、太衝、合谷

Acute pediatric fright wind, convulsions of the limbs: Yìn Táng 印堂 (M-HN-3), Bǎi Huì 百會 (Du 20), Rén Zhōng 人中 (Du 26), Zhōng Chōng 中衝 (PC 9), Dà Dūn 大敦 (LV 1), Tài Chōng 太衝 (LV 3), Hé Gǔ 合谷 (LI 4).

小兒慢脾風，目直視，手足搐，口吐沫：大敦、脾俞、百會、上星、人中

Chronic pediatric spleen wind, forward-staring eyes, convulsions of the limbs, foaming at the mouth: Dà Dūn 大敦 (LV 1), Pí Shū 脾俞 (UB 20), Bǎi Huì 百會 (Du 20), Shàng Xīng 上星 (Du 23), Rén Zhōng 人中 (Du 26).

消渴等症：三消其症不同，消脾，消中，消腎。《素問》云：胃府虛，食斗不能充飢。腎臟渴，飲百杯不能止渴，及房勞不稱心意，此為三消也。乃土燥承渴，不能剋化，故成此病：人中、公孫、脾俞、中脘、關衝、照海（治飲不止渴）、太谿（治房勞不稱心）、三里（治食不充飢）

Dispersion-thirst and similar patterns: The three dispersion patterns are not the same: spleen dispersion, center dispersion, and kidney dispersion. *Elementary Questions* says: In stomach vacuity, the daily allowance of grain is unable to allay hunger. In kidney thirst, drinking [even] a hundred cups is unable to quench the thirst, and sexual taxation does not satisfy one's wishes. These are the three dispersions. It is dryness of earth [element] that supports the thirst, so [the earth] cannot restrain and transform.[125] That is why it becomes

125. "Restrain and transform" Spleen earth should be able to restrain kidney water, but since the earth is dry, it cannot do the job. The kidneys are without constraint so sexual taxation and thirst occur. The spleen's own job is transformation, so even though the patient eats a lot, food essence is

this disease: Rén Zhōng 人中 (Du 26), Gōng Sūn 公孫 (SP 4), Pí Shū 脾俞 (UB 20), Zhōng Wǎn 中脘 (Ren 12), Guān Chōng 關衝 (SJ 1), Zhào Hǎi 照海 (KI 6) (to treat drinking that does not quench thirst), Tài Xī 太谿 (KI 3) (to treat sexual taxation that does not satisfy the heart), Sān Lǐ 三里 (ST 36) (to treat eating that does not allay hunger).

黑痧，腹痛頭疼，發熱惡寒，腰背強痛，不得睡臥：百勞 、天府 、委中 、十宣

Black sand [*shā* 痧],[126] abdomnial pain, headache, fever, aversion to cold, stiffness and pain of the back, insomnia: Bǎi Láo 百勞 (M-HN-30), Tiān Fǔ 天府 (LU 3), Wěi Zhōng 委中 (UB 40), Shí Xuān 十宣 (M-UE-1).

白痧，腹痛吐瀉，四肢厥冷，十指甲黑，不得睡臥：大陵 、百勞 、大敦 、十宣

White sand, abdominal pain, vomiting and diarrhea, reversal cold of the four limbs, the ten fingernails are black, insomnia: Dà Líng 大陵 (PC 7), Bǎi Láo 百勞 (M-HN-30), Dà Dūn 大敦 (LV 1), Shí Xuān 十宣 (M-UE-1).

黑白痧，頭疼發汗，口渴，大腸泄瀉，惡寒，四肢厥冷，名絞腸痧，或腸鳴腹響：委中 、膻中 、百會 、丹田 、大敦 、竅陰 、十宣

Black and white sand, headache, sweating, thirst, large intestine diarrhea, aversion to cold, reversal cold of the four limbs. This is called intestine-gripping sand, or intestinal rumbling and abdominal sounds: Wěi Zhōng 委中 (UB 40), Dàn Zhōng 膻中 (Ren 17), Bǎi Huì 百會 (Du 20), Dān Tián 丹田 (Ren 4), Dà Dūn 大敦 (LV 1), Qiào Yīn 竅陰 (GB 44), Shí Xuān 十宣 (M-UE-1).

楊氏治症：
Master Yáng's treatment of patterns:

血迷血暈：人中

Blood stupor or blood dizziness: Rén Zhōng 人中 (Du 26).

胸膈痞結：湧泉 、少商 、膻中 、內關

Glomus binding up the chest and diaphragm: Yǒng Quán 湧泉 (KI 1), Shào Shāng 少商 (LU

---

not transformed and the patient will become thin.

126. Sand is a type of papule that is caused by external contraction and accompanied by fever.

11), Dàn Zhōng 膻中 (Ren 17), Nèi Guān 內關 (PC 6).

臍腹疼痛：膻中、大敦、中府、少澤、太淵、三陰交

Pain in the umbilicus and abdomen: Dàn Zhōng 膻中 (Ren 17), Dà Dūn 大敦 (LV 1), Zhōng Fǔ 中府 (LU 1), Shào Zé 少澤 (SI 1), Tài Yuān 太淵 (LU 9), Sān Yīn Jiāo 三陰交 (SP 6).

心中煩悶：陰陵、內關

Vexation and oppression in the heart: Yīn Líng 陰陵 (SP 9), Nèi Guān 內關 (PC 6).

耳內蟬鳴：少衝、聽會、中衝、商陽

Tinnitus [like the sounds of] cicadas inside the ears: Shào Chōng 少衝 (HT 9), Tīng Huì 聽會 (GB 2), Zhōng Chōng 中衝 (PC 9), Shāng Yáng 商陽 (LI 1).

鼻流濁污：上星、內關、列缺、曲池、合谷

Running nose with turbid filth: Shàng Xīng 上星 (Du 23), Nèi Guān 內關 (PC 6), Liè Quē 列缺 (LU 7), Qū Chí 曲池 (LI 11), Hé Gǔ 合谷 (LI 4).

傷寒發熱：曲差、內關、列缺、經渠、合谷

Cold damage with fever: Qū Chā 曲差 (UB 4), Nèi Guān 內關 (PC 6), Liè Quē 列缺 (LU 7), Jīng Qú 經渠 (LU 8), Hé Gǔ 合谷 (LI 4).

陰蹻脈
Yīn Qiāo Mài

考穴：照海二穴，腎經。足內踝下陷中，令人穩坐，兩足底相合取之。針一寸二分，主臟腑病，與列缺主客相應。

Examining the point: The two points of Zhào Hǎi 照海 (KI 6) are on the kidney channel. They are in the depression below the medial malleolus. To find it, make the person sit stably with the bottoms of the feet united with each other. Needle it 1.2 *cùn* [deep]. It is indicated for diseases of the viscera and bowels. It responds to Liè Quē 列缺 (LU 7) as host and guest.

針灸大成・卷之五

治病：〔西江月〕

　　喉塞小便淋瀝，膀胱氣痛腸鳴，
　　食黃酒積腹臍并，嘔瀉胃翻便緊。
　　難產昏迷積塊，腸風下血常頻，
　　膈中快氣氣核侵，照海有功必定。

Disease treatment: (West River Moon):

Throat blockage, dribbling rough urination;
urinary bladder qì pain, intestinal rumbling;
Food and yellow wine accumulations
together in the abdomen and umbilicus;
vomiting and diarrhea, stomach reflux, hard stool.
Difficult childbirth, stupor, accumulation lumps;
frequent intestinal wind bleeding;
Depressed qì in the diaphragm, qì nodes invading;
Zhào Hǎi 照海 (KI 6) **has efficacy and will stabilize this.**

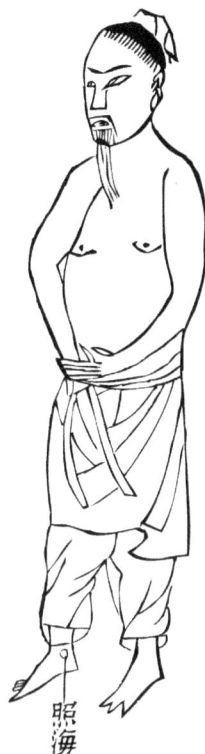

照海

凡治後症，必先取照海為主，次取各穴應之（徐氏）：

Generally to treat the following patterns, you must first select Zhào Hǎi 照海 (KI 6)
as the host and next select each point that responds to it:
（Master Xú）

小便淋瀝不通：陰陵泉、三陰交、關衝、合谷

Dribbling urination with flow stoppage: Yīn Líng Quán 陰陵泉 (SP 9), **Sān Yīn Jiāo** 三陰交
(SP 6), **Guān Chōng** 關衝 (SJ 1), **Hé Gǔ** 合谷 (LI 4).

小腹冷痛，小便頻數：氣海、關元、腎俞、三陰交

Cold pain of the lower abdomen, frequent urination: Qì Hǎi 氣海 (Ren 6), **Guān Yuán** 關元
(Ren 4), **Shèn Shū** 腎俞 (UB 23), **Sān Yīn Jiāo** 三陰交 (SP 6).

膀胱七疝，奔豚等症：大敦、蘭門、丹田、三陰交、湧泉、章門、大陵

Urinary bladder seven *shàn* 疝 (mountings)[127] and running piglet class of patterns: Dà Dūn

---

127. The earliest reference for this section is from *Zhēn Jīng Zhǐ Nán*《針經指南》Dòu
Hànqīng's 竇漢卿 (Compass for the Acupuncture Classic). It lists *páng guāng qì tòng* 膀胱氣痛
(urinary bladder qì pain) instead of urinary bladder seven *shàn* 疝 (mountings).

大敦 (LV 1), Lán Mén 蘭門 (Orchid Gate),[128] Dān Tián 丹田 (Ren 4), Sān Yīn Jiāo 三陰交 (SP 6), Yǒng Quán 湧泉 (KI 1), Zhāng Mén 章門 (LV 13), Dà Líng 大陵 (PC 7).

偏墜水腎，腫大如升：大敦、曲泉、然谷、三陰交、歸來、蘭門、膀胱俞、腎俞（橫紋可灸七壯）

Unilateral sagging of the water kidney,[129] swollen as big as a shēng 升:[130] Dà Dūn 大敦 (LV 1), Qū Quán 曲泉 (LV 8), Rán Gǔ 然谷 (KI 2), Sān Yīn Jiāo 三陰交 (SP 6), Guī Lái 歸來 (ST 29), Lán Mén 蘭門 (Orchid Gate), Páng Guāng Shū 膀胱俞 (UB 28), Shèn Shū 腎俞 (UB 23) (you can apply seven cones of moxibustion at the transverse crease).

乳絃疝氣，發時衝心痛：帶脈、湧泉、太谿、大敦

Breast strings[131] and shàn 疝 (mounting) qì; when it occurs, it surges up to the heart causing pain: Dài Mài 帶脈 (GB 26), Yǒng Quán 湧泉 (KI 1), Tài Xī 太谿 (KI 3), Dà Dūn 大敦 (LV 1).

小便淋血不止，陰器痛：陰谷、湧泉、三陰交

Incessant dribbling [lín 淋] of bloody urine, genital pain: Yīn Gǔ 陰谷 (KI 10), Yǒng Quán 湧泉 (KI 1), Sān Yīn Jiāo 三陰交 (SP 6).

遺精白濁，小便頻數：關元、白環俞、太谿、三陰交

Seminal emission with white turbidity, frequent urination: Guān Yuán 關元 (Ren 4), Bái Huán Shū 白還俞 (UB 30), Tài Xī 太谿 (KI 3), Sān Yīn Jiāo 三陰交 (SP 6).

夜夢鬼交，遺精不禁：中極、膏肓、心俞、然谷、腎俞

Dreaming of intercourse with ghosts, seminal emission: Zhōng Jí 中極 (Ren 3), Gāo Huāng 膏肓 (UB 43), Xīn Shū 心俞 (UB 15), Rán Gǔ 然谷 (KI 2), Shèn Shū 腎俞 (UB 23).

---

128. Yáng (following the *Great Completion*) says in Volume 7 that Lán Mén 蘭門 (Orchid Gate) is three *cùn* to the two sides of Qū Quán 曲泉 (LV 8) on a vessel. This is likely to be an error. Other books say Lán Mén is three *cùn* to the two sides of Qū Gǔ 曲骨 (Ren 2). According to Yáng, Lán Mén treats the urinary bladder, the seven *shàn* 疝 (mountings), and running piglet.

129. *Piān zhuì* 偏墜 Unilateral sagging means one testicle hangs lower. *Shuǐ shèn* 水腎 Water kidney probably should read *mù shèn* 木腎 wooden kidney. Wooden kidney means the testicles are greatly swollen and hard as a piece of wood. There may also be numbness and tingling.

130. A *shēng* 升 is a unit of volume equivalent to a little over a liter during the *Míng* Dynasty.

131. *Xián* 疢 or *xián* 絃 strings are a type of mass.

婦人難產，子掬母心，不能下，胎衣不去：巨闕、合谷、三陰交、至陰（灸效）

Difficult childbirth, the child holds onto the mother's heart so it is unable to descend, retention of the placenta: Jù Què 巨闕 (Ren 14), Hé Gǔ 合谷 (LI 4), Sān Yīn Jiāo 三陰交 (SP 6), Zhì Yīn 至陰 (UB 67) (moxibustion is effective).

女人大便不通：申脈、陰陵泉、三陰交、太谿

Female constipation: Shēn Mài 申脈 (UB 62), Yīn Líng Quán 陰陵泉 (SP 9), Sān Yīn Jiāo 三陰交 (SP 6), Tài Xī 太谿 (KI 3).

婦人產後臍腹痛，惡露不已：水分、關元、膏肓、三陰交

Postpartum pain in the umbilicus and abdomen, incessant flow of lochia: Shuǐ Fēn 水分 (Ren 9), Guān Yuán 關元 (Ren 4), Gāo Huāng 膏肓 (UB 43), Sān Yīn Jiāo 三陰交 (SP 6).

婦人脾氣，血蠱，水蠱，氣蠱，石蠱：膻中、水分（治水）、關元、氣海、三里、行間（治血）、公孫（治氣）、內庭（治石）、支溝、三陰交

Female spleen qì, blood *gǔ* 血蠱, water *gǔ* 水蠱, qì *gǔ* 氣蠱, stone *gǔ* 石蠱: Dàn Zhōng 膻中 (Ren 17), Shuǐ Fēn 水分 (Ren 9) (treats water), Guān Yuán 關元 (Ren 4), Qì Hǎi 氣海 (Ren 6), Sān Lǐ 三里 (ST 36), Xíng Jiān 行間 (LV 2) (treats blood), Gōng Sūn 公孫 (SP 4) (treats qì), Nèi Tíng 內庭 (ST 44) (treats stone), Zhī Gōu 支溝 (SJ 6), Sān Yīn Jiāo 三陰交 (SP 6).

女人血分，單腹氣喘：下脘、膻中、氣海、三里、行間

Female blood aspect, simple abdomen panting:[132] **Xià Wǎn 下脘 (Ren 10), Dàn Zhōng 膻中 (Ren 17), Qì Hǎi 氣海 (Ren 6), Sān Lǐ 三里 (ST 36), Xíng Jiān 行間 (LV 2).**

女人血氣勞倦，五心煩熱，肢體皆痛，頭目昏沉：腎俞、百會、膏肓、曲池、合谷、絕骨

Female blood-qì taxation fatigue, vexing heat of the five hearts, pain in all the limbs, dazed head and eyes: Shèn Shū 腎俞 (UB 23), Bǎi Huì 百會 (Du 20), Gāo Huāng 膏肓 (UB 43), Qū Chí 曲池 (LI 11), Hé Gǔ 合谷 (LI 4), Jué Gǔ 絕骨 (GB 39).

---

132. This was written well before the development of the four aspects of warm disease (defense, qì, construction, and blood), so "blood aspect" refers to something else. The *Great Completion* has the same passage, but Dòu Hànqīng 竇漢卿 lists *fù rén xuè yūn* 婦人血暈 (female blood dizziness), as associated with lungs and kidneys, and *fù rén xuè jī* 婦人血積 (female blood accumulation), as associated with the kidneys and heart. Since this entry also includes panting, perhaps it is related to the former.

老人虛損，手足轉筋，不能舉動：承山、陽陵泉、臨泣、太衝、尺澤、合谷

Vacuity detriment in the elderly, cramping of the limbs, inability to move around: Chéng Shān 承山 (UB 57), Yáng Líng Quán 陽陵泉 (GB 34), Lín Qì 臨泣 (GB 41), Tài Chōng 太衝 (LV 3), Chǐ Zé 尺澤 (LU 5), Hé Gǔ 合谷 (LI 4).

霍亂吐瀉，手足轉筋：京骨、三里、承山、曲池、腕骨、尺澤、陽陵泉

Sudden turmoil [cholera] with vomiting and diarrhea, cramping of the limbs: Jīng Gǔ 京骨 (UB 64), Sān Lǐ 三里 (ST 36), Chéng Shān 承山 (UB 57), Qū Chí 曲池 (LI 11), Wàn Gǔ 腕骨 (SI 4), Chǐ Zé 尺澤 (LU 5), Yáng Líng Quán 陽陵泉 (GB 34).

寒濕腳氣，發熱大痛：太衝、委中、三陰交

Cold-damp leg qì, fever and great pain: Tài Chōng 太衝 (LV 3), Wěi Zhōng 委中 (UB 40), Sān Yīn Jiāo 三陰交 (SP 6).

腎虛，腳氣紅腫，大熱不退：氣衝、太谿、公孫、三陰交、血海、委中

Kidney vacuity, leg qì with redness and swelling, great fever that does not abate: Qì Chōng 氣衝 (ST 30), Tài Xī 太谿 (KI 3), Gōng Sūn 公孫 (SP 4), Sān Yīn Jiāo 三陰交 (SP 6), Xuè Hǎi 血海 (SP 10), Wěi Zhōng 委中 (UB 40).

乾腳氣，膝頭并內踝及五指疼痛：膝關、崑崙、絕骨、委中、陽陵泉、三陰交

Dry leg qì, pain in the knee and medial malleolus as well as the five toes: Xī Guān 膝關 (LV 7), Kūn Lún 崑崙 (UB 60), Jué Gǔ 絕骨 (GB 39), Wěi Zhōng 委中 (UB 40), Yáng Líng Quán 陽陵泉 (GB 34), Sān Yīn Jiāo 三陰交 (SP 6).

渾身脹滿，浮腫生水：氣海、三里、曲池、合谷、內庭、行間、三陰交

Distention and fullness of the entire body, puffy swelling engendering water: Qì Hǎi 氣海 (Ren 6), Sān Lǐ 三里 (ST 36), Qū Chí 曲池 (LI 11), Hé Gǔ 合谷 (LI 4), Nèi Tíng 內庭 (ST 44), Xíng Jiān 行間 (LV 2), Sān Yīn Jiāo 三陰交 (SP 6).

單腹蠱脹，氣喘不息：膻中、氣海、水分、三里、行間、三陰交

Simple abdominal *gǔ* 蠱 distention, incessant panting: Dàn Zhōng 膻中 (Ren 17), Qì Hǎi 氣海 (Ren 6), Shuǐ Fēn 水分 (Ren 9), Sān Lǐ 三里 (ST 36), Xíng Jiān 行間 (LV 2), Sān Yīn Jiāo 三陰交 (SP 6).

心腹脹大如盆：中脘 膻中 、水分 、三陰交

Great distention in the heart region and abdomen, like a basin: Zhōng Wǎn 中脘 (Ren 12), Dàn Zhōng 膻中 (Ren 17), Shuǐ Fēn 水分 (Ren 9), Sān Yīn Jiāo 三陰交 (SP 6).

四肢面目浮腫，大不退：人中 、合谷 、三里 、臨泣 、曲池 、三陰交

Puffy swelling of the four limbs, face, and eyes, great fever[133] which does not abate: Rén Zhōng 人中 (Du 26), Hé Gǔ 合谷 (LI 4), Sān Lǐ 三里 (ST 36), Lín Qì 臨泣 (GB 41), Qū Chí 曲池 (LI 11), Sān Yīn Jiāo 三陰交 (SP 6).

婦人虛損形瘦，赤白帶下：百勞 、腎俞 、關元 、三陰交

Female vacuity detriment with a thin body, red and white vaginal discharge: Bǎi Láo 百勞 (M-HN-30), Shèn Shū 腎俞 (UB 23), Guān Yuán 關元 (Ren 4), Sān Yīn Jiāo 三陰交 (SP 6).

女人子宮久冷，不受胎孕：中樞 、三陰交 、子宮

Enduring cold of the uterus, infertility: Zhōng Jí 中極 (Ren 3), Sān Yīn Jiāo 三陰交 (SP 6), Zǐ Gōng 子宮 (M-CA-18).

女人經水正行，頭暈，小腹痛：陽交 、內庭 、合谷

Dizzy head, pain in the lower abdomen at the time of the female menstrual flow: Yīn Jiāo 陰交 (Ren 7),[134] Nèi Tíng 內庭 (ST 44), Hé Gǔ 合谷 (LI 4).

室女月水不調，臍腹疼痛：腎俞 、三陰交 、關元

Irregular monthly flow in maidens, pain in the umbilicus and abdomen: Shèn Shū 腎俞 (UB 23), Sān Yīn Jiāo 三陰交 (SP 6), Guān Yuán 關元 (Ren 4).

婦人產難，不能分娩：合谷 、三陰交 、獨陰

Difficult childbirth, unable to deliver: Hé Gǔ 合谷 (LI 4), Sān Yīn Jiāo 三陰交 (SP 6), Dú Yīn 獨陰 (Solo Yīn).[135]

---

133. The *Great Compendium* lacks the word *rè* 熱 (heat or fever). However, it is in the *Great Completion*, which was Yáng's source for this section.

134. The *Great Compendium* says Yáng Jiāo 陽交 (GB 35). However, the *Great Completion*, which was Yáng's source for this section, has Yīn Jiāo 陰交 (Ren 7) which makes more sense.

135. Yáng says in Volume 7 that Dú Yīn 獨陰 is below the second toe in the center of the horizontal crease. It treats small intestine *shàn* (mounting) qì 疝氣, and helps expel a dead fetus or the placenta. Apply five cones of moxibustion. However, a note in the *Great Completion* says that Dú

楊氏治症：
Master Yáng's treatment of patterns:

氣血兩蠱：行間、關元、水分、公孫、氣海、臨泣

Dual qì-blood *gǔ* 蠱: Xíng Jiān 行間 (LV 2), Guān Yuán 關元 (Ren 4), Shuǐ Fēn 水分 (Ren 9), Gōng Sūn 公孫 (SP 4), Qì Hǎi 氣海 (Ren 6), Lín Qì 臨泣 (GB 41).

五心煩熱：內關、湧泉、十宣、大陵、合谷、四花

Vexing heat of the five hearts: Nèi Guān 內關 (PC 6), Yǒng Quán 湧泉 (KI 1), Shí Xuān 十宣 (M-UE-1), Dà Líng 大陵 (PC 7), Hé Gǔ 合谷 (LI 4), Sì Huā 四花 (the Four Flowers). [136]

氣攻胸痛：通里、大陵

Qì attacking the chest with pain: Tōng Lǐ 通里 (HT 5), Dà Líng 大陵 (PC 7).

心內怔忡：心俞、內關、神門

Fearful throbbing inside the heart: Xīn Shū 心俞 (UB 15), Nèi Guān 內關 (PC 6), Shén Mén 神門 (HT 7).

咽喉閉塞：少商、風池、照海

Throat blockage: Shào Shāng 少商 (LU 11), Fēng Chí 風池 (GB 20), Zhào Hǎi 照海 (KI 6).

虛陽自脫：心俞、然谷、腎俞、中極、三陰交

Spontaneously desertion of vacuous yáng: Xīn Shū 心俞 (UB 15), Rán Gǔ 然谷 (KI 2), Shèn Shū 腎俞 (UB 23), Zhōng Jí 中極 (Ren 3), Sān Yīn Jiāo 三陰交 (SP 6).

右八法，先刺主症之穴，隨病左右上下所在，取諸應穴，仍循捫導引，按法祛除。如病未已，必求合穴，須要停針待氣，使上下相接，快然無所苦，而後出針，或用艾灸亦可，在乎臨時機變，不可專拘於針也。

In the above eight methods, first needle the indicated point for the pattern. Based on the location of the disease, left or right, above or below, apply treatment to the various corre-

---

Yīn 獨陰 is another name for Zhì Yīn 至陰 (UB 67).

136. Yáng writes elsewhere that the Four Flowers are Gé Shū 膈俞 (UB 17) and Dǎn Shū 膽俞 (UB 19). Moxibustion is used with these points.

sponding points. You still need to use channel rubbing palpation and conduction exercise [*dǎo yǐn* 導引]. Eliminate [evils] in accordance with the models. If the disease does not recover, you must try combining points. It is absolutely necessary to retain the needle and wait for the qì. Make upper and lower join with each other. Remove the needles when the patient is comfortable and there is nothing that is [still] suffering. Sometimes you can also use mugwort moxibustion. Be versatile during clinical practice; you cannot focus on or constrain yourself with acupuncture.

八法手訣歌 (《聚英》)
Eight Methods Hand [Technique] Rhymed Formula Song
(*Gatherings* – Jù Yīng)[137]

春夏先深而後淺，秋冬先淺而後深，
隨處按之呼吸輕，迎而吸之尋內關 。
補虛瀉實公孫是，列缺次當照海深，
臨泣外關和上下，後谿申脈用金針 。
先深後淺行陰數，前三後二卻是陰，
先淺後深陽數法，前二後三陽數定 。
臨泣公孫腸中病，脊頭腰背申脈攻，
照海咽喉並小腹，內關行處治心疼 。
後谿前上外肩背，列缺針時脈氣通，
急按慢提陰氣升，急提慢按陽氣降 。
取陽取陰皆六數，達人刺處有奇功 。

In spring and summer, first [needle] deep and later shallow;
in autumn and winter, first shallow and later deep,
Press following along the site, lightly exhaling and inhaling;
face it and inhale, seeking Nèi Guān 內關 (PC 6).

Supplement vacuity, drain repletion, this is Gōng Sūn 公孫 (SP 4);
[needle] deeply Liè Quē 列缺 (LU 7) followed by Zhào Hǎi 照海 (KI 6),
Lín Qì 臨泣 (GB 41) and Wài Guān 外關 (SJ 5) harmonize upper and lower;
use the golden needle[138] on Hòu Xī 後谿 (SI 3) and Shēn Mài 申脈 (UB 62).

First deep, later shallow, move [the needle] a yīn number [of times];
before three, after two, this is yīn,

---

137. From *Zhēn Jiǔ Jù Yīng*《針灸聚英》(Gatherings from Eminent Acupuncturists), Volume 4.

138. Some editions have *shén zhēn* 神針 (spirit needle) instead of *jīn zhēn* 金針 (golden needle).

First shallow, later deep, is the method of yáng numbers;
before two, after three, the yáng number is determined.

Lín Qì 臨泣 (GB 41) and Gōng Sūn 公孫 (SP 4) for diseases in the intestines;
for spine, head, and back, Shēn Mài 申脈 (UB 62) is effective,
Zhào Hǎi 照海 (KI 6) for the throat and lower abdomen;
the site where Nèi Guān 內關 (PC 6) goes treats heart pain.

Distal Hòu Xī 後谿 (SI 3) ascends to the lateral shoulder and upper back;
when Liè Quē 列缺 (LU 7) is needled vessel qì passes freely,
Quickly press and slowly lift to bring yīn qì upward;
quickly lift and slowly press to bring yáng qì downward.

Select yáng, select yīn, both the number 6;
an intelligent person needling the site will have extraordinary results.

Translator's note:
This poem lists the eight confluence points and mentions some of the conditions they treat. It also describes needling techniques. These techniques are explained in more detail in Volume 4 of the *Great Compendium*.

The Stems and Branches and the Chinese Calendar

Introduction

The stems and branches are the ancient Chinese units for judging the qualities of time. In the past, they were an important consideration for medical treatment. This is documented from the *Yellow Emperor's Inner Cannon* (Hàn dynasty) through the Míng dynasty, the time of the *Great Compendium*. Their medical usage continued, although declining, through the Qīng dynasty and on into the 20th century. Some physicians still use them for this purpose today. Knowledge of the stems and branches and a good foundation in the Chinese calendar are necessary for reading ancient Chinese medical books, including the *Great Compendium*. This appendix discusses the stems and branches and the Chinese calendar to provide the background for understanding the references to time in books such as the *Great Compendium*.

The 22 characters that comprise the ten stems and the twelve branches are some of the oldest Chinese characters. They are found on the oracle bones, making them more than 4,000 years old. These two sets of characters represent the cycles of heaven and earth which have a profound effect on our well-being. They are based on yīn-yáng and the five elements, but have many other correspondences as well.

Most Westerners do not know that the Chinese have always had a solar calendar as well as the more common lunar one. This appendix will also explain these two sides of the Chinese calendar, as well as the Chinese view of the four or five seasons.

The Stems and Branches

Nature consists of regular cycles that never cease. Day follows night, night follows day. The moon waxes and wanes and waxes again. The year progresses through four seasons. The stems and branches also represent the passage of time and a system of order. They imply the natural processes of sprouting, growing, thriving, declining, and dying. They mark the passing of time in cycles and describe the qualities of different time periods.

The Ten Heavenly Stems (十天干)

The ten stems represent the qì of heaven. The number ten represents completion or perfection; therefore it is an appropriate number for heaven. The stems repeat in a cyclical fashion similar to a ten-day week.

The stems consist of:

The Ten Heavenly Stems (十天干)				
Chinese	Pinyin	Number	Element	Organ
甲	Jiǎ	1	Yáng Wood	Gall Bladder
乙	Yǐ	2	Yīn Wood	Liver
丙	Bǐng	3	Yáng Fire	Small Intestine
丁	Dīng	4	Yīn Fire	Heart
戊	Wù	5	Yáng Earth	Stomach
己	Jǐ	6	Yīn Earth	Spleen
庚	Gēng	7	Yáng Metal	Large Intestine
辛	Xīn	8	Yīn Metal	Lungs
壬	Rén	9	Yáng Water	Urinary Bladder
癸	Guǐ	10	Yīn Water	Kidneys

Notice the following patterns:
- The nature of each stem is yīn or yáng. They alternate yáng and yīn, beginning with yáng for Stem 1.
- Yáng stems are always associated with odd numbers and yīn stems with even numbers.
- The stems run in the generating order of the five elements, beginning with wood, as wood represents birth and beginnings.
- Two stems belong to each of the five elements: one yīn and one yáng. These two stems of the same element are adjacent to each other: yáng wood stem, then yīn wood stem, yáng fire stem, then yīn fire stem, etc.
- An organ is associated with each of the stems. It is the organ with the same associations of yīn-yáng and element.

針
灸
大
成
·
卷
之
五

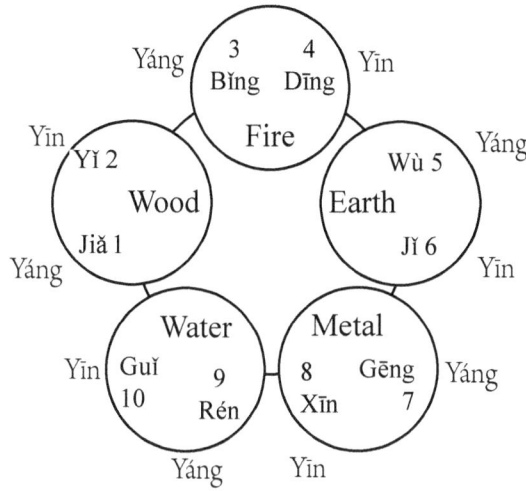

This diagram shows the five elements and their associated stems.

The Twelve Earthly Branches (十二地支)

The earthly branches flow in a cycle of twelve. They represent the qì of the earth. Each branch corresponds with an element and with an animal of the so-called Chinese zodiac.

The Twelve Earthly Branches (十二地支)				
Chinese	Branch	Number	Animal	Element
子	Zǐ	1	Rat	Yáng Water
丑	Chǒu	2	Ox	Yīn Earth
寅	Yín	3	Tiger	Yáng Wood
卯	Mǎo	4	Rabbit	Yīn Wood
辰	Chén	5	Dragon	Yáng Earth
巳	Sì	6	Snake	Yīn Fire
午	Wǔ	7	Horse	Yáng Fire
未	Wèi	8	Sheep	Yīn Earth
申	Shēn	9	Monkey	Yáng Metal
酉	Yǒu	10	Rooster	Yīn Metal
戌	Xū	11	Dog	Yáng Earth
亥	Hài	12	Pig	Yīn Water

Notice the following:

- The branches alternate between yáng and yīn, as do the stems. The odd-numbered branches are yáng and the even-numbered branches are yīn.
- Two branches exist for every element except earth, which has four.
- The four earth element branches separate the other elements. This is because the qì of the earthly branches, unlike the heavenly stems, returns to the center (earth) before transforming into the next element. This can be seen more easily in the diagram below.

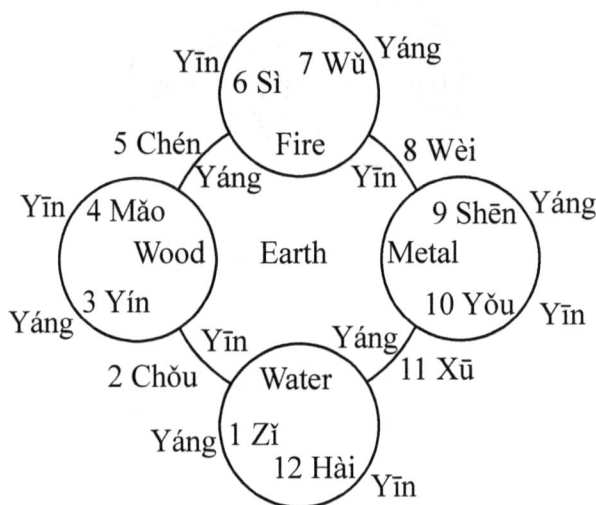

Do not confuse the stem wù (戊) with the branch wǔ (午). Notice that they have different Chinese characters and also different tones. Another area of possible confusion is the third branch, yín (寅). The Pinyin is the same as for the yīn (陰) of yīn-yáng, but the tone and the character are different. You should also be careful not to confuse the ten heavenly stems with the twelve earthly branches. They are different data sets and are used differently.

The number twelve represents the dimension of time. We have 12 months in a year, and 12 double-hours in a day,[1] so each branch represents one month and one two-hour period, shown in the diagram below. Notice that the Chinese day starts at 11 p.m. of the prior evening, not at midnight as it does in the West. The branches and their two-hour periods are also associated with acu-moxa channels.

---

1. The Chinese traditionally had twelve double-hours in a day. See below.

針
灸
大
成
·
卷
之
五

The Twelve Earthly Branches (十二地支)				
Branch	**Number**	**Month**	**Hour**	**Channel**
Zǐ	1	11th	11pm-1am	Gall Bladder
Chǒu	2	12th	1-3am	Liver
Yín	3	1st	3-5am	Lungs
Mǎo	4	2nd	5-7am	Large Intestine
Chén	5	3rd	7-9am	Stomach
Sì	6	4th	9-11am	Spleen
Wǔ	7	5th	11am-1pm	Heart
Wèi	8	6th	1-3pm	Small Intestine
Shēn	9	7th	3-5pm	Urinary Bladder
Yǒu	10	8th	5-7pm	Kidneys
Xū	11	9th	7-9pm	Pericardium
Hài	12	10th	9-11pm	Triple Burner

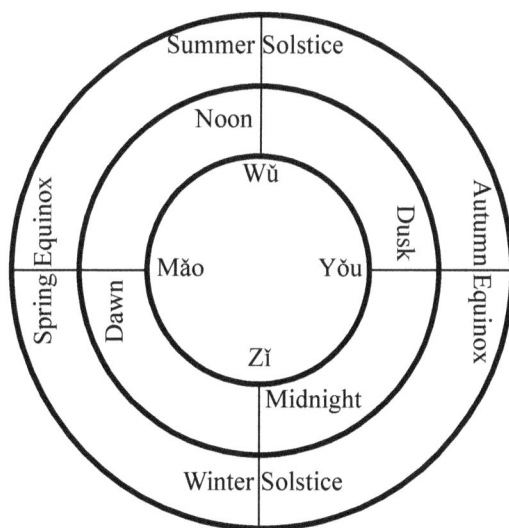

The first branch, zǐ, rules at the period containing both midnight and the winter solstice. This is the time when yīn is the strongest.

Zǐ corresponds to the water element. The branches start with water at the bottom of the cycle when yīn is at its maximum and right at the moment that yáng begins to increase again. The earthly branches start with water while the heavenly stems begin with wood. This is because the earth's qì is more yīn than heaven's and the branches belong to the earth. Water, overall, is more yīn than wood.

The third branch yín corresponds to the wood element, representing spring, birth, and beginnings. This also corresponds to the first month of the Chinese calendar and marks the beginning of spring. Because the first month corresponds to the third branch, the first branch, zǐ, represents the eleventh month (the time of the winter solstice).

The Cycle of Sixty

The stems flow from heaven while the branches flow from earth, and in between, both affect humanity.

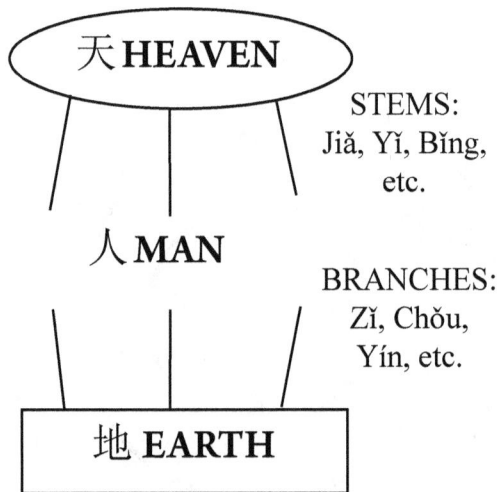

天 **HEAVEN**

STEMS:
Jiǎ, Yǐ, Bǐng,
etc.

人 **MAN**

BRANCHES:
Zǐ, Chǒu,
Yín, etc.

地 **EARTH**

The stems and branches progress in parallel cycles. When the ten stems and twelve branches combine, they become a greater cycle of 60. This cycle of sixty (also known as the sexagenary cycle) consists of six cycles of the stems and five cycles of the branches. Yīn stems always combine with yīn branches and yáng stems always combine with yáng branches.

The combinations progress as follows:

Stem 1 Branch 1 both yáng
Stem 2 Branch 2 both yīn
Stem 3 Branch 3 both yáng
Stem 4 Branch 4 both yīn
Stem 5 Branch 5 both yáng
Stem 6 Branch 6 both yīn
Stem 7 Branch 7 both yáng
Stem 8 Branch 8 both yīn
Stem 9 Branch 9 both yáng
Stem 10 Branch 10 both yīn
Stem 1 Branch 11 both yáng
Stem 2 Branch 12 both yīn
Stem 3 Branch 1 both yáng etc.

This cycle counts the progression of years, months, days, and hours as the stems and branches apply to these four units of time.

針
灸
大
成
·
卷
之
五

The following table shows the cycle of sixty and its associations:

#	Stem/ Branch		Elements	#	Stem/ Branch		Elements
1	S1B1	Jiǎ Zǐ	Yáng Wood Water	31	S1B7	Jiǎ Wǔ	Yáng Wood Fire
2	S2B2	Yǐ Chǒu	Yīn Wood Earth	32	S2B8	Yi Wei	Yīn Wood Earth
3	S3B3	Bǐng Yín	Yáng Fire Wood	33	S3B9	Bǐng Shēn	Yáng Fire Metal
4	S4B4	Dīng Mǎo	Yīn Fire Wood	34	S4B10	Dīng Yǒu	Yīn Fire Metal
5	S5B5	Wù Chén	Yáng Earth Earth	35	S5B11	Wù Xū	Yáng Earth Earth
6	S6B6	Jǐ Sì	Yīn Earth Fire	36	S6B12	Jǐ Hài	Yīn Earth Water
7	S7B7	Gēng Wǔ	Yáng Metal Fire	37	S7B1	Gēng Zǐ	Yáng Metal Water
8	S8B8	Xīn Wèi	Yīn Metal Earth	38	S8B2	Xīn Chǒu	Yīn Metal Earth
9	S9B9	Rén Shēn	Yáng Water Metal	39	S9B3	Rén Yín	Yáng Water Wood
10	S10B10	Guǐ Yǒu	Yīn Water Metal	40	S10B4	Guǐ Mǎo	Yīn Water Wood
11	S1B11	Jiǎ Xū	Yáng Wood Earth	41	S1B5	Jiǎ Chén	Yáng Wood Earth
12	S2B12	Yǐ Hài	Yīn Wood Water	42	S2B6	Yǐ Sì	Yīn Wood Fire
13	S3B1	Bing Zǐ	Yáng Fire Water	43	S3B7	Bǐng Wǔ	Yáng Fire Fire
14	S4B2	Dīng Chǒu	Yīn Fire Earth	44	S4B8	Dīng Wèi	Yīn Fire Earth
15	S5B3	Wù Yín	Yáng Earth Wood	45	S5B9	Wù Shēn	Yáng Earth Metal
16	S6B4	Jǐ Mǎo	Yīn Earth Wood	46	S6B10	Jǐ Yǒu	Yīn Earth Metal
17	S7B5	Gēng Chén	Yáng Metal Earth	47	S7B11	Gēng Xū	Yáng Metal Earth
18	S8B6	Xīn Sì	Yīn Metal Fire	48	S8B12	Xīn Hài	Yīn Metal Water
19	S9B7	Rén Wǔ	Yáng Water Fire	49	S9B1	Rén Zǐ	Yáng Water Water
20	S10B8	Guǐ Wèi	Yīn Water Earth	50	S10B2	Guǐ Chǒu	Yīn Water Earth
21	S1B9	Jiǎ Shēn	Yáng Wood Metal	51	S1B3	Jiǎ Yín	Yáng Wood Wood
22	S2B10	Yǐ Yǒu	Yīn Wood Metal	52	S2B4	Yǐ Mǎo	Yīn Wood Wood
23	S3B11	Bǐng Xū	Yáng Fire Earth	53	S3B5	Bǐng Chén	Yáng Fire Earth
24	S4B12	Dīng Hài	Yīn Fire Water	54	S4B6	Dīng Sì	Yīn Fire Fire
25	S5B1	Wù Zǐ	Yáng Earth Water	55	S5B7	Wù Wǔ	Yáng Earth Fire
26	S6B2	Jǐ Chǒu	Yīn Earth Earth	56	S6B8	Jǐ Wèi	Yīn Earth Earth
27	S7B3	Gēng Yín	Yáng Metal Wood	57	S7B9	Gēng Shēn	Yáng Metal Metal
28	S8B4	Xīn Mǎo	Yīn Metal Wood	58	S8B10	Xīn Yǒu	Yīn Metal Metal
29	S9B5	Rén Chén	Yáng Water Earth	59	S9B11	Rén Xū	Yáng Water Earth
30	S10B6	Guǐ Sì	Yīn Water Fire	60	S10B12	Guǐ Hài	Yīn Water Water

As an example, let's look at number 29 in the Cycle of Sixty. It contains Stem 9 (rén) and Branch 5 (chén), abbreviated in the chart as 'S9B5.' This is a yáng combination because 9 and 5 are both odd, or yáng. Rén is yáng water and chén is yáng earth; therefore we call the combination yáng water and earth.

When a stem and branch for a time period are given, the stem is always listed first and the branch comes second.

Each year, month, day, and double-hour has a stem and a branch, or a position in the cycle of sixty. For example, there is a sixty year cycle, as well as a sixty day cycle. Examples of the medical use of the stems and branches include choosing acu-moxa points by the time of day, and medical day selection (determining which days various procedures are to be avoided or which days treatment is especially effective).

Relationships of the Stems and Branches

The stems and branches have various relationships. For example, in choosing points based on the time and date, the points originally calculated for one day stem may also be used on a day with the stem that "unites" with the original day.

A Relationship of the Stems

The most important stem relationship is called the **Five Unities** (wǔ hé 五合).

The Five Unities (wǔ hé 五合)					
Stem	**#**	**Element**	**Stem**	**#**	**Element**
Jiǎ 甲	1	Yáng Wood	Jǐ 己	6	Yīn Earth
Yǐ 乙	2	Yīn Wood	Gēng 庚	7	Yáng Metal
Bǐng 丙	3	Yáng Fire	Xīn 辛	8	Yīn Metal
Dīng 丁	4	Yīn Fire	Rén 壬	9	Yáng Water
Wù 戊	5	Yáng Earth	Guǐ 癸	10	Yīn Water

The two stems that are in the same row in the above table have a special attraction to each other. Note that stem 1 and stem 6 are a pair, stem 2 and stem 7, stem 3 and stem 8, etc. All paired stems have a difference of 5 in their stem numbers. This is called the Five Unities because there are five pairs that unite with each other.

Notice that in each pair, one stem is yīn while the other is yáng. The element of the yáng stem controls the element of the yīn stem. While a control relationship usually causes friction, there is attraction here. In Chinese literature, this was compared to the relationship between husband and wife, where the husband (yáng) controls the wife (yīn). The stereotype may have changed today, but the attraction between these pairs of stems remains.

In fact, if the two attracted stems meet each other, they can combine to produce another element. This can be compared to the husband and wife producing a baby.

The Five Combinations				
Stem		**Stem**		**Element**
Jiǎ 甲		Jǐ 己		Earth
Yǐ 乙	**combines with**	Gēng 庚	**to create**	Metal
Bǐng 丙		Xīn 辛		Water
Dīng 丁		Rén 壬		Wood
Wù 戊		Guǐ 癸		Fire

To summarize the Five Unities of the stems:
- When a yáng stem dominates a yīn stem, this is the relationship called the five unities. They generate a new element together.

Relationships of the Branches

The branches have more types of relationships than the stems. We will describe a few here.

The branches can be placed in a circle, like the face of a clock, with zǐ at 6 o'clock, and wǔ at 12 o'clock:

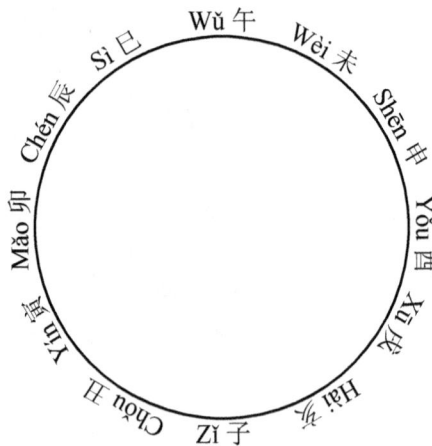

Oppositions (liù chōng 六衝)

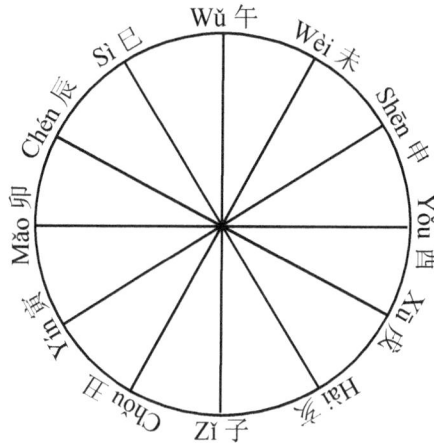

Branches that are across from each other in the above diagram are 'in opposition.' In most cases, this means that they are incompatible, causing friction, or even harming each other. Most of the pairs of opposing branches have a control relationship when the elements are examined. However, in some cases this relationship is significant without implying disharmony.

OPPOSITIONS	
Zǐ 子	Wǔ 午
Chǒu 丑	Wèi 未
Yín 寅	Shēn 申
Mǎo 卯	Yǒu 酉
Chén 辰	Xū 戌
Sì 巳	Hài 亥
Wǔ 午	Zǐ 子
Wèi 未	Chǒu 丑
Shēn 申	Yín 寅
Yǒu 酉	Mǎo 卯
Xū 戌	Chén 辰
Hài 亥	Sì 巳

The Three Unities (sān hé 三合)

Like the Five Unities of the stems, the Three Unities is a relationship of attraction between branches with the ability to transform to another element when the three meet up.

When the branches are placed around a clock face, one can draw equilateral triangles to make four groups of three branches each.

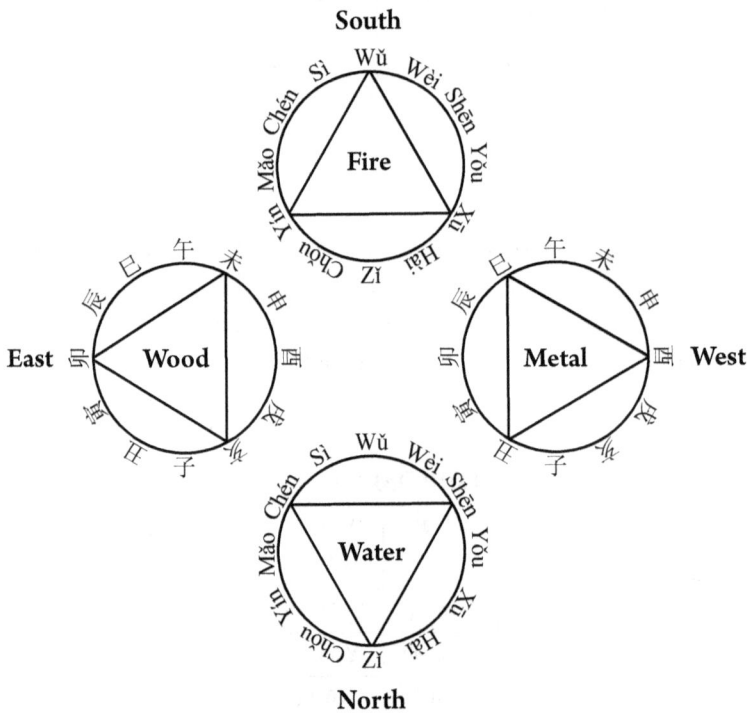

Each triangle points in one of the four main directions. The four directions are north (zǐ), east (mǎo), south (wǔ), and west (yǒu). This is the member of the group of three that defines the group. For example, the south (wǔ branch) relates to the fire element, so the combination containing wǔ transforms to fire. Note that classically, Chinese maps have south at the top.

Example: Shēn, zǐ, and chén are one group of the Three Unities. Zǐ is located in the north direction, so it defines the transformation of this group as water.

The Three Unities				
Branches			**Element**	**Direction**
Shēn 申	Zǐ 子	Chén 辰	Water	North
Sì 巳	Yǒu 酉	Chǒu 丑	Metal	West
Yín 寅	Wǔ 午	Xū 戌	Fire	South
Hài 亥	Mǎo 卯	Wèi 未	Wood	East

The Three Meetings (sān huì 三會)

The Three Meetings are related to the four seasons. Since each season has three months, the branches of the three months of a season have a relationship. For example, the three months of spring are yín, mǎo, and chén. Yín and mǎo are the wood months, and chén is an earth month at the end of the season. When these three branches meet up, they make very strong wood qì. The situation is the same with the other seasons.

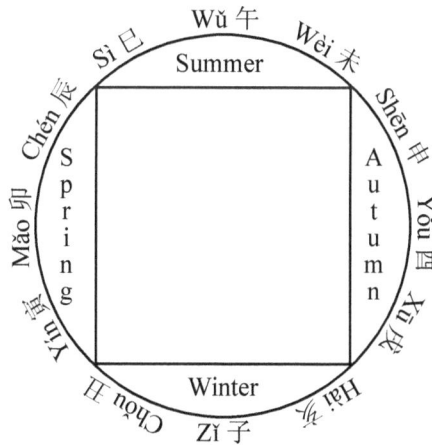

For a discussion of the Chinese view of the four seasons, see below. The Chinese seasons begin and end at different times than the Western seasons.

The Three Unities		
Branches	**Make**	**Season**
Hài 亥, Zǐ 子, Chǒu 丑	Water	Winter
Yín 寅, Mǎo 卯, Chén 辰	Wood	Spring
Sì 巳, Wǔ 午, Wèi 未	Fire	Summer
Shēn 申, Yǒu 酉, Xū 戌	Metal	Autumn

There are additional branch relationships and other aspects of stems and branches that are not discussed here. They are omitted in this appendix because they are not used in the *Great Compendium*.

Chinese Calendar Overview

Before we discuss the Chinese calendar, it is best to review information regarding the Western calendar for comparison.

The Western 'Gregorian' Calendar

The Western calendar is called the Gregorian Calendar. It was named after Pope Gregory, who oversaw its development. The Gregorian calendar is a solar calendar because it is based on the earth's rotation around the sun. It consists of 365 days per year, except on leap years when an extra day is added on February 29th.

A leap year occurs every fourth year in most cases. Years ending in two zeros are not leap years (for example, 1900). On years ending in three zeros, a leap day is added (for example, 2000).

These rules keep the months in their appropriate season. Without leap years, the months would creep out of their assigned seasons because the earth takes approximately 365-1/4 days to circle the sun. The extra quarter day adds up with time, affecting the accuracy of the calendar. Inserting a leap day periodically compensates for this quarter-day discrepancy.

The Chinese Luni-Solar Calendar

The Chinese developed a luni-solar calendar, based on the phases of the moon, as well as the position of the earth relative to the sun. Twelve lunar months make up a year: this leaves the calendar about ten days short of a solar year. To correct this, a leap month is added periodically. In this way, the first month of the Chinese lunar calendar appears at the expected time and aligns the lunar calendar with the four seasons. The seasons are based on the relationship between the earth and the sun. That is part of the reason the Chinese calendar is called luni-solar: it has both lunar and solar aspects to it.

Each lunar month begins on the new moon day and lasts for 29 or 30 days, as it takes about 29-1/2 days from new moon to new moon as seen from the earth. Chinese months have no special names. They are simply referred to as the first month, the second month, the third month, etc.

The Chinese also developed a more detailed solar aspect to their calendar called the 'twenty-four solar terms.' Both the solar and lunar aspects of the Chinese calendar are discussed below.

Conversion Between the Calendars

In this appendix, names such as 'January' refer to the Gregorian calendar. Numbered months, such as the '11th month,' refer to the Chinese calendar.

A *Ten-Thousand-Year Calendar* (《萬年曆》) is a book that allows you to look up any date over a number of years and convert it from one calendar to another. This is a necessary tool for Chinese astrology, Feng Shui, and Day Selection. The data for the current time and date is also necessary for using chrono-acupuncture and some of the other techniques discussed in the *Great Compendium*.

Below, aspects of the Chinese calendar regarding the year, month, day, and hour are explained.

The Year

Every year has its own stem and branch. The year stem and branch repeat every 60 years.

- The same stem-branch combination is used for a particular year whether you are using the solar or the lunar calendar.
- However the start date for the year will vary, depending on whether you are using the lunar or solar calendar.
  - In the lunar calendar, the year begins on the first day of the first lunar month. This is the general day for celebrating the Chinese New Year. See below.
  - If you are using the *twenty-four solar terms* (the Chinese solar calendar), the first day of the year is most often on February 4th. See below.
- This means that whether using the Chinese solar or lunar calendar, the beginning of the Western year (January and the beginning of February) still belongs to the end of the previous year in the Chinese calendar.

The stem and the branch for a year are easy to calculate. If you know the stem-branch for any year, you can count up or down through the cycle of sixty to calculate the stem-branch for any other year. Below is a table covering the years 2010 through 2043.

The Cycle of Sixty					
Year	Cycle of Sixty		Year	Cycle of Sixty	
2010	27	Gēng Yín	2027	44	Dīng Wèi
2011	28	Xīn Mǎo	2028	45	Wù Shēn
2012	29	Rén Chén	2029	46	Jǐ Yǒu
2013	30	Guǐ Sì	2030	47	Gēng Xū
2014	31	Jiǎ Wǔ	2031	48	Xīn Hài
2015	32	Yǐ Wei	2032	49	Rén Zǐ
2016	33	Bǐng Shēn	2033	50	Guǐ Chǒu
2017	34	Dīng Yǒu	2034	51	Jiǎ Yín
2018	35	Wù Xū	2035	52	Yǐ Mǎo
2019	36	Jǐ Hài	2036	53	Bǐng Chén
2020	37	Gēng Zǐ	2037	54	Dīng Sì
2021	38	Xīn Chǒu	2038	55	Wù Wǔ
2022	39	Rén Yín	2039	56	Jǐ Wèi
2023	40	Guǐ Mǎo	2040	57	Gēng Shēn
2024	41	Jiǎ Chén	2041	58	Xīn Yǒu
2025	42	Yǐ Sì	2042	59	Rén Xū
2026	43	Bǐng Wǔ	2043	60	Guǐ Hài

Months: The Lunar Aspect of the Chinese Calendar

In the Chinese lunar calendar, one year consists of 12 or 13 lunar months. A lunar month begins on the day of the new moon. The new moon is the phase of the moon occurring when it passes between the earth and the sun. At that time, the moon is not visible or visible only as a narrow crescent at sunset.

The full moon takes place on the 15th day of the lunar month.

A short lunar month is 29 days and a long lunar month is 30 days. Lunar months vary in length because it takes about 29-1/2 days for the moon to complete one cycle from new moon to new moon from the perspective of planet earth.

When using the lunar calendar, it is easy to know the phase of the moon: On the first, it is a new moon. From the 2nd to the 14th, the moon is waxing. On the 15th, the moon is full. From the 16th through the 29th or 30th, the moon is waning.

A leap month is added about seven times in 19 years in order to keep the calendar 'in accord with heaven.' Certain solar events must always take place at specific times in the lunar calendar. For example, the winter solstice must always take place in the 11th lunar month. When a leap month is added, it must be put in the place that will keep the solstices, equinoxes, and new years day within the correct months.

The Solar Aspect of the Chinese Calendar, also known as the Twenty-Four Solar Terms

The twenty-four solar terms (èr shí sì jié qi 二十四節氣) are twenty-four periods of 15 or 16 days, making up one year. They are defined by solar markers: the solstices and equinoxes. Technically, they are twenty-four equal divisions of the sun's ecliptic. Each term is 15 degrees of longitude, measured along the horizon.

Solstice: Either of two times of the year when the sun is at its greatest distance from the celestial equator. The summer solstice in the Northern Hemisphere occurs about June 21, when the sun is in the zenith at the tropic of Cancer; the winter solstice occurs about December 21, when the sun is over the tropic of Capricorn. The summer solstice is the longest day of the year and the winter solstice is the shortest.

Equinox: Either of the two times during a year when the sun crosses the celestial equator and when the length of day and night are approximately equal; the vernal equinox is in spring and the autumnal equinox is in the fall.

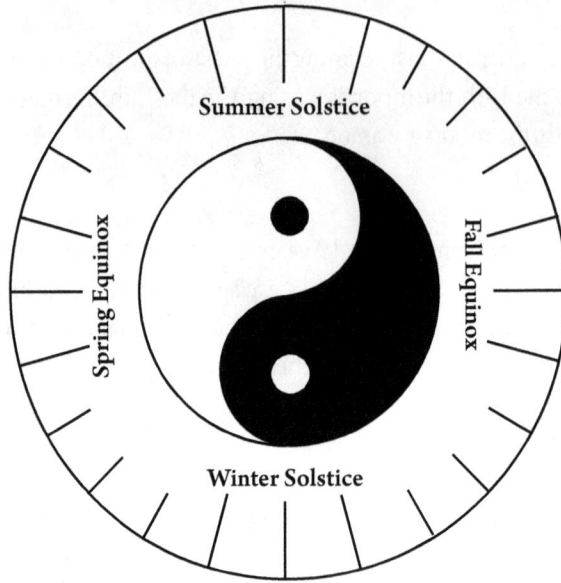

The twenty-four solar terms are:

The Twenty-Four Solar Terms				Approximate Start Date	Chinese Month
	Term	Pinyin	Meaning		
1	立春	Lì Chūn	Spring Commences	Feb 4-5	First
2	雨水	Yǔ Shuǐ	Rain Water	Feb 19-20	
3	驚蟄	Jīng Zhí	Insects Awaken	Mar 5-6	Second
4	春分	Chūn Fēn	Spring Equinox	Mar 21-22	
5	清明	Qīng Míng	Pure Brightness	Apr 4-6	Third
6	穀雨	Gǔ Yǔ	Grain Rain	Apr 20-21	
7	立夏	Lì Xià	Summer Commences	May 5-6	Fourth
8	小滿	Xiǎo Mǎn	Grain Sprouting	May 21-22	
9	芒種	Máng Zhǒng	Grain in Ear	Jun 5-7	Fifth
10	夏至	Xià Zhì	Summer Solstice	Jun 21-22	
11	小暑	Xiǎo Shǔ	Little Heat	Jul 7-8	Sixth
12	大暑	Dà Shǔ	Great Heat	Jul 23-24	
13	立秋	Lì Qiū	Autumn Commences	Aug 7-8	Seventh
14	處暑	Chǔ Shǔ	Heat Finishes	Aug 23-24	
15	白露	Bái Lù	Clear Dew	Sep 7-9	Eighth
16	秋分	Qiū Fēn	Autumn Equinox	Sep 23-24	

17	寒露	Hán Lù	Cold Dew	Oct 8-9	Ninth
18	霜降	Shuāng Jiàng	Frost Descends	Oct 23-24	
19	立冬	Lì Dōng	Winter Commences	Nov 7-8	Tenth
20	小雪	Xiǎo Xuě	Little Snow	Nov 22-23	
21	大雪	Dà Xuě	Great Snow	Dec 7-8	Eleventh
22	冬至	Dōng Zhì	Winter Solstice	Dec 22-23	
23	小寒	Xiǎo Hán	Little Cold	Jan 5-6	Twelfth
24	大寒	Dà Hán	Great Cold	Jan 20-21	

The dates (in our Western calendar) of these solar terms vary within a day or two because our calendar adds a leap day every four years. This makes for a little 'wobble' between the two calendars.

There are two solar terms within one solar month. The twelve solar months start near the beginning (between the 4th and the 9th day) of the Western month.

Spring Commences (Lì Chūn) is the first day of spring, and also the solar Chinese new year. It falls on February 4th or 5th every year. When using the Chinese solar calendar, consider a date before February 4th as belonging to the previous year.

There is never a leap month in the Chinese solar calendar. This is because the solar year is divided evenly into 12 or 24 divisions. Think about this like a pie. If the pie is already cut into eight sections, but seven people show up, there is a remainder. Something must be done with the leftover pie. In some ways, this resembles the lunar calendar. However, if the host waits until the guests show up, and then divides the pie into the exact number of slices so that each guest has an equal share, there is no remainder. This is more like the solar calendar.

These twelve solar months each have a stem and branch. The branch for any given month is the same every year. For example, the fourth month, beginning on May 5th or 6th, always has the branch, sì 巳. However, the stem changes from year to year. See below.

The Stem and Branch of the Month

The 1st month of the year is yín 寅, the 3rd branch. The branch yín corresponds with yáng wood. Wood is the element associated with spring. Chinese new year is associated with spring, the time of birth and new beginnings.

Seasonal beginnings are calculated differently in the Chinese calendar than in the west. In the west, the solstices and equinoxes are considered the first day of a season. The Chinese consider these astronomical events to be the midpoint of a season. Therefore, Chinese spring begins about six weeks prior to Western spring, in the beginning of February. The Chinese view of the seasons will be discussed in more detail below.

The stem for a month will vary from year to year, as there are ten stems and twelve months. The month stem is calculated using the year stem and the month branch. Find the number or branch of the Chinese month in question in the month column on the left. Then read the column with the year stem on the right. The intersection of the month row and the year stem column gives the stem and branch of the month.

The Month Stem and Branch						
Month		Year Stem				
Number	Branch	Jiǎ or Jǐ	Yǐ or Gēng	Bǐng or Xīn	Dīng or Rén	Wù or Guǐ
1	Yín	Bǐng Yín	Wù Yín	Gēng Yín	Rén Yín	Jiǎ Yín
2	Mǎo	Dīng Mǎo	Jǐ Mǎo	Xīn Mǎo	Guǐ Mǎo	Yǐ Mǎo
3	Chén	Wù Chén	Gēng Chén	Rén Chén	Jiǎ Chén	Bǐng Chén
4	Sì	Jǐ Sì	Xīn Sì	Guǐ Sì	Yǐ Sì	Dīng Sì
5	Wǔ	Gēng Wǔ	Rén Wǔ	Jiǎ Wǔ	Bǐng Wǔ	Wù Wǔ
6	Wèi	Xīn Wèi	Guǐ Wèi	Yǐ Wèi	Dīng Wèi	Jǐ Wèi
7	Shēn	Rén Shēn	Jiǎ Shēn	Bǐng Shēn	Wù Shēn	Gēng Shēn
8	Yǒu	Guǐ Yǒu	Yǐ Yǒu	Dīng Yǒu	Jǐ Yǒu	Xīn Yǒu
9	Xū	Jiǎ Xū	Bǐng Xū	Wù Xū	Gēng Xū	Rén Xū
10	Hài	Yǐ Hài	Dīng Hài	Jǐ Hài	Xīn Hài	Guǐ Hài
11	Zǐ	Bǐng Zǐ	Wù Zǐ	Gēng Zǐ	Rén Zǐ	Jiǎ Zǐ
12	Chǒu	Dīng Chǒu	Jǐ Chǒu	Xīn Chǒu	Guǐ Chǒu	Yǐ Chǒu

For example, what is the stem of a shēn (7th) month in a guǐ yǒu year? Follow the 7th month row over to the last column. This is the column for a wù or a guǐ stem year. Therefore, it is the column for a guǐ yǒu year. We find that the shēn month is a gēng shēn month in a guǐ stem year.

Note that the year stems paired in each column are in the relationship of the Five Unities. For example, jiǎ and jǐ unite with each other, as jiǎ is yáng wood and jǐ is yīn earth. This is because the 60 month cycle will repeat every five years. See the section on the Five Unities above.

This table is the same whether using the lunar months or the solar months of the 24 Solar Terms. Only the start date of each month changes.

The Day Stem and Branch

Each day has its own stem and branch. This daily stem and branch combination is the same in both the lunar and the solar calendar. The easiest way to find the day stem and branch is to look it up in the *Ten-Thousand Year Calendar*. Please see appendix b.

針
灸
大
成
·
卷
之
五

The day stem and/or branch are important for calculating open points and for medical day selection.

Time Periods

The Chinese divide the day into 12 two-hour periods or 'double-hours,' each associated with one branch. The branch of any given double-hour is always the same from day to day. For example, noon always falls within the wù branch time period. This is illustrated in the table below:

Branch	Branch #	Double Hour	
Zǐ	1	23:00-01:00	11pm-1am
Chǒu	2	01:00-03:00	1-3am
Yín	3	03:00-05:00	3-5am
Mǎo	4	05:00-07:00	5-7am
Chén	5	07:00-09:00	7-9am
Sì	6	09:00-11:00	9-11am
Wǔ	7	11:00-13:00	11am-1pm
Wèi	8	13:00-15:00	1-3pm
Shēn	9	15:00-17:00	3-5pm
Yǒu	10	17:00-19:00	5-7pm
Xū	11	19:00-21:00	7-9pm
Hài	12	21:00-23:00	9-11pm

Notice that the day starts with the first branch, zǐ, at 11 pm of the evening before. Therefore, if we are concerned with 11:18 pm on September 16th (Western calendar), we would say the hour corresponds to the first branch, zǐ, on September 17th.

Always use local time. We do not need to convert the hour to Greenwich Mean Time, Beijing time or any other standard. We are only concerned with the time according to the local position of the sun. The time when the sun is most closely perpendicular overhead (noon) is always wǔ (午), the 7th hour.

A calculation can also be done to make local time more accurate based on longitude. This calculation does include the use of Greenwich Mean Time, but only as a tool to derive a more accurate local time. This will be briefly discussed below.

We must consider Daylight Savings Time (DST) if it is in effect. DST is used in the warmer months in most of the United States. The government mandates that we move the clock forward an hour for this half of the year. This is an artificial time, as the sun does not jump to a new position when a government says to change the clocks. Because it does not reflect sun time, we need to correct for Daylight Savings Time by 'falling back,' or subtracting one hour from the time on the clock.

For example, if it is 4:30 p.m. on a summer day in a location that uses DST, we need to correct the time to 3:30 p.m. This is 'falling back' one hour.

The branches (not the stems) repeat for the twelve double-hours on a daily basis. For example, 6 a.m. is always during a mǎo branch time. The sixty-hour cycle (using the stems and branches combined) repeats every five days because sixty two-hour periods make 120 hours, or five days.

The stem of a double-hour will change from day to day. You must know the stem of the day in order to find the stem of the hour. In the table that follows, there are five columns on the right, one for each of the five days it takes to complete a sixty-hour cycle. The same column is used for a jiǎ stem day and a jǐ stem day, an yǐ stem day and gēng stem day, etc. This table is basically the same as the table for finding the month stem. The only difference is that here we are using the day stem and the hour branch instead of the year stem and the month branch.

The Double-Hour Stems and Branches						
Double-Hour		**Day Stem**				
Time	Branch	Jiǎ or Jǐ	Yǐ or Gēng	Bǐng or Xīn	Dīng or Rén	Wù or Guǐ
11p-1a	Zǐ	Jiǎ Zǐ	Bǐng Zǐ	Wù Zǐ	Gēng Zǐ	Rén Zǐ
1-3a	Chǒu	Yǐ Chǒu	Dīng Chǒu	Jǐ Chǒu	Xīn Chǒu	Guǐ Chǒu
3-5a	Yín	Bǐng Yín	Wù Yín	Gēng Yín	Rén Yín	Jiǎ Yín
5-7a	Mǎo	Dīng Mǎo	Jǐ Mǎo	Xīn Mǎo	Guǐ Mǎo	Yǐ Mǎo
7-9a	Chén	Wù Chén	Gēng Chén	Rén Chén	Jiǎ Chén	Bǐng Chén
9-11a	Sì	Jǐ Sì	Xīn Sì	Guǐ Sì	Yǐ Sì	Dīng Sì
11a-1p	Wǔ	Gēng Wǔ	Rén Wǔ	Jiǎ Wǔ	Bǐng Wǔ	Wù Wǔ
1-3p	Wèi	Xīn Wèi	Guǐ Wèi	Yǐ Wèi	Dīng Wèi	Jǐ Wèi
3-5p	Shēn	Rén Shēn	Jiǎ Shēn	Bǐng Shēn	Wù Shēn	Gēng Shēn
5-7p	Yǒu	Guǐ Yǒu	Yǐ Yǒu	Dīng Yǒu	Jǐ Yǒu	Xīn Yǒu
7-9p	Xū	Jiǎ Xū	Bǐng Xū	Wù Xū	Gēng Xū	Rén Xū
9-11p	Hài	Yǐ Hài	Dīng Hài	Jǐ Hài	Xīn Hài	Guǐ Hài

Note: Correct for Daylight Savings Time, if necessary.

For example, if you want to find the stem and branch for 4 p.m. on a certain day, you must first find the stem for that day. If it is a xīn stem day, then you would look in the third column from the right in the above table, the one that is labeled 'bǐng or xīn.' Follow that column down until you find the row that is labeled 3-5p. It says that 4 p.m. on a xīn day is bǐng shēn. Remember, 4 p.m. is always a shēn branch hour, regardless of the day stem.

Another example: 8:26 a.m. on a gēng wù day. Follow the 'Yǐ or Gēng' column down because gēng is the day stem. Follow the 7-9 a.m. row across because 8:26 a.m. is within that time period. The two-hour time period in which 8:26 a.m. falls on a gēng stem day is gēng chén.

Sometimes this same table is used, but with the yín branch hour as the first row. That is called the Five Tigers Method because the yín branch is associated with the tiger. This above table is called the Five Zǐ Method because the first row belongs to the zǐ branch.

The Accuracy of Local Time

The world is divided into 24 time zones. If there were a clock for every time zone together in the same room, they would each show a different hour, but the minute hand of the clocks would all be in the same position. This is not the reality of sun time. The time according to the sun varies by minutes within a time zone. We just agree to make the whole time zone the same time to avoid confusion, and to have a standard time within a geographic area.

Greenwich Mean Time (GMT) is the standard time on which all zones base their clocks. We can calculate from Greenwich Mean Time to improve accuracy because it is the one place that uses local sun time. All other time zones are derived from Greenwich Mean Time, not on their own local sun time.

One can calculate local sun time, including minutes, using the longitude of a location. Each degree of longitude is equal to four minutes of time. Fifteen degrees of longitude equals one hour of time difference. Hence, most time zones are 15 degrees wide.

It is beyond the scope of this appendix to describe the method of rectifying local time. However, if you know you are in a time zone that has odd boundaries due to political considerations, you may want to research how to find a more accurate 'sun time' for your location. Otherwise, if you choose points according to the time, your selection will be in error.

A Chinese View of the Four Seasons

The Chinese view the seasons in a different light than we do in the West. In the West, we say that the first day of spring is on the spring equinox, around March 21st. Summer begins on the summer solstice, around June 21st. Fall begins on the autumn equinox, around September 23rd. Winter begins on the winter solstice, around December 22nd. These dates are approximate, and may vary by a day, depending on the exact time of the solstices or equinoxes in any given year.

In China, the seasons were traditionally calculated using the solstices and equinoxes as the mid-point of the season, not the beginning. This makes a Chinese season arrive about six weeks earlier than it does in the West.

For an example of this calculation: there are 89 days between December 22nd (the winter solstice) and March 21st (the spring equinox) in a non-leap year. Half of 89 is 44 or 45 days. February 4th, considered to be the first day of spring, is 45 days after the winter solstice, halfway between the landmarks. The same calculation may be made for the other seasons.

The Seasons	First day (approximate date) of the season in:	
	China	The West
Spring	February 4th	March 21st
Summer	May 5th	June 21st
Fall	August 7th	September 23rd
Winter	November 7th	December 22nd

As you already know, spring belongs to the wood element, summer belongs to fire, fall belongs to metal, and winter belongs to water. But what about earth?

If the average year of 365 days is divided by 5 (for the five elements), you get 73 days. If you divide a year by four seasons, you get about 91 days per season. The difference between 91 days per season and 73 days per element is 18 days. The last 18 days of each season, then, is a buffer period relating to the earth element. You can see this in the following table:

The Seasons with an Earth Buffer in between		
Season	Starts	Element
SPRING	February 4th	Wood
earth buffer	April 17th	Earth
SUMMER	May 5th	Fire
earth buffer	July 20th	Earth
FALL	August 7th	Metal
earth buffer	October 20th	Earth
WINTER	November 7th	Water
earth buffer	January 17th	Earth

This arrangement is similar to the element of the branches for the twelve months:

Month	Branch	Element	Season
1st	Yín	Wood	Spring
2nd	Mǎo		
3rd	Chén	Earth	
4th	Sì	Fire	Summer
5th	Wǔ		
6th	Wèi	Earth	
7th	Shēn	Metal	Autumn
8th	Yǒu		
9th	Xū	Earth	
10th	Hài	Water	Winter
11th	Zǐ		
12th	Chǒu	Earth	

As you can see in the above table, the first two months in any season have the same element as the season. The third month of a season is an earth buffer month. This is the most common way we will view the seasons.

There is a second way that earth may be dealt with, as far as the seasons go: sometimes the Chinese used five seasons, adding 'late summer' as an independent season related to the earth element. This was related to the climate in China:

Wood relates to wind, which is predominant in the spring.
Fire relates to heat, which is predominant in the summer.
Earth relates to dampness, which is predominant as rain in the 'late summer.'
Metal relates to dryness, which is predominant in the autumn.
Water relates to cold, which is predominant in winter.

Once again, the average year of 365 days divided by 5 (for five seasons) is 73 days. Now we have five consecutive seasons of 73 days each. This gives us the following (the calculation is based on the solar terms):

The Five Seasons (including Late Summer)			
Season	**Starts**	**Calculation**	**Element**
Spring	January 20th	1st day of Great Cold	Wood
Summer	April 3rd	13th day after Spring Equinox	Fire
Late Summer	June 16th	10th day after Grain in Ear	Earth
Fall	August 30th	7th day after Heat Finishes	Metal
Winter	November 11th	4th day after Winter Commences	Water

These dates come out of the *Yellow Emperor's Inner Canon, Elementary Questions.*

While the dates of the Chinese seasons may seem quite early to the Westerner, remember how early the first flowers, such as crocus, appear as the first sign of spring. Think how soon the first really warm day comes, when you can go outside without a jacket; surely this is the genesis of summer. The fall harvest can begin at the end of August or beginning of September. And in many places the first frost of winter shows up in November. The Chinese appear more attune to the first sign of a season, than to fullness of it, as we do in the West.

Guide to Using the Calendar Pages

In the following pages, one year goes across two facing sheets.

- The top row contains the year with its stem and branch.
- The second and third rows are headings for the twelve lunar months (plus a leap month if necessary) and the stem and branch of the month.
- The first day of the first lunar month is Chinese lunar new year.
- Because the Chinese lunar year begins at a different time than the Western new year, the fourth row shows when the Western year changes.
- Next there are 30 numbered rows. These show the day of the lunar month. The first day of the lunar month is the new moon day. The 15th day of the lunar month is the full moon day. Some months have 29 days and others have 30 days.
- The bottom four rows show the twenty-four solar terms.

  o The Jié 節 are the terms than come at the beginning of the Western month. The Jié are considered the beginning of the Chinese solar "month." They are also highlighted in the calendar above. For example, Lì Chūn 立春 is "Spring Commences." It occurs on February 4th in most years, so under Lì Chūn, it says 2/4 and the exact time it occurs. In the calendar above, 2/4 is highlighted. This sometimes occurs in the same column and sometimes in an adjacent column. Note for example, that 2/4 is highlighted in the year 2012 as the 13th day of the first month.

  o The Qì 氣 are the solar terms that come in the second half of the Western month.

- Each day according to the Western calendar is recorded as month/day. January 23rd of the Western Gregorian calendar is written as 1/23.
- The stem and branch for the day is recorded next to it.
- The stem is always written before the branch.

Example: April 15th, 2012

- Turn to the pages for 2012.
- Locate 4/15.
- It is in the 3rd month column and the 25th day row. So it is the 25th day of the third lunar month. We know the moon was waning at the time because it is after the 15th day of the lunar month.
- April 15th, 2012 is a Bǐng Wǔ day. If we want to use Midnight-Noon Flowing and Pooling points, we now know it is a Bǐng day. If we want to use the Eight Methods of the Mystical Tortoise, we see it is a Bǐng Wǔ day.
- April 15th, 2012 is in a Jiǎ Chén month, and a Rén Chén year.
- April 15th, 2012 occurs in the solar term called Qīng Míng 清明 (Jié) because it is after April 4th, the first day of Qing Ming that year, and before Gǔ Yǔ 穀雨 (Qì) which occurs on April 20th, 2012.

	YEAR: 2010 Gēng Yín -- First six months.										
	1ST MONTH		2ND MONTH		3RD MONTH		4TH MONTH		5TH MONTH		6TH MONTH
	Wù Yín		Jǐ Mǎo		Gēng Chén		Xīn Sì		Rén Wǔ		Guǐ Wèi
1	2/14	Yǐ Wèi	3/16	Yǐ Chǒu	4/14	Jiǎ Wǔ	5/14	Jiǎ Zǐ	6/12	Guǐ Sì	7/12	Guǐ Hài
2	2/15	Bǐng Shēn	3/17	Bǐng Yín	4/15	Yǐ Wèi	5/15	Yǐ Chǒu	6/13	Jiǎ Wǔ	7/13	Jiǎ Zǐ
3	2/16	Dīng Yǒu	3/18	Dīng Mǎo	4/16	Bǐng Shēn	5/16	Bǐng Yín	6/14	Yǐ Wèi	7/14	Yǐ Chǒu
4	2/17	Wù Xū	3/19	Wù Chén	4/17	Dīng Yǒu	5/17	Dīng Mǎo	6/15	Bǐng Shēn	7/15	Bǐng Yín
5	2/18	Jǐ Hài	3/20	Jǐ Sì	4/18	Wù Xū	5/18	Wù Chén	6/16	Dīng Yǒu	7/16	Dīng Mǎo
6	2/19	Gēng Zǐ	3/21	Gēng Wǔ	4/19	Jǐ Hài	5/19	Jǐ Sì	6/17	Wù Xū	7/17	Wù Chén
7	2/20	Xīn Chǒu	3/22	Xīn Wèi	4/20	Gēng Zǐ	5/20	Gēng Wǔ	6/18	Jǐ Hài	7/18	Jǐ Sì
8	2/21	Rén Yín	3/23	Rén Shēn	4/21	Xīn Chǒu	5/21	Xīn Wèi	6/19	Gēng Zǐ	7/19	Gēng Wǔ
9	2/22	Guǐ Mǎo	3/24	Guǐ Yǒu	4/22	Rén Yín	5/22	Rén Shēn	6/20	Xīn Chǒu	7/20	Xīn Wèi
10	2/23	Jiǎ Chén	3/25	Jiǎ Xū	4/23	Guǐ Mǎo	5/23	Guǐ Yǒu	6/21	Rén Yín	7/21	Rén Shēn
11	2/24	Yǐ Sì	3/26	Yǐ Hài	4/24	Jiǎ Chén	5/24	Jiǎ Xū	6/22	Guǐ Mǎo	7/22	Guǐ Yǒu
12	2/25	Bǐng Wǔ	3/27	Bǐng Zǐ	4/25	Yǐ Sì	5/25	Yǐ Hài	6/23	Jiǎ Chén	7/23	Jiǎ Xū
13	2/26	Dīng Wèi	3/28	Dīng Chǒu	4/26	Bǐng Wǔ	5/26	Bǐng Zǐ	6/24	Yǐ Sì	7/24	Yǐ Hài
14	2/27	Wù Shēn	3/29	Wù Yín	4/27	Dīng Wèi	5/27	Dīng Chǒu	6/25	Bǐng Wǔ	7/25	Bǐng Zǐ
15	2/28	Jǐ Yǒu	3/30	Jǐ Mǎo	4/28	Wù Shēn	5/28	Wù Yín	6/26	Dīng Wèi	7/26	Dīng Chǒu
16	3/1	Gēng Xū	3/31	Gēng Chén	4/29	Jǐ Yǒu	5/29	Jǐ Mǎo	6/27	Wù Shēn	7/27	Wù Yín
17	3/2	Xīn Hài	4/1	Xīn Sì	4/30	Gēng Xū	5/30	Gēng Chén	6/28	Jǐ Yǒu	7/28	Jǐ Mǎo
18	3/3	Rén Zǐ	4/2	Rén Wǔ	5/1	Xīn Hài	5/31	Xīn Sì	6/29	Gēng Xū	7/29	Gēng Chén
19	3/4	Guǐ Chǒu	4/3	Guǐ Wèi	5/2	Rén Zǐ	6/1	Rén Wǔ	6/30	Xīn Hài	7/30	Xīn Sì
20	3/5	Jiǎ Yín	4/4	Jiǎ Shēn	5/3	Guǐ Chǒu	6/2	Guǐ Wèi	7/1	Rén Zǐ	7/31	Rén Wǔ
21	3/6	Yǐ Mǎo	4/5	Yǐ Yǒu	5/4	Jiǎ Yín	6/3	Jiǎ Shēn	7/2	Guǐ Chǒu	8/1	Guǐ Wèi
22	3/7	Bǐng Chén	4/6	Bǐng Xū	5/5	Yǐ Mǎo	6/4	Yǐ Yǒu	7/3	Jiǎ Yín	8/2	Jiǎ Shēn
23	3/8	Dīng Sì	4/7	Dīng Hài	5/6	Bǐng Chén	6/5	Bǐng Xū	7/4	Yǐ Mǎo	8/3	Yǐ Yǒu
24	3/9	Wù Wǔ	4/8	Wù Zǐ	5/7	Dīng Sì	6/6	Dīng Hài	7/5	Bǐng Chén	8/4	Bǐng Xū
25	3/10	Jǐ Wèi	4/9	Jǐ Chǒu	5/8	Wù Wǔ	6/7	Wù Zǐ	7/6	Dīng Sì	8/5	Dīng Hài
26	3/11	Gēng Shēn	4/10	Gēng Yín	5/9	Jǐ Wèi	6/8	Jǐ Chǒu	7/7	Wù Wǔ	8/6	Wù Zǐ
27	3/12	Xīn Yǒu	4/11	Xīn Mǎo	5/10	Gēng Shēn	6/9	Gēng Yín	7/8	Jǐ Wèi	8/7	Jǐ Chǒu
28	3/13	Rén Xū	4/12	Rén Chén	5/11	Xīn Yǒu	6/10	Xīn Mǎo	7/9	Gēng Shēn	8/8	Gēng Yín
29	3/14	Guǐ Hài	4/13	Guǐ Sì	5/12	Rén Xū	6/11	Rén Chén	7/10	Xīn Yǒu	8/9	Xīn Mǎo
30	3/15	Jiǎ Zǐ			5/13	Guǐ Hài			7/11	Rén Xū		
Jie	Li Chun		Jing Zhi		Qing Ming		Li Xia		Mang Zhong		Xiao Shu	
	2/4	6:42a	3/6	12:52a	4/5	5:55a	5/5	11:29p	6/6	3:51a	7/7	2:14p
Qi	Yu Shui		Chun Fen		Gu Yu		Xiao Man		Xia Zhi		Da Shu	
	2/19	2:35a	3/21	1:48a	4/20	1:07p	5/21	12:29p	6/21	8:35p	7/23	7:28a

206

針灸大成 · 卷之五

YEAR: 2010 Gēng Yín -- Last six months.												
7TH MONTH		8TH MONTH		9TH MONTH		10TH MONTH		11TH MONTH		12TH MONTH		
Jiǎ Shēn		Yǐ Yǒu		Bǐng Xū		Dīng Hài		Wù Zǐ		Jǐ Chǒu		
								2010 - 2011				
8/10	Rén Chén	9/8	Xīn Yǒu	10/8	Xīn Mǎo	11/6	Gēng Shēn	12/6	Gēng Yín	1/4	Jǐ Wèi	1
8/11	Guǐ Sì	9/9	Rén Xū	10/9	Rén Chén	11/7	Xīn Yǒu	12/7	Xīn Mǎo	1/5	Gēng Shēn	2
8/12	Jiǎ Wǔ	9/10	Guǐ Hài	10/10	Guǐ Sì	11/8	Rén Xū	12/8	Rén Chén	1/6	Xīn Yǒu	3
8/13	Yǐ Wèi	9/11	Jiǎ Zǐ	10/11	Jiǎ Wǔ	11/9	Guǐ Hài	12/9	Guǐ Sì	1/7	Rén Xū	4
8/14	Bǐng Shēn	9/12	Yǐ Chǒu	10/12	Yǐ Wèi	11/10	Jiǎ Zǐ	12/10	Jiǎ Wǔ	1/8	Guǐ Hài	5
8/15	Dīng Yǒu	9/13	Bǐng Yín	10/13	Bǐng Shēn	11/11	Yǐ Chǒu	12/11	Yǐ Wèi	1/9	Jiǎ Zǐ	6
8/16	Wù Xū	9/14	Dīng Mǎo	10/14	Dīng Yǒu	11/12	Bǐng Yín	12/12	Bǐng Shēn	1/10	Yǐ Chǒu	7
8/17	Jǐ Hài	9/15	Wù Chén	10/15	Wù Xū	11/13	Dīng Mǎo	12/13	Dīng Yǒu	1/11	Bǐng Yín	8
8/18	Gēng Zǐ	9/16	Jǐ Sì	10/16	Jǐ Hài	11/14	Wù Chén	12/14	Wù Xū	1/12	Dīng Mǎo	9
8/19	Xīn Chǒu	9/17	Gēng Wǔ	10/17	Gēng Zǐ	11/15	Jǐ Sì	12/15	Jǐ Hài	1/13	Wù Chén	10
8/20	Rén Yín	9/18	Xīn Wèi	10/18	Xīn Chǒu	11/16	Gēng Wǔ	12/16	Gēng Zǐ	1/14	Jǐ Sì	11
8/21	Guǐ Mǎo	9/19	Rén Shēn	10/19	Rén Yín	11/17	Xīn Wèi	12/17	Xīn Chǒu	1/15	Gēng Wǔ	12
8/22	Jiǎ Chén	9/20	Guǐ Yǒu	10/20	Guǐ Mǎo	11/18	Rén Shēn	12/18	Rén Yín	1/16	Xīn Wèi	13
8/23	Yǐ Sì	9/21	Jiǎ Xū	10/21	Jiǎ Chén	11/19	Guǐ Yǒu	12/19	Guǐ Mǎo	1/17	Rén Shēn	14
8/24	Bǐng Wǔ	9/22	Yǐ Hài	10/22	Yǐ Sì	11/20	Jiǎ Xū	12/20	Jiǎ Chén	1/18	Guǐ Yǒu	15
8/25	Dīng Wèi	9/23	Bǐng Zǐ	10/23	Bǐng Wǔ	11/21	Yǐ Hài	12/21	Yǐ Sì	1/19	Jiǎ Xū	16
8/26	Wù Shēn	9/24	Dīng Chǒu	10/24	Dīng Wèi	11/22	Bǐng Zǐ	12/22	Bǐng Wǔ	1/20	Yǐ Hài	17
8/27	Jǐ Yǒu	9/25	Wù Yín	10/25	Wù Shēn	11/23	Dīng Chǒu	12/23	Dīng Wèi	1/21	Bǐng Zǐ	18
8/28	Gēng Xū	9/26	Jǐ Mǎo	10/26	Jǐ Yǒu	11/24	Wù Yín	12/24	Wù Shēn	1/22	Dīng Chǒu	19
8/29	Xīn Hài	9/27	Gēng Chén	10/27	Gēng Xū	11/25	Jǐ Mǎo	12/25	Jǐ Yǒu	1/23	Wù Yín	20
8/30	Rén Zǐ	9/28	Xīn Sì	10/28	Xīn Hài	11/26	Gēng Chén	12/26	Gēng Xū	1/24	Jǐ Mǎo	21
8/31	Guǐ Chǒu	9/29	Rén Wǔ	10/29	Rén Zǐ	11/27	Xīn Sì	12/27	Xīn Hài	1/25	Gēng Chén	22
9/1	Jiǎ Yín	9/30	Guǐ Wèi	10/30	Guǐ Chǒu	11/28	Rén Wǔ	12/28	Rén Zǐ	1/26	Xīn Sì	23
9/2	Yǐ Mǎo	10/1	Jiǎ Shēn	10/31	Jiǎ Yín	11/29	Guǐ Wèi	12/29	Guǐ Chǒu	1/27	Rén Wǔ	24
9/3	Bǐng Chén	10/2	Yǐ Yǒu	11/1	Yǐ Mǎo	11/30	Jiǎ Shēn	12/30	Jiǎ Yín	1/28	Guǐ Wèi	25
9/4	Dīng Sì	10/3	Bǐng Xū	11/2	Bǐng Chén	12/1	Yǐ Yǒu	12/31	Yǐ Mǎo	1/29	Jiǎ Shēn	26
9/5	Wù Wǔ	10/4	Dīng Hài	11/3	Dīng Sì	12/2	Bǐng Xū	1/1	Bǐng Chén	1/30	Yǐ Yǒu	27
9/6	Jǐ Wèi	10/5	Wù Zǐ	11/4	Wù Wǔ	12/3	Dīng Hài	1/2	Dīng Sì	1/31	Bǐng Xū	28
9/7	Gēng Shēn	10/6	Jǐ Chǒu	11/5	Jǐ Wèi	12/4	Wù Zǐ	1/3	Wù Wǔ	2/1	Dīng Hài	29
		10/7	Gēng Yín			12/5	Jǐ Chǒu			2/2	Wù Zǐ	30
Li Qiu		Bai Lu		Han Lu		Li Dong		Da Xue		Xiao Han		Jie
8/7	11:57p	9/8	2:41a	10/8	6:05p	11/7	9:01p	12/7	1:41p	1/6	12:50a	
Chu Shu		Qiu Fen		Shuang Jiang		Xiao Xue		Dong Zhi		Da Han		Qi
8/23	2:24p	9/23	11:48a	10/23	8:54p	11/22	6:16p	12/22	7:29a	1/20	6:07p	

	1ST MONTH		2ND MONTH		3RD MONTH		4TH MONTH		5TH MONTH		6TH MONTH	
	Gēng Yín		Xīn Mǎo		Rén Chén		Guǐ Sì		Jiǎ Wǔ		Yǐ Wèi	
1	2/3	Jǐ Chǒu	3/5	Jǐ Wèi	4/3	Wù Zǐ	5/3	Wù Wǔ	6/2	Wù Zǐ	7/1	Dīng Sì
2	2/4	Gēng Yín	3/6	Gēng Shēn	4/4	Jǐ Chǒu	5/4	Jǐ Wèi	6/3	Jǐ Chǒu	7/2	Wù Wǔ
3	2/5	Xīn Mǎo	3/7	Xīn Yǒu	4/5	Gēng Yín	5/5	Gēng Shēn	6/4	Gēng Yín	7/3	Jǐ Wèi
4	2/6	Rén Chén	3/8	Rén Xū	4/6	Xīn Mǎo	5/6	Xīn Yǒu	6/5	Xīn Mǎo	7/4	Gēng Shēn
5	2/7	Guǐ Sì	3/9	Guǐ Hài	4/7	Rén Chén	5/7	Rén Xū	6/6	Rén Chén	7/5	Xīn Yǒu
6	2/8	Jiǎ Wǔ	3/10	Jiǎ Zǐ	4/8	Guǐ Sì	5/8	Guǐ Hài	6/7	Guǐ Sì	7/6	Rén Xū
7	2/9	Yǐ Wèi	3/11	Yǐ Chǒu	4/9	Jiǎ Wǔ	5/9	Jiǎ Zǐ	6/8	Jiǎ Wǔ	7/7	Guǐ Hài
8	2/10	Bǐng Shēn	3/12	Bǐng Yín	4/10	Yǐ Wèi	5/10	Yǐ Chǒu	6/9	Yǐ Wèi	7/8	Jiǎ Zǐ
9	2/11	Dīng Yǒu	3/13	Dīng Mǎo	4/11	Bǐng Shēn	5/11	Bǐng Yín	6/10	Bǐng Shēn	7/9	Yǐ Chǒu
10	2/12	Wù Xū	3/14	Wù Chén	4/12	Dīng Yǒu	5/12	Dīng Mǎo	6/11	Dīng Yǒu	7/10	Bǐng Yín
11	2/13	Jǐ Hài	3/15	Jǐ Sì	4/13	Wù Xū	5/13	Wù Chén	6/12	Wù Xū	7/11	Dīng Mǎo
12	2/14	Gēng Zǐ	3/16	Gēng Wǔ	4/14	Jǐ Hài	5/14	Jǐ Sì	6/13	Jǐ Hài	7/12	Wù Chén
13	2/15	Xīn Chǒu	3/17	Xīn Wèi	4/15	Gēng Zǐ	5/15	Gēng Wǔ	6/14	Gēng Zǐ	7/13	Jǐ Sì
14	2/16	Rén Yín	3/18	Rén Shēn	4/16	Xīn Chǒu	5/16	Xīn Wèi	6/15	Xīn Chǒu	7/14	Gēng Wǔ
15	2/17	Guǐ Mǎo	3/19	Guǐ Yǒu	4/17	Rén Yín	5/17	Rén Shēn	6/16	Rén Yín	7/15	Xīn Wèi
16	2/18	Jiǎ Chén	3/20	Jiǎ Xū	4/18	Guǐ Mǎo	5/18	Guǐ Yǒu	6/17	Guǐ Mǎo	7/16	Rén Shēn
17	2/19	Yǐ Sì	3/21	Yǐ Hài	4/19	Jiǎ Chén	5/19	Jiǎ Xū	6/18	Jiǎ Chén	7/17	Guǐ Yǒu
18	2/20	Bǐng Wǔ	3/22	Bǐng Zǐ	4/20	Yǐ Sì	5/20	Yǐ Hài	6/19	Yǐ Sì	7/18	Jiǎ Xū
19	2/21	Dīng Wèi	3/23	Dīng Chǒu	4/21	Bǐng Wǔ	5/21	Bǐng Zǐ	6/20	Bǐng Wǔ	7/19	Yǐ Hài
20	2/22	Wù Shēn	3/24	Wù Yín	4/22	Dīng Wèi	5/22	Dīng Chǒu	6/21	Dīng Wèi	7/20	Bǐng Zǐ
21	2/23	Jǐ Yǒu	3/25	Jǐ Mǎo	4/23	Wù Shēn	5/23	Wù Yín	6/22	Wù Shēn	7/21	Dīng Chǒu
22	2/24	Gēng Xū	3/26	Gēng Chén	4/24	Jǐ Yǒu	5/24	Jǐ Mǎo	6/23	Jǐ Yǒu	7/22	Wù Yín
23	2/25	Xīn Hài	3/27	Xīn Sì	4/25	Gēng Xū	5/25	Gēng Chén	6/24	Gēng Xū	7/23	Jǐ Mǎo
24	2/26	Rén Zǐ	3/28	Rén Wǔ	4/26	Xīn Hài	5/26	Xīn Sì	6/25	Xīn Hài	7/24	Gēng Chén
25	2/27	Guǐ Chǒu	3/29	Guǐ Wèi	4/27	Rén Zǐ	5/27	Rén Wǔ	6/26	Rén Zǐ	7/25	Xīn Sì
26	2/28	Jiǎ Yín	3/30	Jiǎ Shēn	4/28	Guǐ Chǒu	5/28	Guǐ Wèi	6/27	Guǐ Chǒu	7/26	Rén Wǔ
27	3/1	Yǐ Mǎo	3/31	Yǐ Yǒu	4/29	Jiǎ Yín	5/29	Jiǎ Shēn	6/28	Jiǎ Yín	7/27	Guǐ Wèi
28	3/2	Bǐng Chén	4/1	Bǐng Xū	4/30	Yǐ Mǎo	5/30	Yǐ Yǒu	6/29	Yǐ Mǎo	7/28	Jiǎ Shēn
29	3/3	Dīng Sì	4/2	Dīng Hài	5/1	Bǐng Chén	5/31	Bǐng Xū	6/30	Bǐng Chén	7/29	Yǐ Yǒu
30	3/4	Wù Wǔ			5/2	Dīng Sì	6/1	Dīng Hài			7/30	Bǐng Xū
Jie	Li Chun		Jing Zhi		Qing Ming		Li Xia		Mang Zhong		Xiao Shu	
	2/4	12:32p	3/6	6:43a	4/5	11:46a	5/6	5:20a	6/6	9:43a	7/7	8:06p
Qi	Yu Shui		Chun Fen		Gu Yu		Xiao Man		Xia Zhi		Da Shu	
	2/19	8:24a	3/21	7:37a	4/20	6:56p	5/21	6:18p	6/22	2:24a	7/23	1:17p

YEAR: 2011 Xīn Mǎo -- First six months.

針灸大成・卷之五

YEAR: 2011 Xīn Mǎo -- Last six months.												
7TH MONTH		8TH MONTH		9TH MONTH		10TH MONTH		11TH MONTH		12TH MONTH		
Bǐng Shēn		Dīng Yǒu		Wù Xū		Jǐ Hài		Gēng Zǐ		Xīn Chǒu		
										2011 - 2012		
7/31	Dīng Hài	8/29	Bǐng Chén	9/27	Yǐ Yǒu	10/27	Yǐ Mǎo	11/25	Jiǎ Shēn	12/25	Jiǎ Yín	1
8/1	Wù Zǐ	8/30	Dīng Sì	9/28	Bǐng Xū	10/28	Bǐng Chén	11/26	Yǐ Yǒu	12/26	Yǐ Mǎo	2
8/2	Jǐ Chǒu	8/31	Wù Wǔ	9/29	Dīng Hài	10/29	Dīng Sì	11/27	Bǐng Xū	12/27	Bǐng Chén	3
8/3	Gēng Yín	9/1	Jǐ Wèi	9/30	Wù Zǐ	10/30	Wù Wǔ	11/28	Dīng Hài	12/28	Dīng Sì	4
8/4	Xīn Mǎo	9/2	Gēng Shēn	10/1	Jǐ Chǒu	10/31	Jǐ Wèi	11/29	Wù Zǐ	12/29	Wù Wǔ	5
8/5	Rén Chén	9/3	Xīn Yǒu	10/2	Gēng Yín	11/1	Gēng Shēn	11/30	Jǐ Chǒu	12/30	Jǐ Wèi	6
8/6	Guǐ Sì	9/4	Rén Xū	10/3	Xīn Mǎo	11/2	Xīn Yǒu	12/1	Gēng Yín	12/31	Gēng Shēn	7
8/7	Jiǎ Wǔ	9/5	Guǐ Hài	10/4	Rén Chén	11/3	Rén Xū	12/2	Xīn Mǎo	1/1	Xīn Yǒu	8
8/8	Yǐ Wèi	9/6	Jiǎ Zǐ	10/5	Guǐ Sì	11/4	Guǐ Hài	12/3	Rén Chén	1/2	Rén Xū	9
8/9	Bǐng Shēn	9/7	Yǐ Chǒu	10/6	Jiǎ Wǔ	11/5	Jiǎ Zǐ	12/4	Guǐ Sì	1/3	Guǐ Hài	10
8/10	Dīng Yǒu	9/8	Bǐng Yín	10/7	Yǐ Wèi	11/6	Yǐ Chǒu	12/5	Jiǎ Wǔ	1/4	Jiǎ Zǐ	11
8/11	Wù Xū	9/9	Dīng Mǎo	10/8	Bǐng Shēn	11/7	Bǐng Yín	12/6	Yǐ Wèi	1/5	Yǐ Chǒu	12
8/12	Jǐ Hài	9/10	Wù Chén	10/9	Dīng Yǒu	11/8	Dīng Mǎo	12/7	Bǐng Shēn	1/6	Bǐng Yín	13
8/13	Gēng Zǐ	9/11	Jǐ Sì	10/10	Wù Xū	11/9	Wù Chén	12/8	Dīng Yǒu	1/7	Dīng Mǎo	14
8/14	Xīn Chǒu	9/12	Gēng Wǔ	10/11	Jǐ Hài	11/10	Jǐ Sì	12/9	Wù Xū	1/8	Wù Chén	15
8/15	Rén Yín	9/13	Xīn Wèi	10/12	Gēng Zǐ	11/11	Gēng Wǔ	12/10	Jǐ Hài	1/9	Jǐ Sì	16
8/16	Guǐ Mǎo	9/14	Rén Shēn	10/13	Xīn Chǒu	11/12	Xīn Wèi	12/11	Gēng Zǐ	1/10	Gēng Wǔ	17
8/17	Jiǎ Chén	9/15	Guǐ Yǒu	10/14	Rén Yín	11/13	Rén Shēn	12/12	Xīn Chǒu	1/11	Xīn Wèi	18
8/18	Yǐ Sì	9/16	Jiǎ Xū	10/15	Guǐ Mǎo	11/14	Guǐ Yǒu	12/13	Rén Yín	1/12	Rén Shēn	19
8/19	Bǐng Wǔ	9/17	Yǐ Hài	10/16	Jiǎ Chén	11/15	Jiǎ Xū	12/14	Guǐ Mǎo	1/13	Guǐ Yǒu	20
8/20	Dīng Wèi	9/18	Bǐng Zǐ	10/17	Yǐ Sì	11/16	Yǐ Hài	12/15	Jiǎ Chén	1/14	Jiǎ Xū	21
8/21	Wù Shēn	9/19	Dīng Chǒu	10/18	Bǐng Wǔ	11/17	Bǐng Zǐ	12/16	Yǐ Sì	1/15	Yǐ Hài	22
8/22	Jǐ Yǒu	9/20	Wù Yín	10/19	Dīng Wèi	11/18	Dīng Chǒu	12/17	Bǐng Wǔ	1/16	Bǐng Zǐ	23
8/23	Gēng Xū	9/21	Jǐ Mǎo	10/20	Wù Shēn	11/19	Wù Yín	12/18	Dīng Wèi	1/17	Dīng Chǒu	24
8/24	Xīn Hài	9/22	Gēng Chén	10/21	Jǐ Yǒu	11/20	Jǐ Mǎo	12/19	Wù Shēn	1/18	Wù Yín	25
8/25	Rén Zǐ	9/23	Xīn Sì	10/22	Gēng Xū	11/21	Gēng Chén	12/20	Jǐ Yǒu	1/19	Jǐ Mǎo	26
8/26	Guǐ Chǒu	9/24	Rén Wǔ	10/23	Xīn Hài	11/22	Xīn Sì	12/21	Gēng Xū	1/20	Gēng Chén	27
8/27	Jiǎ Yín	9/25	Guǐ Wèi	10/24	Rén Zǐ	11/23	Rén Wǔ	12/22	Xīn Hài	1/21	Xīn Sì	28
8/28	Yǐ Mǎo	9/26	Jiǎ Shēn	10/25	Guǐ Chǒu	11/24	Guǐ Wèi	12/23	Rén Zǐ	1/22	Rén Wǔ	29
				10/26	Jiǎ Yín			12/24	Guǐ Chǒu			30
Li Qiu		Bai Lu		Han Lu		Li Dong		Da Xue		Xiao Han		Jie
8/8	5:49a	9/8	8:33a	10/8	11:57p	11/8	2:52a	12/7	7:32p	1/6	6:41a	
Chu Shu		Qiu Fen		Shuang Jiang		Xiao Xue		Dong Zhi		Da Han		Qi
8/23	8:13p	9/23	5:37p	10/24	2:43a	11/23	12:05a	12/22	1:18p	1/20	11:56p	

YEAR: 2012 Rén Chén -- First six months.														
	1ST MONTH		2ND MONTH		3RD MONTH		4TH MONTH		LEAP MONTH		5Th MONTH		6TH MONTH	
	Rén Yín		Guǐ Mǎo		Jiǎ Chén		Yǐ Sì				Bǐng Wǔ		Dīng Wèi	
1	1/23	Guǐ Wèi	2/22	Guǐ Chǒu	3/22	Rén Wǔ	4/21	Rén Zǐ	5/21	Rén Wǔ	6/19	Xīn Hài	7/19	Xīn Sì
2	1/24	Jiǎ Shēn	2/23	Jiǎ Yín	3/23	Guǐ Wèi	4/22	Guǐ Chǒu	5/22	Guǐ Wèi	6/20	Rén Zǐ	7/20	Rén Wǔ
3	1/25	Yǐ Yǒu	2/24	Yǐ Mǎo	3/24	Jiǎ Shēn	4/23	Jiǎ Yín	5/23	Jiǎ Shēn	6/21	Guǐ Chǒu	7/21	Guǐ Wèi
4	1/26	Bǐng Xū	2/25	Bǐng Chén	3/25	Yǐ Yǒu	4/24	Yǐ Mǎo	5/24	Yǐ Yǒu	6/22	Jiǎ Yín	7/22	Jiǎ Shēn
5	1/27	Dīng Hài	2/26	Dīng Sì	3/26	Bǐng Xū	4/25	Bǐng Chén	5/25	Bǐng Xū	6/23	Yǐ Mǎo	7/23	Yǐ Yǒu
6	1/28	Wù Zǐ	2/27	Wù Wǔ	3/27	Dīng Hài	4/26	Dīng Sì	5/26	Dīng Hài	6/24	Bǐng Chén	7/24	Bǐng Xū
7	1/29	Jǐ Chǒu	2/28	Jǐ Wèi	3/28	Wù Zǐ	4/27	Wù Wǔ	5/27	Wù Zǐ	6/25	Dīng Sì	7/25	Dīng Hài
8	1/30	Gēng Yín	2/29	Gēng Shēn	3/29	Jǐ Chǒu	4/28	Jǐ Wèi	5/28	Jǐ Chǒu	6/26	Wù Wǔ	7/26	Wù Zǐ
9	1/31	Xīn Mǎo	3/1	Xīn Yǒu	3/30	Gēng Yín	4/29	Gēng Shēn	5/29	Gēng Yín	6/27	Jǐ Wèi	7/27	Jǐ Chǒu
10	2/1	Rén Chén	3/2	Rén Xū	3/31	Xīn Mǎo	4/30	Xīn Yǒu	5/30	Xīn Mǎo	6/28	Gēng Shēn	7/28	Gēng Yín
11	2/2	Guǐ Sì	3/3	Guǐ Hài	4/1	Rén Chén	5/1	Rén Xū	5/31	Rén Chén	6/29	Xīn Yǒu	7/29	Xīn Mǎo
12	2/3	Jiǎ Wǔ	3/4	Jiǎ Zǐ	4/2	Guǐ Sì	5/2	Guǐ Hài	6/1	Guǐ Sì	6/30	Rén Xū	7/30	Rén Chén
13	2/4	Yǐ Wèi	3/5	Yǐ Chǒu	4/3	Jiǎ Wǔ	5/3	Jiǎ Zǐ	6/2	Jiǎ Wǔ	7/1	Guǐ Hài	7/31	Guǐ Sì
14	2/5	Bǐng Shēn	3/6	Bǐng Yín	4/4	Yǐ Wèi	5/4	Yǐ Chǒu	6/3	Yǐ Wèi	7/2	Jiǎ Zǐ	8/1	Jiǎ Wǔ
15	2/6	Dīng Yǒu	3/7	Dīng Mǎo	4/5	Bǐng Shēn	5/5	Bǐng Yín	6/4	Bǐng Shēn	7/3	Yǐ Chǒu	8/2	Yǐ Wèi
16	2/7	Wù Xū	3/8	Wù Chén	4/6	Dīng Yǒu	5/6	Dīng Mǎo	6/5	Dīng Yǒu	7/4	Bǐng Yín	8/3	Bǐng Shēn
17	2/8	Jǐ Hài	3/9	Jǐ Sì	4/7	Wù Xū	5/7	Wù Chén	6/6	Wù Xū	7/5	Dīng Mǎo	8/4	Dīng Yǒu
18	2/9	Gēng Zǐ	3/10	Gēng Wǔ	4/8	Jǐ Hài	5/8	Jǐ Sì	6/7	Jǐ Hài	7/6	Wù Chén	8/5	Wù Xū
19	2/10	Xīn Chǒu	3/11	Xīn Wèi	4/9	Gēng Zǐ	5/9	Gēng Wǔ	6/8	Gēng Zǐ	7/7	Jǐ Sì	8/6	Jǐ Hài
20	2/11	Rén Yín	3/12	Rén Shēn	4/10	Xīn Chǒu	5/10	Xīn Wèi	6/9	Xīn Chǒu	7/8	Gēng Wǔ	8/7	Gēng Zǐ
21	2/12	Guǐ Mǎo	3/13	Guǐ Yǒu	4/11	Rén Yín	5/11	Rén Shēn	6/10	Rén Yín	7/9	Xīn Wèi	8/8	Xīn Chǒu
22	2/13	Jiǎ Chén	3/14	Jiǎ Xū	4/12	Guǐ Mǎo	5/12	Guǐ Yǒu	6/11	Guǐ Mǎo	7/10	Rén Shēn	8/9	Rén Yín
23	2/14	Yǐ Sì	3/15	Yǐ Hài	4/13	Jiǎ Chén	5/13	Jiǎ Xū	6/12	Jiǎ Chén	7/11	Guǐ Yǒu	8/10	Guǐ Mǎo
24	2/15	Bǐng Wǔ	3/16	Bǐng Zǐ	4/14	Yǐ Sì	5/14	Yǐ Hài	6/13	Yǐ Sì	7/12	Jiǎ Xū	8/11	Jiǎ Chén
25	2/16	Dīng Wèi	3/17	Dīng Chǒu	4/15	Bǐng Wǔ	5/15	Bǐng Zǐ	6/14	Bǐng Wǔ	7/13	Yǐ Hài	8/12	Yǐ Sì
26	2/17	Wù Shēn	3/18	Wù Yín	4/16	Dīng Wèi	5/16	Dīng Chǒu	6/15	Dīng Wèi	7/14	Bǐng Zǐ	8/13	Bǐng Wǔ
27	2/18	Jǐ Yǒu	3/19	Jǐ Mǎo	4/17	Wù Shēn	5/17	Wù Yín	6/16	Wù Shēn	7/15	Dīng Chǒu	8/14	Dīng Wèi
28	2/19	Gēng Xū	3/20	Gēng Chén	4/18	Jǐ Yǒu	5/18	Jǐ Mǎo	6/17	Jǐ Yǒu	7/16	Wù Yín	8/15	Wù Shēn
29	2/20	Xīn Hài	3/21	Xīn Sì	4/19	Gēng Xū	5/19	Gēng Chén	6/18	Gēng Xū	7/17	Jǐ Mǎo	8/16	Jǐ Yǒu
30	2/21	Rén Zǐ			4/20	Xīn Hài	5/20	Xīn Sì			7/18	Gēng Chén		
Jie	Li Chun		Jing Zhi		Qing Ming		Li Xia				Mang Zhong		Xiao Shu	
	2/4	6:40p	3/5	12:28p	4/4	5:16p	5/5	10:40a			6/5	2:50p	7/7	1:21a
Qi	Yu Shui		Chun Fen		Gu Yu		Xiao Man				Xia Zhi		Da Shu	
	2/19	2:25p	3/20	1:20p	4/20	12:25a	5/20	11:40p			6/21	7:45a	7/22	6:51p

針灸大成 · 卷之五

	YEAR: 2012 Rén Chén -- Last six months.											
7TH MONTH		**8TH MONTH**		**9TH MONTH**		**10TH MONTH**		**11TH MONTH**		**12TH MONTH**		
Wù Shēn		Jǐ Yǒu		Gēng Xū		Xīn Hài		Rén Zǐ		Guǐ Chǒu		
										2011 - 2012		
8/17	Gēng Xū	9/16	Gēng Chén	10/15	Jǐ Yǒu	11/14	Jǐ Mǎo	12/13	Wù Shēn	1/12	Wù Yín	1
8/18	Xīn Hài	9/17	Xīn Sì	10/16	Gēng Xū	11/15	Gēng Chén	12/14	Jǐ Yǒu	1/13	Jǐ Mǎo	2
8/19	Rén Zǐ	9/18	Rén Wǔ	10/17	Xīn Hài	11/16	Xīn Sì	12/15	Gēng Xū	1/14	Gēng Chén	3
8/20	Guǐ Chǒu	9/19	Guǐ Wèi	10/18	Rén Zǐ	11/17	Rén Wǔ	12/16	Xīn Hài	1/15	Xīn Sì	4
8/21	Jiǎ Yín	9/20	Jiǎ Shēn	10/19	Guǐ Chǒu	11/18	Guǐ Wèi	12/17	Rén Zǐ	1/16	Rén Wǔ	5
8/22	Yǐ Mǎo	9/21	Yǐ Yǒu	10/20	Jiǎ Yín	11/19	Jiǎ Shēn	12/18	Guǐ Chǒu	1/17	Guǐ Wèi	6
8/23	Bǐng Chén	9/22	Bǐng Xū	10/21	Yǐ Mǎo	11/20	Yǐ Yǒu	12/19	Jiǎ Yín	1/18	Jiǎ Shēn	7
8/24	Dīng Sì	9/23	Dīng Hài	10/22	Bǐng Chén	11/21	Bǐng Xū	12/20	Yǐ Mǎo	1/19	Yǐ Yǒu	8
8/25	Wù Wǔ	9/24	Wù Zǐ	10/23	Dīng Sì	11/22	Dīng Hài	12/21	Bǐng Chén	1/20	Bǐng Xū	9
8/26	Jǐ Wèi	9/25	Jǐ Chǒu	10/24	Wù Wǔ	11/23	Wù Zǐ	12/22	Dīng Sì	1/21	Dīng Hài	10
8/27	Gēng Shēn	9/26	Gēng Yín	10/25	Jǐ Wèi	11/24	Jǐ Chǒu	12/23	Wù Wǔ	1/22	Wù Zǐ	11
8/28	Xīn Yǒu	9/27	Xīn Mǎo	10/26	Gēng Shēn	11/25	Gēng Yín	12/24	Jǐ Wèi	1/23	Jǐ Chǒu	12
8/29	Rén Xū	9/28	Rén Chén	10/27	Xīn Yǒu	11/26	Xīn Mǎo	12/25	Gēng Shēn	1/24	Gēng Yín	13
8/30	Guǐ Hài	9/29	Guǐ Sì	10/28	Rén Xū	11/27	Rén Chén	12/26	Xīn Yǒu	1/25	Xīn Mǎo	14
8/31	Jiǎ Zǐ	9/30	Jiǎ Wǔ	10/29	Guǐ Hài	11/28	Guǐ Sì	12/27	Rén Xū	1/26	Rén Chén	15
9/1	Yǐ Chǒu	10/1	Yǐ Wèi	10/30	Jiǎ Zǐ	11/29	Jiǎ Wǔ	12/28	Guǐ Hài	1/27	Guǐ Sì	16
9/2	Bǐng Yín	10/2	Bǐng Shēn	10/31	Yǐ Chǒu	11/30	Yǐ Wèi	12/29	Jiǎ Zǐ	1/28	Jiǎ Wǔ	17
9/3	Dīng Mǎo	10/3	Dīng Yǒu	11/1	Bǐng Yín	12/1	Bǐng Shēn	12/30	Yǐ Chǒu	1/29	Yǐ Wèi	18
9/4	Wù Chén	10/4	Wù Xū	11/2	Dīng Mǎo	12/2	Dīng Yǒu	12/31	Bǐng Yín	1/30	Bǐng Shēn	19
9/5	Jǐ Sì	10/5	Jǐ Hài	11/3	Wù Chén	12/3	Wù Xū	1/1	Dīng Mǎo	1/31	Dīng Yǒu	20
9/6	Gēng Wǔ	10/6	Gēng Zǐ	11/4	Jǐ Sì	12/4	Jǐ Hài	1/2	Wù Chén	2/1	Wù Xū	21
9/7	Xīn Wèi	10/7	Xīn Chǒu	11/5	Gēng Wǔ	12/5	Gēng Zǐ	1/3	Jǐ Sì	2/2	Jǐ Hài	22
9/8	Rén Shēn	10/8	Rén Yín	11/6	Xīn Wèi	12/6	Xīn Chǒu	1/4	Gēng Wǔ	2/3	Gēng Zǐ	23
9/9	Guǐ Yǒu	10/9	Guǐ Mǎo	11/7	Rén Shēn	12/7	Rén Yín	1/5	Xīn Wèi	2/4	Xīn Chǒu	24
9/10	Jiǎ Xū	10/10	Jiǎ Chén	11/8	Guǐ Yǒu	12/8	Guǐ Mǎo	1/6	Rén Shēn	2/5	Rén Yín	25
9/11	Yǐ Hài	10/11	Yǐ Sì	11/9	Jiǎ Xū	12/9	Jiǎ Chén	1/7	Guǐ Yǒu	2/6	Guǐ Mǎo	26
9/12	Bǐng Zǐ	10/12	Bǐng Wǔ	11/10	Yǐ Hài	12/10	Yǐ Sì	1/8	Jiǎ Xū	2/7	Jiǎ Chén	27
9/13	Dīng Chǒu	10/13	Dīng Wèi	11/11	Bǐng Zǐ	12/11	Bǐng Wǔ	1/9	Yǐ Hài	2/8	Yǐ Sì	28
9/14	Wù Yín	10/14	Wù Shēn	11/12	Dīng Chǒu	12/12	Dīng Wèi	1/10	Bǐng Zǐ	2/9	Bǐng Wǔ	29
9/15	Jǐ Mǎo			11/13	Wù Yín			1/11	Dīng Chǒu			30
Li Qiu		Bai Lu		Han Lu		Li Dong		Da Xue		Xiao Han		Jie
8/7	11:26a	9/7	2:44p	10/8	6:42a	11/7	9:56a	12/7	2:32a	1/5	1:16p	
Chu Shu		Qiu Fen		Shuang Jiang		Xiao Xue		Dong Zhi		Da Han		Qi
8/23	2:16a	9/23	12:18a	10/23	9:52a	11/22	7:19p	12/21	8:16p	1/20	6:26a	

YEAR: 2013 Guǐ Sì -- First six months.												
	1ST MONTH		2ND MONTH		3RD MONTH		4TH MONTH		5TH MONTH		6TH MONTH	
	Jiǎ Yín		Yǐ Mǎo		Bǐng Chén		Dīng Sì		Wù Wǔ		Jǐ Wèi	
1	2/10	Dīng Wèi	3/12	Dīng Chǒu	4/10	Bǐng Wǔ	5/10	Bǐng Zǐ	6/9	Bǐng Wǔ	7/8	Yǐ Hài
2	2/11	Wù Shēn	3/13	Wù Yín	4/11	Dīng Wèi	5/11	Dīng Chǒu	6/10	Dīng Wèi	7/9	Bǐng Zǐ
3	2/12	Jǐ Yǒu	3/14	Jǐ Mǎo	4/12	Wù Shēn	5/12	Wù Yín	6/11	Wù Shēn	7/10	Dīng Chǒu
4	2/13	Gēng Xū	3/15	Gēng Chén	4/13	Jǐ Yǒu	5/13	Jǐ Mǎo	6/12	Jǐ Yǒu	7/11	Wù Yín
5	2/14	Xīn Hài	3/16	Xīn Sì	4/14	Gēng Xū	5/14	Gēng Chén	6/13	Gēng Xū	7/12	Jǐ Mǎo
6	2/15	Rén Zǐ	3/17	Rén Wǔ	4/15	Xīn Hài	5/15	Xīn Sì	6/14	Xīn Hài	7/13	Gēng Chén
7	2/16	Guǐ Chǒu	3/18	Guǐ Wèi	4/16	Rén Zǐ	5/16	Rén Wǔ	6/15	Rén Zǐ	7/14	Xīn Sì
8	2/17	Jiǎ Yín	3/19	Jiǎ Shēn	4/17	Guǐ Chǒu	5/17	Guǐ Wèi	6/16	Guǐ Chǒu	7/15	Rén Wǔ
9	2/18	Yǐ Mǎo	3/20	Yǐ Yǒu	4/18	Jiǎ Yín	5/18	Jiǎ Shēn	6/17	Jiǎ Yín	7/16	Guǐ Wèi
10	2/19	Bǐng Chén	3/21	Bǐng Xū	4/19	Yǐ Mǎo	5/19	Yǐ Yǒu	6/18	Yǐ Mǎo	7/17	Jiǎ Shēn
11	2/20	Dīng Sì	3/22	Dīng Hài	4/20	Bǐng Chén	5/20	Bǐng Xū	6/19	Bǐng Chén	7/18	Yǐ Yǒu
12	2/21	Wù Wǔ	3/23	Wù Zǐ	4/21	Dīng Sì	5/21	Dīng Hài	6/20	Dīng Sì	7/19	Bǐng Xū
13	2/22	Jǐ Wèi	3/24	Jǐ Chǒu	4/22	Wù Wǔ	5/22	Wù Zǐ	6/21	Wù Wǔ	7/20	Dīng Hài
14	2/23	Gēng Shēn	3/25	Gēng Yín	4/23	Jǐ Wèi	5/23	Jǐ Chǒu	6/22	Jǐ Wèi	7/21	Wù Zǐ
15	2/24	Xīn Yǒu	3/26	Xīn Mǎo	4/24	Gēng Shēn	5/24	Gēng Yín	6/23	Gēng Shēn	7/22	Jǐ Chǒu
16	2/25	Rén Xū	3/27	Rén Chén	4/25	Xīn Yǒu	5/25	Xīn Mǎo	6/24	Xīn Yǒu	7/23	Gēng Yín
17	2/26	Guǐ Hài	3/28	Guǐ Sì	4/26	Rén Xū	5/26	Rén Chén	6/25	Rén Xū	7/24	Xīn Mǎo
18	2/27	Jiǎ Zǐ	3/29	Jiǎ Wǔ	4/27	Guǐ Hài	5/27	Guǐ Sì	6/26	Guǐ Hài	7/25	Rén Chén
19	2/28	Yǐ Chǒu	3/30	Yǐ Wèi	4/28	Jiǎ Zǐ	5/28	Jiǎ Wǔ	6/27	Jiǎ Zǐ	7/26	Guǐ Sì
20	3/1	Bǐng Yín	3/31	Bǐng Shēn	4/29	Yǐ Chǒu	5/29	Yǐ Wèi	6/28	Yǐ Chǒu	7/27	Jiǎ Wǔ
21	3/2	Dīng Mǎo	4/1	Dīng Yǒu	4/30	Bǐng Yín	5/30	Bǐng Shēn	6/29	Bǐng Yín	7/28	Yǐ Wèi
22	3/3	Wù Chén	4/2	Wù Xū	5/1	Dīng Mǎo	5/31	Dīng Yǒu	6/30	Dīng Mǎo	7/29	Bǐng Shēn
23	3/4	Jǐ Sì	4/3	Jǐ Hài	5/2	Wù Chén	6/1	Wù Xū	7/1	Wù Chén	7/30	Dīng Yǒu
24	3/5	Gēng Wǔ	4/4	Gēng Zǐ	5/3	Jǐ Sì	6/2	Jǐ Hài	7/2	Jǐ Sì	7/31	Wù Xū
25	3/6	Xīn Wèi	4/5	Xīn Chǒu	5/4	Gēng Wǔ	6/3	Gēng Zǐ	7/3	Gēng Wǔ	8/1	Jǐ Hài
26	3/7	Rén Shēn	4/6	Rén Yín	5/5	Xīn Wèi	6/4	Xīn Chǒu	7/4	Xīn Wèi	8/2	Gēng Zǐ
27	3/8	Guǐ Yǒu	4/7	Guǐ Mǎo	5/6	Rén Shēn	6/5	Rén Yín	7/5	Rén Shēn	8/3	Xīn Chǒu
28	3/9	Jiǎ Xū	4/8	Jiǎ Chén	5/7	Guǐ Yǒu	6/6	Guǐ Mǎo	7/6	Guǐ Yǒu	8/4	Rén Yín
29	3/10	Yǐ Hài	4/9	Yǐ Sì	5/8	Jiǎ Xū	6/7	Jiǎ Chén	7/7	Jiǎ Xū	8/5	Guǐ Mǎo
30	3/11	Bǐng Zǐ			5/9	Yǐ Hài	6/8	Yǐ Sì			8/6	Jiǎ Chén
Jie	Li Chun		Jing Zhi		Qing Ming		Li Xia		Mang Zhong		Xiao Shu	
	2/4	12:31a	3/5	6:19p	4/4	11:05a	5/5	4:28p	6/5	8:44p	7/7	7:09a
Qi	Yu Shui		Chun Fen		Gu Yu		Xiao Man		Xia Zhi		Da Shu	
	2/18	8:15p	3/20	7:09p	4/20	6:14a	5/21	5:29a	6/21	1:33p	7/23	12:40a

針灸大成・卷之五

YEAR: 2013 Guǐ Sì -- Last six months.												
7TH MONTH		8TH MONTH		9TH MONTH		10TH MONTH		11TH MONTH		12TH MONTH		
Gēng Shēn		Xīn Yǒu		Rén Xū		Guǐ Hài		Jiǎ Zǐ		Yǐ Chǒu		
								2013		**2014**		
8/7	Yǐ Sì	9/5	Jiǎ Xū	10/5	Jiǎ Chén	11/3	Guǐ Yǒu	12/3	Guǐ Mǎo	1/1	Rén Shēn	1
8/8	Bǐng Wǔ	9/6	Yǐ Hài	10/6	Yǐ Sì	11/4	Jiǎ Xū	12/4	Jiǎ Chén	1/2	Guǐ Yǒu	2
8/9	Dīng Wèi	9/7	Bǐng Zǐ	10/7	Bǐng Wǔ	11/5	Yǐ Hài	12/5	Yǐ Sì	1/3	Jiǎ Xū	3
8/10	Wù Shēn	9/8	Dīng Chǒu	10/8	Dīng Wèi	11/6	Bǐng Zǐ	12/6	Bǐng Wǔ	1/4	Yǐ Hài	4
8/11	Jǐ Yǒu	9/9	Wù Yín	10/9	Wù Shēn	11/7	Dīng Chǒu	12/7	Dīng Wèi	1/5	Bǐng Zǐ	5
8/12	Gēng Xū	9/10	Jǐ Mǎo	10/10	Jǐ Yǒu	11/8	Wù Yín	12/8	Wù Shēn	1/6	Dīng Chǒu	6
8/13	Xīn Hài	9/11	Gēng Chén	10/11	Gēng Xū	11/9	Jǐ Mǎo	12/9	Jǐ Yǒu	1/7	Wù Yín	7
8/14	Rén Zǐ	9/12	Xīn Sì	10/12	Xīn Hài	11/10	Gēng Chén	12/10	Gēng Xū	1/8	Jǐ Mǎo	8
8/15	Guǐ Chǒu	9/13	Rén Wǔ	10/13	Rén Zǐ	11/11	Xīn Sì	12/11	Xīn Hài	1/9	Gēng Chén	9
8/16	Jiǎ Yín	9/14	Guǐ Wèi	10/14	Guǐ Chǒu	11/12	Rén Wǔ	12/12	Rén Zǐ	1/10	Xīn Sì	10
8/17	Yǐ Mǎo	9/15	Jiǎ Shēn	10/15	Jiǎ Yín	11/13	Guǐ Wèi	12/13	Guǐ Chǒu	1/11	Rén Wǔ	11
8/18	Bǐng Chén	9/16	Yǐ Yǒu	10/16	Yǐ Mǎo	11/14	Jiǎ Shēn	12/14	Jiǎ Yín	1/12	Guǐ Wèi	12
8/19	Dīng Sì	9/17	Bǐng Xū	10/17	Bǐng Chén	11/15	Yǐ Yǒu	12/15	Yǐ Mǎo	1/13	Jiǎ Shēn	13
8/20	Wù Wǔ	9/18	Dīng Hài	10/18	Dīng Sì	11/16	Bǐng Xū	12/16	Bǐng Chén	1/14	Yǐ Yǒu	14
8/21	Jǐ Wèi	9/19	Wù Zǐ	10/19	Wù Wǔ	11/17	Dīng Hài	12/17	Dīng Sì	1/15	Bǐng Xū	15
8/22	Gēng Shēn	9/20	Jǐ Chǒu	10/20	Jǐ Wèi	11/18	Wù Zǐ	12/18	Wù Wǔ	1/16	Dīng Hài	16
8/23	Xīn Yǒu	9/21	Gēng Yín	10/21	Gēng Shēn	11/19	Jǐ Chǒu	12/19	Jǐ Wèi	1/17	Wù Zǐ	17
8/24	Rén Xū	9/22	Xīn Mǎo	10/22	Xīn Yǒu	11/20	Gēng Yín	12/20	Gēng Shēn	1/18	Jǐ Chǒu	18
8/25	Guǐ Hài	9/23	Rén Chén	10/23	Rén Xū	11/21	Xīn Mǎo	12/21	Xīn Yǒu	1/19	Gēng Yín	19
8/26	Jiǎ Zǐ	9/24	Guǐ Sì	10/24	Guǐ Hài	11/22	Rén Chén	12/22	Rén Xū	1/20	Xīn Mǎo	20
8/27	Yǐ Chǒu	9/25	Jiǎ Wǔ	10/25	Jiǎ Zǐ	11/23	Guǐ Sì	12/23	Guǐ Hài	1/21	Rén Chén	21
8/28	Bǐng Yín	9/26	Yǐ Wèi	10/26	Yǐ Chǒu	11/24	Jiǎ Wǔ	12/24	Jiǎ Zǐ	1/22	Guǐ Sì	22
8/29	Dīng Mǎo	9/27	Bǐng Shēn	10/27	Bǐng Yín	11/25	Yǐ Wèi	12/25	Yǐ Chǒu	1/23	Jiǎ Wǔ	23
8/30	Wù Chén	9/28	Dīng Yǒu	10/28	Dīng Mǎo	11/26	Bǐng Shēn	12/26	Bǐng Yín	1/24	Yǐ Wèi	24
8/31	Jǐ Sì	9/29	Wù Xū	10/29	Wù Chén	11/27	Dīng Yǒu	12/27	Dīng Mǎo	1/25	Bǐng Shēn	25
9/1	Gēng Wǔ	9/30	Jǐ Hài	10/30	Jǐ Sì	11/28	Wù Xū	12/28	Wù Chén	1/26	Dīng Yǒu	26
9/2	Xīn Wèi	10/1	Gēng Zǐ	10/31	Gēng Wǔ	11/29	Jǐ Hài	12/29	Jǐ Sì	1/27	Wù Xū	27
9/3	Rén Shēn	10/2	Xīn Chǒu	11/1	Xīn Wèi	11/30	Gēng Zǐ	12/30	Gēng Wǔ	1/28	Jǐ Hài	28
9/4	Guǐ Yǒu	10/3	Rén Yín	11/2	Rén Shēn	12/1	Xīn Chǒu	12/31	Xīn Wèi	1/29	Gēng Zǐ	29
		10/4	Guǐ Mǎo			12/2	Rén Yín			1/30	Xīn Chǒu	30
Li Qiu		Bai Lu		Han Lu		Li Dong		Da Xue		Xiao Han		Jie
8/7	5:14p	9/7	8:33p	10/8	12:31p	11/7	3:45p	12/7	8:21a	1/6	8:07p	
Chu Shu		Qiu Fen		Shuang Jiang		Xiao Xue		Dong Zhi		Da Han		Qi
8/23	8:05a	9/23	6:22a	10/23	3:41p	11/22	1:08p	12/22	2:05a	1/20	12:15p	

YEAR: 2014 Jiǎ Wǔ -- First six months.											
1ST MONTH		2ND MONTH		3RD MONTH		4TH MONTH		5TH MONTH		6TH MONTH	
Bǐng Yín		Dīng Mǎo		Wù Chén		Jǐ Sì		Gēng Wǔ		Xīn Wèi	
1	1/31 Rén Yín	3/1 Xīn Wèi		3/31 Xīn Chǒu		4/29 Gēng Wǔ		5/29 Gēng Zǐ		6/27 Jǐ Sì	
2	2/1 Guǐ Mǎo	3/2 Rén Shēn		4/1 Rén Yín		4/30 Xīn Wèi		5/30 Xīn Chǒu		6/28 Gēng Wǔ	
3	2/2 Jiǎ Chén	3/3 Guǐ Yǒu		4/2 Guǐ Mǎo		5/1 Rén Shēn		5/31 Rén Yín		6/29 Xīn Wèi	
4	2/3 Yǐ Sì	3/4 Jiǎ Xū		4/3 Jiǎ Chén		5/2 Guǐ Yǒu		6/1 Guǐ Mǎo		6/30 Rén Shēn	
5	2/4 Bǐng Wǔ	3/5 Yǐ Hài		4/4 Yǐ Sì		5/3 Jiǎ Xū		6/2 Jiǎ Chén		7/1 Guǐ Yǒu	
6	2/5 Dīng Wèi	3/6 Bǐng Zǐ		4/5 Bǐng Wǔ		5/4 Yǐ Hài		6/3 Yǐ Sì		7/2 Jiǎ Xū	
7	2/6 Wù Shēn	3/7 Dīng Chǒu		4/6 Dīng Wèi		5/5 Bǐng Zǐ		6/4 Bǐng Wǔ		7/3 Yǐ Hài	
8	2/7 Jǐ Yǒu	3/8 Wù Yín		4/7 Wù Shēn		5/6 Dīng Chǒu		6/5 Dīng Wèi		7/4 Bǐng Zǐ	
9	2/8 Gēng Xū	3/9 Jǐ Mǎo		4/8 Jǐ Yǒu		5/7 Wù Yín		6/6 Wù Shēn		7/5 Dīng Chǒu	
10	2/9 Xīn Hài	3/10 Gēng Chén		4/9 Gēng Xū		5/8 Jǐ Mǎo		6/7 Jǐ Yǒu		7/6 Wù Yín	
11	2/10 Rén Zǐ	3/11 Xīn Sì		4/10 Xīn Hài		5/9 Gēng Chén		6/8 Gēng Xū		7/7 Jǐ Mǎo	
12	2/11 Guǐ Chǒu	3/12 Rén Wǔ		4/11 Rén Zǐ		5/10 Xīn Sì		6/9 Xīn Hài		7/8 Gēng Chén	
13	2/12 Jiǎ Yín	3/13 Guǐ Wèi		4/12 Guǐ Chǒu		5/11 Rén Wǔ		6/10 Rén Zǐ		7/9 Xīn Sì	
14	2/13 Yǐ Mǎo	3/14 Jiǎ Shēn		4/13 Jiǎ Yín		5/12 Guǐ Wèi		6/11 Guǐ Chǒu		7/10 Rén Wǔ	
15	2/14 Bǐng Chén	3/15 Yǐ Yǒu		4/14 Yǐ Mǎo		5/13 Jiǎ Shēn		6/12 Jiǎ Yín		7/11 Guǐ Wèi	
16	2/15 Dīng Sì	3/16 Bǐng Xū		4/15 Bǐng Chén		5/14 Yǐ Yǒu		6/13 Yǐ Mǎo		7/12 Jiǎ Shēn	
17	2/16 Wù Wǔ	3/17 Dīng Hài		4/16 Dīng Sì		5/15 Bǐng Xū		6/14 Bǐng Chén		7/13 Yǐ Yǒu	
18	2/17 Jǐ Wèi	3/18 Wù Zǐ		4/17 Wù Wǔ		5/16 Dīng Hài		6/15 Dīng Sì		7/14 Bǐng Xū	
19	2/18 Gēng Shēn	3/19 Jǐ Chǒu		4/18 Jǐ Wèi		5/17 Wù Zǐ		6/16 Wù Wǔ		7/15 Dīng Hài	
20	2/19 Xīn Yǒu	3/20 Gēng Yín		4/19 Gēng Shēn		5/18 Jǐ Chǒu		6/17 Jǐ Wèi		7/16 Wù Zǐ	
21	2/20 Rén Xū	3/21 Xīn Mǎo		4/20 Xīn Yǒu		5/19 Gēng Yín		6/18 Gēng Shēn		7/17 Jǐ Chǒu	
22	2/21 Guǐ Hài	3/22 Rén Chén		4/21 Rén Xū		5/20 Xīn Mǎo		6/19 Xīn Yǒu		7/18 Gēng Yín	
23	2/22 Jiǎ Zǐ	3/23 Guǐ Sì		4/22 Guǐ Hài		5/21 Rén Chén		6/20 Rén Xū		7/19 Xīn Mǎo	
24	2/23 Yǐ Chǒu	3/24 Jiǎ Wǔ		4/23 Jiǎ Zǐ		5/22 Guǐ Sì		6/21 Guǐ Hài		7/20 Rén Chén	
25	2/24 Bǐng Yín	3/25 Yǐ Wèi		4/24 Yǐ Chǒu		5/23 Jiǎ Wǔ		6/22 Jiǎ Zǐ		7/21 Guǐ Sì	
26	2/25 Dīng Mǎo	3/26 Bǐng Shēn		4/25 Bǐng Yín		5/24 Yǐ Wèi		6/23 Yǐ Chǒu		7/22 Jiǎ Wǔ	
27	2/26 Wù Chén	3/27 Dīng Yǒu		4/26 Dīng Mǎo		5/25 Bǐng Shēn		6/24 Bǐng Yín		7/23 Yǐ Wèi	
28	2/27 Jǐ Sì	3/28 Wù Xū		4/27 Wù Chén		5/26 Dīng Yǒu		6/25 Dīng Mǎo		7/24 Bǐng Shēn	
29	2/28 Gēng Wǔ	3/29 Jǐ Hài		4/28 Jǐ Sì		5/27 Wù Xū		6/26 Wù Chén		7/25 Dīng Yǒu	
30		3/30 Gēng Zǐ				5/28 Jǐ Hài				7/26 Wù Xū	
Jie	Li Chun	Jing Zhi		Qing Ming		Li Xia		Mang Zhong		Xiao Shu	
	2/4 6:21a	3/6 12:07a		4/5 4:54a		5/5 10:16p		6/6 2:32a		7/7 12:57p	
Qi	Yu Shui	Chun Fen		Gu Yu		Xiao Man		Xia Zhi		Da Shu	
	2/19 2:04a	3/21 12:57a		4/20 12:12p		5/21 12:17p		6/21 7:21p		7/23 6:27a	

214

針灸大成 · 卷之五

YEAR: 2014 Jiǎ Wǔ -- Last six months.														
7TH MONTH		8TH MONTH		9TH MONTH		LEAP MONTH		10TH MONTH		11TH MONTH		12TH MONTH		
Rén Shēn		Guǐ Yǒu		Jiǎ Xū				Yǐ Hài		Bǐng Zǐ		Dīng Chǒu		
								2014 - 2015						
7/27	Jǐ Hài	8/25	Wù Chén	9/24	Wù Xū	10/24	Wù Chén	11/22	Dīng Yǒu	12/22	Dīng Mǎo	1/20	Bǐng Shēn	1
7/28	Gēng Zǐ	8/26	Jǐ Sì	9/25	Jǐ Hài	10/25	Jǐ Sì	11/23	Wù Xū	12/23	Wù Chén	1/21	Dīng Yǒu	2
7/29	Xīn Chǒu	8/27	Gēng Wǔ	9/26	Gēng Zǐ	10/26	Gēng Wǔ	11/24	Jǐ Hài	12/24	Jǐ Sì	1/22	Wù Xū	3
7/30	Rén Yín	8/28	Xīn Wèi	9/27	Xīn Chǒu	10/27	Xīn Wèi	11/25	Gēng Zǐ	12/25	Gēng Wǔ	1/23	Jǐ Hài	4
7/31	Guǐ Mǎo	8/29	Rén Shēn	9/28	Rén Yín	10/28	Rén Shēn	11/26	Xīn Chǒu	12/26	Xīn Wèi	1/24	Gēng Zǐ	5
8/1	Jiǎ Chén	8/30	Guǐ Yǒu	9/29	Guǐ Mǎo	10/29	Guǐ Yǒu	11/27	Rén Yín	12/27	Rén Shēn	1/25	Xīn Chǒu	6
8/2	Yǐ Sì	8/31	Jiǎ Xū	9/30	Jiǎ Chén	10/30	Jiǎ Xū	11/28	Guǐ Mǎo	12/28	Guǐ Yǒu	1/26	Rén Yín	7
8/3	Bǐng Wǔ	9/1	Yǐ Hài	10/1	Yǐ Sì	10/31	Yǐ Hài	11/29	Jiǎ Chén	12/29	Jiǎ Xū	1/27	Guǐ Mǎo	8
8/4	Dīng Wèi	9/2	Bǐng Zǐ	10/2	Bǐng Wǔ	11/1	Bǐng Zǐ	11/30	Yǐ Sì	12/30	Yǐ Hài	1/28	Jiǎ Chén	9
8/5	Wù Shēn	9/3	Dīng Chǒu	10/3	Dīng Wèi	11/2	Dīng Chǒu	12/1	Bǐng Wǔ	12/31	Bǐng Zǐ	1/29	Yǐ Sì	10
8/6	Jǐ Yǒu	9/4	Wù Yín	10/4	Wù Shēn	11/3	Wù Yín	12/2	Dīng Wèi	1/1	Dīng Chǒu	1/30	Bǐng Wǔ	11
8/7	Gēng Xū	9/5	Jǐ Mǎo	10/5	Jǐ Yǒu	11/4	Jǐ Mǎo	12/3	Wù Shēn	1/2	Wù Yín	1/31	Dīng Wèi	12
8/8	Xīn Hài	9/6	Gēng Chén	10/6	Gēng Xū	11/5	Gēng Chén	12/4	Jǐ Yǒu	1/3	Jǐ Mǎo	2/1	Wù Shēn	13
8/9	Rén Zǐ	9/7	Xīn Sì	10/7	Xīn Hài	11/6	Xīn Sì	12/5	Gēng Xū	1/4	Gēng Chén	2/2	Jǐ Yǒu	14
8/10	Guǐ Chǒu	9/8	Rén Wǔ	10/8	Rén Zǐ	11/7	Rén Wǔ	12/6	Xīn Hài	1/5	Xīn Sì	2/3	Gēng Xū	15
8/11	Jiǎ Yín	9/9	Guǐ Wèi	10/9	Guǐ Chǒu	11/8	Guǐ Wèi	12/7	Rén Zǐ	1/6	Rén Wǔ	2/4	Xīn Hài	16
8/12	Yǐ Mǎo	9/10	Jiǎ Shēn	10/10	Jiǎ Yín	11/9	Jiǎ Shēn	12/8	Guǐ Chǒu	1/7	Guǐ Wèi	2/5	Rén Zǐ	17
8/13	Bǐng Chén	9/11	Yǐ Yǒu	10/11	Yǐ Mǎo	11/10	Yǐ Yǒu	12/9	Jiǎ Yín	1/8	Jiǎ Shēn	2/6	Guǐ Chǒu	18
8/14	Dīng Sì	9/12	Bǐng Xū	10/12	Bǐng Chén	11/11	Bǐng Xū	12/10	Yǐ Mǎo	1/9	Yǐ Yǒu	2/7	Jiǎ Yín	19
8/15	Wù Wǔ	9/13	Dīng Hài	10/13	Dīng Sì	11/12	Dīng Hài	12/11	Bǐng Chén	1/10	Bǐng Xū	2/8	Yǐ Mǎo	20
8/16	Jǐ Wèi	9/14	Wù Zǐ	10/14	Wù Wǔ	11/13	Wù Zǐ	12/12	Dīng Sì	1/11	Dīng Hài	2/9	Bǐng Chén	21
8/17	Gēng Shēn	9/15	Jǐ Chǒu	10/15	Jǐ Wèi	11/14	Jǐ Chǒu	12/13	Wù Wǔ	1/12	Wù Zǐ	2/10	Dīng Sì	22
8/18	Xīn Yǒu	9/16	Gēng Yín	10/16	Gēng Shēn	11/15	Gēng Yín	12/14	Jǐ Wèi	1/13	Jǐ Chǒu	2/11	Wù Wǔ	23
8/19	Rén Xū	9/17	Xīn Mǎo	10/17	Xīn Yǒu	11/16	Xīn Mǎo	12/15	Gēng Shēn	1/14	Gēng Yín	2/12	Jǐ Wèi	24
8/20	Guǐ Hài	9/18	Rén Chén	10/18	Rén Xū	11/17	Rén Chén	12/16	Xīn Yǒu	1/15	Xīn Mǎo	2/13	Gēng Shēn	25
8/21	Jiǎ Zǐ	9/19	Guǐ Sì	10/19	Guǐ Hài	11/18	Guǐ Sì	12/17	Rén Xū	1/16	Rén Chén	2/14	Xīn Yǒu	26
8/22	Yǐ Chǒu	9/20	Jiǎ Wǔ	10/20	Jiǎ Zǐ	11/19	Jiǎ Wǔ	12/18	Guǐ Hài	1/17	Guǐ Sì	2/15	Rén Xū	27
8/23	Bǐng Yín	9/21	Yǐ Wèi	10/21	Yǐ Chǒu	11/20	Yǐ Wèi	12/19	Jiǎ Zǐ	1/18	Jiǎ Wǔ	2/16	Guǐ Hài	28
8/24	Dīng Mǎo	9/22	Bǐng Shēn	10/22	Bǐng Yín	11/21	Bǐng Shēn	12/20	Yǐ Chǒu	1/19	Yǐ Wèi	2/17	Jiǎ Zǐ	29
		9/23	Dīng Yǒu	10/23	Dīng Mǎo			12/21	Bǐng Yín			2/18	Yǐ Chǒu	30
Li Qiu		Bai Lu		Han Lu				Li Dong		Da Xue		Xiao Han		Jie
8/7	11:02p	9/8	2:21a	10/8	6:20p			11/7	9:36p	12/7	2:11p	1/6	12:57a	
Chu Shu		Qiu Fen		Shuang Jiang				Xiao Xue		Dong Zhi		Da Han		Qi
8/23	1:53p	9/23	11:51a	10/23	9:30p			11/22	6:58p	12/22	7:50a	1/20	6:05p	

215

YEAR: 2015 Yǐ Wèi -- First six months.											
	1ST MONTH		2ND MONTH		3RD MONTH		4TH MONTH		5TH MONTH		6TH MONTH
	Wù Yín		Jǐ Mǎo		Gēng Chén		Xīn Sì		Rén Wǔ		Guǐ Wèi
1	2/19	Bǐng Yín	3/20	Yǐ Wèi	4/19	Yǐ Chǒu	5/18	Jiǎ Wǔ	6/16	Guǐ Hài	7/16	Guǐ Sì
2	2/20	Dīng Mǎo	3/21	Bǐng Shēn	4/20	Bǐng Yín	5/19	Yǐ Wèi	6/17	Jiǎ Zǐ	7/17	Jiǎ Wǔ
3	2/21	Wù Chén	3/22	Dīng Yǒu	4/21	Dīng Mǎo	5/20	Bǐng Shēn	6/18	Yǐ Chǒu	7/18	Yǐ Wèi
4	2/22	Jǐ Sì	3/23	Wù Xū	4/22	Wù Chén	5/21	Dīng Yǒu	6/19	Bǐng Yín	7/19	Bǐng Shēn
5	2/23	Gēng Wǔ	3/24	Jǐ Hài	4/23	Jǐ Sì	5/22	Wù Xū	6/20	Dīng Mǎo	7/20	Dīng Yǒu
6	2/24	Xīn Wèi	3/25	Gēng Zǐ	4/24	Gēng Wǔ	5/23	Jǐ Hài	6/21	Wù Chén	7/21	Wù Xū
7	2/25	Rén Shēn	3/26	Xīn Chǒu	4/25	Xīn Wèi	5/24	Gēng Zǐ	6/22	Jǐ Sì	7/22	Jǐ Hài
8	2/26	Guǐ Yǒu	3/27	Rén Yín	4/26	Rén Shēn	5/25	Xīn Chǒu	6/23	Gēng Wǔ	7/23	Gēng Zǐ
9	2/27	Jiǎ Xū	3/28	Guǐ Mǎo	4/27	Guǐ Yǒu	5/26	Rén Yín	6/24	Xīn Wèi	7/24	Xīn Chǒu
10	2/28	Yǐ Hài	3/29	Jiǎ Chén	4/28	Jiǎ Xū	5/27	Guǐ Mǎo	6/25	Rén Shēn	7/25	Rén Yín
11	3/1	Bǐng Zǐ	3/30	Yǐ Sì	4/29	Yǐ Hài	5/28	Jiǎ Chén	6/26	Guǐ Yǒu	7/26	Guǐ Mǎo
12	3/2	Dīng Chǒu	3/31	Bǐng Wǔ	4/30	Bǐng Zǐ	5/29	Yǐ Sì	6/27	Jiǎ Xū	7/27	Jiǎ Chén
13	3/3	Wù Yín	4/1	Dīng Wèi	5/1	Dīng Chǒu	5/30	Bǐng Wǔ	6/28	Yǐ Hài	7/28	Yǐ Sì
14	3/4	Jǐ Mǎo	4/2	Wù Shēn	5/2	Wù Yín	5/31	Dīng Wèi	6/29	Bǐng Zǐ	7/29	Bǐng Wǔ
15	3/5	Gēng Chén	4/3	Jǐ Yǒu	5/3	Jǐ Mǎo	6/1	Wù Shēn	6/30	Dīng Chǒu	7/30	Dīng Wèi
16	3/6	Xīn Sì	4/4	Gēng Xū	5/4	Gēng Chén	6/2	Jǐ Yǒu	7/1	Wù Yín	7/31	Wù Shēn
17	3/7	Rén Wǔ	4/5	Xīn Hài	5/5	Xīn Sì	6/3	Gēng Xū	7/2	Jǐ Mǎo	8/1	Jǐ Yǒu
18	3/8	Guǐ Wèi	4/6	Rén Zǐ	5/6	Rén Wǔ	6/4	Xīn Hài	7/3	Gēng Chén	8/2	Gēng Xū
19	3/9	Jiǎ Shēn	4/7	Guǐ Chǒu	5/7	Guǐ Wèi	6/5	Rén Zǐ	7/4	Xīn Sì	8/3	Xīn Hài
20	3/10	Yǐ Yǒu	4/8	Jiǎ Yín	5/8	Jiǎ Shēn	6/6	Guǐ Chǒu	7/5	Rén Wǔ	8/4	Rén Zǐ
21	3/11	Bǐng Xū	4/9	Yǐ Mǎo	5/9	Yǐ Yǒu	6/7	Jiǎ Yín	7/6	Guǐ Wèi	8/5	Guǐ Chǒu
22	3/12	Dīng Hài	4/10	Bǐng Chén	5/10	Bǐng Xū	6/8	Yǐ Mǎo	7/7	Jiǎ Shēn	8/6	Jiǎ Yín
23	3/13	Wù Zǐ	4/11	Dīng Sì	5/11	Dīng Hài	6/9	Bǐng Chén	7/8	Yǐ Yǒu	8/7	Yǐ Mǎo
24	3/14	Jǐ Chǒu	4/12	Wù Wǔ	5/12	Wù Zǐ	6/10	Dīng Sì	7/9	Bǐng Xū	8/8	Bǐng Chén
25	3/15	Gēng Yín	4/13	Jǐ Wèi	5/13	Jǐ Chǒu	6/11	Wù Wǔ	7/10	Dīng Hài	8/9	Dīng Sì
26	3/16	Xīn Mǎo	4/14	Gēng Shēn	5/14	Gēng Yín	6/12	Jǐ Wèi	7/11	Wù Zǐ	8/10	Wù Wǔ
27	3/17	Rén Chén	4/15	Xīn Yǒu	5/15	Xīn Mǎo	6/13	Gēng Shēn	7/12	Jǐ Chǒu	8/11	Jǐ Wèi
28	3/18	Guǐ Sì	4/16	Rén Xū	5/16	Rén Chén	6/14	Xīn Yǒu	7/13	Gēng Yín	8/12	Gēng Shēn
29	3/19	Jiǎ Wǔ	4/17	Guǐ Hài	5/17	Guǐ Sì	6/15	Rén Xū	7/14	Xīn Mǎo	8/13	Xīn Yǒu
30			4/18	Jiǎ Zǐ					7/15	Rén Chén		
Jie	Li Chun		Jing Zhi		Qing Ming		Li Xia		Mang Zhong		Xiao Shu	
	2/4	12:09p	3/6	5:56a	4/5	10:58a	5/6	4:00a	6/6	8:20a	7/7	6:30p
Qi	Yu Shui		Chun Fen		Gu Yu		Xiao Man		Xia Zhi		Da Shu	
	2/19	7:54a	3/21	6:47a	4/20	5:52p	5/21	5:05p	6/22	2:09a	7/23	12:16p

YEAR: 2015 Yǐ Wèi -- Last six months.												
7TH MONTH		8TH MONTH		9TH MONTH		10TH MONTH		11TH MONTH		12TH MONTH		
Jiǎ Shēn		Yǐ Yǒu		Bǐng Xū		Dīng Hài		Wù Zǐ		Jǐ Chǒu		
								2015 - 2016				
8/14	Rén Xū	9/13	Rén Chén	10/13	Rén Xū	11/12	Rén Chén	12/11	Xīn Yǒu	1/10	Xīn Mǎo	1
8/15	Guǐ Hài	9/14	Guǐ Sì	10/14	Guǐ Hài	11/13	Guǐ Sì	12/12	Rén Xū	1/11	Rén Chén	2
8/16	Jiǎ Zǐ	9/15	Jiǎ Wǔ	10/15	Jiǎ Zǐ	11/14	Jiǎ Wǔ	12/13	Guǐ Hài	1/12	Guǐ Sì	3
8/17	Yǐ Chǒu	9/16	Yǐ Wèi	10/16	Yǐ Chǒu	11/15	Yǐ Wèi	12/14	Jiǎ Zǐ	1/13	Jiǎ Wǔ	4
8/18	Bǐng Yín	9/17	Bǐng Shēn	10/17	Bǐng Yín	11/16	Bǐng Shēn	12/15	Yǐ Chǒu	1/14	Yǐ Wèi	5
8/19	Dīng Mǎo	9/18	Dīng Yǒu	10/18	Dīng Mǎo	11/17	Dīng Yǒu	12/16	Bǐng Yín	1/15	Bǐng Shēn	6
8/20	Wù Chén	9/19	Wù Xū	10/19	Wù Chén	11/18	Wù Xū	12/17	Dīng Mǎo	1/16	Dīng Yǒu	7
8/21	Jǐ Sì	9/20	Jǐ Hài	10/20	Jǐ Sì	11/19	Jǐ Hài	12/18	Wù Chén	1/17	Wù Xū	8
8/22	Gēng Wǔ	9/21	Gēng Zǐ	10/21	Gēng Wǔ	11/20	Gēng Zǐ	12/19	Jǐ Sì	1/18	Jǐ Hài	9
8/23	Xīn Wèi	9/22	Xīn Chǒu	10/22	Xīn Wèi	11/21	Xīn Chǒu	12/20	Gēng Wǔ	1/19	Gēng Zǐ	10
8/24	Rén Shēn	9/23	Rén Yín	10/23	Rén Shēn	11/22	Rén Yín	12/21	Xīn Wèi	1/20	Xīn Chǒu	11
8/25	Guǐ Yǒu	9/24	Guǐ Mǎo	10/24	Guǐ Yǒu	11/23	Guǐ Mǎo	12/22	Rén Shēn	1/21	Rén Yín	12
8/26	Jiǎ Xū	9/25	Jiǎ Chén	10/25	Jiǎ Xū	11/24	Jiǎ Chén	12/23	Guǐ Yǒu	1/22	Guǐ Mǎo	13
8/27	Yǐ Hài	9/26	Yǐ Sì	10/26	Yǐ Hài	11/25	Yǐ Sì	12/24	Jiǎ Xū	1/23	Jiǎ Chén	14
8/28	Bǐng Zǐ	9/27	Bǐng Wǔ	10/27	Bǐng Zǐ	11/26	Bǐng Wǔ	12/25	Yǐ Hài	1/24	Yǐ Sì	15
8/29	Dīng Chǒu	9/28	Dīng Wèi	10/28	Dīng Chǒu	11/27	Dīng Wèi	12/26	Bǐng Zǐ	1/25	Bǐng Wǔ	16
8/30	Wù Yín	9/29	Wù Shēn	10/29	Wù Yín	11/28	Wù Shēn	12/27	Dīng Chǒu	1/26	Dīng Wèi	17
8/31	Jǐ Mǎo	9/30	Jǐ Yǒu	10/30	Jǐ Mǎo	11/29	Jǐ Yǒu	12/28	Wù Yín	1/27	Wù Shēn	18
9/1	Gēng Chén	10/1	Gēng Xū	10/31	Gēng Chén	11/30	Gēng Xū	12/29	Jǐ Mǎo	1/28	Jǐ Yǒu	19
9/2	Xīn Sì	10/2	Xīn Hài	11/1	Xīn Sì	12/1	Xīn Hài	12/30	Gēng Chén	1/29	Gēng Xū	20
9/3	Rén Wǔ	10/3	Rén Zǐ	11/2	Rén Wǔ	12/2	Rén Zǐ	12/31	Xīn Sì	1/30	Xīn Hài	21
9/4	Guǐ Wèi	10/4	Guǐ Chǒu	11/3	Guǐ Wèi	12/3	Guǐ Chǒu	1/1	Rén Wǔ	1/31	Rén Zǐ	22
9/5	Jiǎ Shēn	10/5	Jiǎ Yín	11/4	Jiǎ Shēn	12/4	Jiǎ Yín	1/2	Guǐ Wèi	2/1	Guǐ Chǒu	23
9/6	Yǐ Yǒu	10/6	Yǐ Mǎo	11/5	Yǐ Yǒu	12/5	Yǐ Mǎo	1/3	Jiǎ Shēn	2/2	Jiǎ Yín	24
9/7	Bǐng Xū	10/7	Bǐng Chén	11/6	Bǐng Xū	12/6	Bǐng Chén	1/4	Yǐ Yǒu	2/3	Yǐ Mǎo	25
9/8	Dīng Hài	10/8	Dīng Sì	11/7	Dīng Hài	**12/7**	Dīng Sì	1/5	Bǐng Xū	**2/4**	Bǐng Chén	26
9/9	Wù Zǐ	**10/9**	Wù Wǔ	**11/8**	Wù Zǐ	12/8	Wù Wǔ	**1/6**	Dīng Hài	2/5	Dīng Sì	27
9/10	Jǐ Chǒu	10/10	Jǐ Wèi	11/9	Jǐ Chǒu	12/9	Jǐ Wèi	1/7	Wù Zǐ	2/6	Wù Wǔ	28
9/11	Gēng Yín	10/11	Gēng Shēn	11/10	Gēng Yín	12/10	Gēng Shēn	1/8	Jǐ Chǒu	2/7	Jǐ Wèi	29
9/12	Xīn Mǎo	10/12	Xīn Yǒu	11/11	Xīn Mǎo			1/9	Gēng Yín			30
Li Qiu		Bai Lu		Han Lu		Li Dong		Da Xue		Xiao Han		Jie
8/8	4:51a	9/8	8:10a	10/9	12:09a	11/8	3:25a	12/7	8:01p	1/6	6:47a	
Chu Shu		Qiu Fen		Shuang Jiang		Xiao Xue		Dong Zhi		Da Han		Qi
8/23	7:51p	9/23	5:45p	10/24	3:20a	11/23	12:48a	12/22	1:45p	1/20	11:50p	

針灸大成 · 卷之五

YEAR: 2016 Bǐng Shēn -- First six months.												
	1ST MONTH		2ND MONTH		3RD MONTH		4TH MONTH		5TH MONTH		6TH MONTH	
	Gēng Yín		Xīn Mǎo		Rén Chén		Guǐ Sì		Jiǎ Wǔ		Yǐ Wèi	
1	2/8	Gēng Shēn	3/9	Gēng Yín	4/7	Jǐ Wèi	5/7	Jǐ Chǒu	6/5	Wù Wǔ	7/4	Dīng Hài
2	2/9	Xīn Yǒu	3/10	Xīn Mǎo	4/8	Gēng Shēn	5/8	Gēng Yín	6/6	Jǐ Wèi	7/5	Wù Zǐ
3	2/10	Rén Xū	3/11	Rén Chén	4/9	Xīn Yǒu	5/9	Xīn Mǎo	6/7	Gēng Shēn	7/6	Jǐ Chǒu
4	2/11	Guǐ Hài	3/12	Guǐ Sì	4/10	Rén Xū	5/10	Rén Chén	6/8	Xīn Yǒu	7/7	Gēng Yín
5	2/12	Jiǎ Zǐ	3/13	Jiǎ Wǔ	4/11	Guǐ Hài	5/11	Guǐ Sì	6/9	Rén Xū	7/8	Xīn Mǎo
6	2/13	Yǐ Chǒu	3/14	Yǐ Wèi	4/12	Jiǎ Zǐ	5/12	Jiǎ Wǔ	6/10	Guǐ Hài	7/9	Rén Chén
7	2/14	Bǐng Yín	3/15	Bǐng Shēn	4/13	Yǐ Chǒu	5/13	Yǐ Wèi	6/11	Jiǎ Zǐ	7/10	Guǐ Sì
8	2/15	Dīng Mǎo	3/16	Dīng Yǒu	4/14	Bǐng Yín	5/14	Bǐng Shēn	6/12	Yǐ Chǒu	7/11	Jiǎ Wǔ
9	2/16	Wù Chén	3/17	Wù Xū	4/15	Dīng Mǎo	5/15	Dīng Yǒu	6/13	Bǐng Yín	7/12	Yǐ Wèi
10	2/17	Jǐ Sì	3/18	Jǐ Hài	4/16	Wù Chén	5/16	Wù Xū	6/14	Dīng Mǎo	7/13	Bǐng Shēn
11	2/18	Gēng Wǔ	3/19	Gēng Zǐ	4/17	Jǐ Sì	5/17	Jǐ Hài	6/15	Wù Chén	7/14	Dīng Yǒu
12	2/19	Xīn Wèi	3/20	Xīn Chǒu	4/18	Gēng Wǔ	5/18	Gēng Zǐ	6/16	Jǐ Sì	7/15	Wù Xū
13	2/20	Rén Shēn	3/21	Rén Yín	4/19	Xīn Wèi	5/19	Xīn Chǒu	6/17	Gēng Wǔ	7/16	Jǐ Hài
14	2/21	Guǐ Yǒu	3/22	Guǐ Mǎo	4/20	Rén Shēn	5/20	Rén Yín	6/18	Xīn Wèi	7/17	Gēng Zǐ
15	2/22	Jiǎ Xū	3/23	Jiǎ Chén	4/21	Guǐ Yǒu	5/21	Guǐ Mǎo	6/19	Rén Shēn	7/18	Xīn Chǒu
16	2/23	Yǐ Hài	3/24	Yǐ Sì	4/22	Jiǎ Xū	5/22	Jiǎ Chén	6/20	Guǐ Yǒu	7/19	Rén Yín
17	2/24	Bǐng Zǐ	3/25	Bǐng Wǔ	4/23	Yǐ Hài	5/23	Yǐ Sì	6/21	Jiǎ Xū	7/20	Guǐ Mǎo
18	2/25	Dīng Chǒu	3/26	Dīng Wèi	4/24	Bǐng Zǐ	5/24	Bǐng Wǔ	6/22	Yǐ Hài	7/21	Jiǎ Chén
19	2/26	Wù Yín	3/27	Wù Shēn	4/25	Dīng Chǒu	5/25	Dīng Wèi	6/23	Bǐng Zǐ	7/22	Yǐ Sì
20	2/27	Jǐ Mǎo	3/28	Jǐ Yǒu	4/26	Wù Yín	5/26	Wù Shēn	6/24	Dīng Chǒu	7/23	Bǐng Wǔ
21	2/28	Gēng Chén	3/29	Gēng Xū	4/27	Jǐ Mǎo	5/27	Jǐ Yǒu	6/25	Wù Yín	7/24	Dīng Wèi
22	2/29	Xīn Sì	3/30	Xīn Hài	4/28	Gēng Chén	5/28	Gēng Xū	6/26	Jǐ Mǎo	7/25	Wù Shēn
23	3/1	Rén Wǔ	3/31	Rén Zǐ	4/29	Xīn Sì	5/29	Xīn Hài	6/27	Gēng Chén	7/26	Jǐ Yǒu
24	3/2	Guǐ Wèi	4/1	Guǐ Chǒu	4/30	Rén Wǔ	5/30	Rén Zǐ	6/28	Xīn Sì	7/27	Gēng Xū
25	3/3	Jiǎ Shēn	4/2	Jiǎ Yín	5/1	Guǐ Wèi	5/31	Guǐ Chǒu	6/29	Rén Wǔ	7/28	Xīn Hài
26	3/4	Yǐ Yǒu	4/3	Yǐ Mǎo	5/2	Jiǎ Shēn	6/1	Jiǎ Yín	6/30	Guǐ Wèi	7/29	Rén Zǐ
27	3/5	Bǐng Xū	4/4	Bǐng Chén	5/3	Yǐ Yǒu	6/2	Yǐ Mǎo	7/1	Jiǎ Shēn	7/30	Guǐ Chǒu
28	3/6	Dīng Hài	4/5	Dīng Sì	5/4	Bǐng Xū	6/3	Bǐng Chén	7/2	Yǐ Yǒu	7/31	Jiǎ Yín
29	3/7	Wù Zǐ	4/6	Wù Wǔ	5/5	Dīng Hài	6/4	Dīng Sì	7/3	Bǐng Xū	8/1	Yǐ Mǎo
30	3/8	Jǐ Chǒu			5/6	Wù Zǐ					8/2	Bǐng Chén
Jie	Li Chun		Jing Zhi		Qing Ming		Li Xia		Mang Zhong		Xiao Shu	
	2/4	6:00p	3/5	11:46a	4/4	4:32p	5/5	9:54a	6/5	2:09p	7/7	12:33a
Qi	Yu Shui		Chun Fen		Gu Yu		Xiao Man		Xia Zhi		Da Shu	
	2/19	1:44p	3/20	12:37p	4/19	11:30a	5/20	10:54p	6/21	6:57a	7/22	6:03p

YEAR: 2016 Bǐng Shēn -- Last six months.											
7TH MONTH		8TH MONTH		9TH MONTH		10TH MONTH		11TH MONTH		12TH MONTH	
Bǐng Shēn		Dīng Yǒu		Wù Xū		Jǐ Hài		Gēng Zǐ		Xīn Chǒu	
										2016 - 2017	
8/3	Dīng Sì	9/1	Bǐng Xū	10/1	Bǐng Chén	10/31	Bǐng Xū	11/29	Yǐ Mǎo	12/29	Yǐ Yǒu	1
8/4	Wù Wǔ	9/2	Dīng Hài	10/2	Dīng Sì	11/1	Dīng Hài	11/30	Bǐng Chén	12/30	Bǐng Xū	2
8/5	Jǐ Wèi	9/3	Wù Zǐ	10/3	Wù Wǔ	11/2	Wù Zǐ	12/1	Dīng Sì	12/31	Dīng Hài	3
8/6	Gēng Shēn	9/4	Jǐ Chǒu	10/4	Jǐ Wèi	11/3	Jǐ Chǒu	12/2	Wù Wǔ	1/1	Wù Zǐ	4
8/7	Xīn Yǒu	9/5	Gēng Yín	10/5	Gēng Shēn	11/4	Gēng Yín	12/3	Jǐ Wèi	1/2	Jǐ Chǒu	5
8/8	Rén Xū	9/6	Xīn Mǎo	10/6	Xīn Yǒu	11/5	Xīn Mǎo	12/4	Gēng Shēn	1/3	Gēng Yín	6
8/9	Guǐ Hài	9/7	Rén Chén	10/7	Rén Xū	11/6	Rén Chén	12/5	Xīn Yǒu	1/4	Xīn Mǎo	7
8/10	Jiǎ Zǐ	9/8	Guǐ Sì	10/8	Guǐ Hài	11/7	Guǐ Sì	12/6	Rén Xū	1/5	Rén Chén	8
8/11	Yǐ Chǒu	9/9	Jiǎ Wǔ	10/9	Jiǎ Zǐ	11/8	Jiǎ Wǔ	12/7	Guǐ Hài	1/6	Guǐ Sì	9
8/12	Bǐng Yín	9/10	Yǐ Wèi	10/10	Yǐ Chǒu	11/9	Yǐ Wèi	12/8	Jiǎ Zǐ	1/7	Jiǎ Wǔ	10
8/13	Dīng Mǎo	9/11	Bǐng Shēn	10/11	Bǐng Yín	11/10	Bǐng Shēn	12/9	Yǐ Chǒu	1/8	Yǐ Wèi	11
8/14	Wù Chén	9/12	Dīng Yǒu	10/12	Dīng Mǎo	11/11	Dīng Yǒu	12/10	Bǐng Yín	1/9	Bǐng Shēn	12
8/15	Jǐ Sì	9/13	Wù Xū	10/13	Wù Chén	11/12	Wù Xū	12/11	Dīng Mǎo	1/10	Dīng Yǒu	13
8/16	Gēng Wǔ	9/14	Jǐ Hài	10/14	Jǐ Sì	11/13	Jǐ Hài	12/12	Wù Chén	1/11	Wù Xū	14
8/17	Xīn Wèi	9/15	Gēng Zǐ	10/15	Gēng Wǔ	11/14	Gēng Zǐ	12/13	Jǐ Sì	1/12	Jǐ Hài	15
8/18	Rén Shēn	9/16	Xīn Chǒu	10/16	Xīn Wèi	11/15	Xīn Chǒu	12/14	Gēng Wǔ	1/13	Gēng Zǐ	16
8/19	Guǐ Yǒu	9/17	Rén Yín	10/17	Rén Shēn	11/16	Rén Yín	12/15	Xīn Wèi	1/14	Xīn Chǒu	17
8/20	Jiǎ Xū	9/18	Guǐ Mǎo	10/18	Guǐ Yǒu	11/17	Guǐ Mǎo	12/16	Rén Shēn	1/15	Rén Yín	18
8/21	Yǐ Hài	9/19	Jiǎ Chén	10/19	Jiǎ Xū	11/18	Jiǎ Chén	12/17	Guǐ Yǒu	1/16	Guǐ Mǎo	19
8/22	Bǐng Zǐ	9/20	Yǐ Sì	10/20	Yǐ Hài	11/19	Yǐ Sì	12/18	Jiǎ Xū	1/17	Jiǎ Chén	20
8/23	Dīng Chǒu	9/21	Bǐng Wǔ	10/21	Bǐng Zǐ	11/20	Bǐng Wǔ	12/19	Yǐ Hài	1/18	Yǐ Sì	21
8/24	Wù Yín	9/22	Dīng Wèi	10/22	Dīng Chǒu	11/21	Dīng Wèi	12/20	Bǐng Zǐ	1/19	Bǐng Wǔ	22
8/25	Jǐ Mǎo	9/23	Wù Shēn	10/23	Wù Yín	11/22	Wù Shēn	12/21	Dīng Chǒu	1/20	Dīng Wèi	23
8/26	Gēng Chén	9/24	Jǐ Yǒu	10/24	Jǐ Mǎo	11/23	Jǐ Yǒu	12/22	Wù Yín	1/21	Wù Shēn	24
8/27	Xīn Sì	9/25	Gēng Xū	10/25	Gēng Chén	11/24	Gēng Xū	12/23	Jǐ Mǎo	1/22	Jǐ Yǒu	25
8/28	Rén Wǔ	9/26	Xīn Hài	10/26	Xīn Sì	11/25	Xīn Hài	12/24	Gēng Chén	1/23	Gēng Xū	26
8/29	Guǐ Wèi	9/27	Rén Zǐ	10/27	Rén Wǔ	11/26	Rén Zǐ	12/25	Xīn Sì	1/24	Xīn Hài	27
8/30	Jiǎ Shēn	9/28	Guǐ Chǒu	10/28	Guǐ Wèi	11/27	Guǐ Chǒu	12/26	Rén Wǔ	1/25	Rén Zǐ	28
8/31	Yǐ Yǒu	9/29	Jiǎ Yín	10/29	Jiǎ Shēn	11/28	Jiǎ Yín	12/27	Guǐ Wèi	1/26	Guǐ Chǒu	29
		9/30	Yǐ Mǎo	10/30	Yǐ Yǒu			12/28	Jiǎ Shēn	1/27	Jiǎ Yín	30
Li Qiu		Bai Lu		Han Lu		Li Dong		Da Xue		Xiao Han		Jie
8/7	10:39a	9/7	1:48p	10/8	5:59a	11/7	9:14a	12/7	1:54a	1/5	12:36p	
Chu Shu		Qiu Fen		Shuang Jiang		Xiao Xue		Dong Zhi		Da Han		Qi
8/23	1:30a	9/22	11:34p	10/23	9:09a	11/22	6:38a	12/21	7:35p	1/20	5:45a	

針灸大成 · 卷之五

	1ST MONTH		2ND MONTH		3RD MONTH		4TH MONTH		5TH MONTH		6TH MONTH		LEAP MONTH	
YEAR: 2017 Dīng Yǒu -- First six months.														
	Rén Yín		Guǐ Mǎo		Jiǎ Chén		Yǐ Sì		Bǐng Wǔ		Dīng Wèi			
1	1/28	Yǐ Mǎo	2/26	Jiǎ Shēn	3/28	Jiǎ Yín	4/26	Guǐ Wèi	5/26	Guǐ Chǒu	6/24	Rén Wǔ	7/23	Xīn Hài
2	1/29	Bǐng Chén	2/27	Yǐ Yǒu	3/29	Yǐ Mǎo	4/27	Jiǎ Shēn	5/27	Jiǎ Yín	6/25	Guǐ Wèi	7/24	Rén Zǐ
3	1/30	Dīng Sì	2/28	Bǐng Xū	3/30	Bǐng Chén	4/28	Yǐ Yǒu	5/28	Yǐ Mǎo	6/26	Jiǎ Shēn	7/25	Guǐ Chǒu
4	1/31	Wù Wǔ	3/1	Dīng Hài	3/31	Dīng Sì	4/29	Bǐng Xū	5/29	Bǐng Chén	6/27	Yǐ Yǒu	7/26	Jiǎ Yín
5	2/1	Jǐ Wèi	3/2	Wù Zǐ	4/1	Wù Wǔ	4/30	Dīng Hài	5/30	Dīng Sì	6/28	Bǐng Xū	7/27	Yǐ Mǎo
6	2/2	Gēng Shēn	3/3	Jǐ Chǒu	4/2	Jǐ Wèi	5/1	Wù Zǐ	5/31	Wù Wǔ	6/29	Dīng Hài	7/28	Bǐng Chén
7	2/3	Xīn Yǒu	3/4	Gēng Yín	4/3	Gēng Shēn	5/2	Jǐ Chǒu	6/1	Jǐ Wèi	6/30	Wù Zǐ	7/29	Dīng Sì
8	2/4	Rén Xū	3/5	Xīn Mǎo	4/4	Xīn Yǒu	5/3	Gēng Yín	6/2	Gēng Shēn	7/1	Jǐ Chǒu	7/30	Wù Wǔ
9	2/5	Guǐ Hài	3/6	Rén Chén	4/5	Rén Xū	5/4	Xīn Mǎo	6/3	Xīn Yǒu	7/2	Gēng Yín	7/31	Jǐ Wèi
10	2/6	Jiǎ Zǐ	3/7	Guǐ Sì	4/6	Guǐ Hài	5/5	Rén Chén	6/4	Rén Xū	7/3	Xīn Mǎo	8/1	Gēng Shēn
11	2/7	Yǐ Chǒu	3/8	Jiǎ Wǔ	4/7	Jiǎ Zǐ	5/6	Guǐ Sì	6/5	Guǐ Hài	7/4	Rén Chén	8/2	Xīn Yǒu
12	2/8	Bǐng Yín	3/9	Yǐ Wèi	4/8	Yǐ Chǒu	5/7	Jiǎ Wǔ	6/6	Jiǎ Zǐ	7/5	Guǐ Sì	8/3	Rén Xū
13	2/9	Dīng Mǎo	3/10	Bǐng Shēn	4/9	Bǐng Yín	5/8	Yǐ Wèi	6/7	Yǐ Chǒu	7/6	Jiǎ Wǔ	8/4	Guǐ Hài
14	2/10	Wù Chén	3/11	Dīng Yǒu	4/10	Dīng Mǎo	5/9	Bǐng Shēn	6/8	Bǐng Yín	7/7	Yǐ Wèi	8/5	Jiǎ Zǐ
15	2/11	Jǐ Sì	3/12	Wù Xū	4/11	Wù Chén	5/10	Dīng Yǒu	6/9	Dīng Mǎo	7/8	Bǐng Shēn	8/6	Yǐ Chǒu
16	2/12	Gēng Wǔ	3/13	Jǐ Hài	4/12	Jǐ Sì	5/11	Wù Xū	6/10	Wù Chén	7/9	Dīng Yǒu	8/7	Bǐng Yín
17	2/13	Xīn Wèi	3/14	Gēng Zǐ	4/13	Gēng Wǔ	5/12	Jǐ Hài	6/11	Jǐ Sì	7/10	Wù Xū	8/8	Dīng Mǎo
18	2/14	Rén Shēn	3/15	Xīn Chǒu	4/14	Xīn Wèi	5/13	Gēng Zǐ	6/12	Gēng Wǔ	7/11	Jǐ Hài	8/9	Wù Chén
19	2/15	Guǐ Yǒu	3/16	Rén Yín	4/15	Rén Shēn	5/14	Xīn Chǒu	6/13	Xīn Wèi	7/12	Gēng Zǐ	8/10	Jǐ Sì
20	2/16	Jiǎ Xū	3/17	Guǐ Mǎo	4/16	Guǐ Yǒu	5/15	Rén Yín	6/14	Rén Shēn	7/13	Xīn Chǒu	8/11	Gēng Wǔ
21	2/17	Yǐ Hài	3/18	Jiǎ Chén	4/17	Jiǎ Xū	5/16	Guǐ Mǎo	6/15	Guǐ Yǒu	7/14	Rén Yín	8/12	Xīn Wèi
22	2/18	Bǐng Zǐ	3/19	Yǐ Sì	4/18	Yǐ Hài	5/17	Jiǎ Chén	6/16	Jiǎ Xū	7/15	Guǐ Mǎo	8/13	Rén Shēn
23	2/19	Dīng Chǒu	3/20	Bǐng Wǔ	4/19	Bǐng Zǐ	5/18	Yǐ Sì	6/17	Yǐ Hài	7/16	Jiǎ Chén	8/14	Guǐ Yǒu
24	2/20	Wù Yín	3/21	Dīng Wèi	4/20	Dīng Chǒu	5/19	Bǐng Wǔ	6/18	Bǐng Zǐ	7/17	Yǐ Sì	8/15	Jiǎ Xū
25	2/21	Jǐ Mǎo	3/22	Wù Shēn	4/21	Wù Yín	5/20	Dīng Wèi	6/19	Dīng Chǒu	7/18	Bǐng Wǔ	8/16	Yǐ Hài
26	2/22	Gēng Chén	3/23	Jǐ Yǒu	4/22	Jǐ Mǎo	5/21	Wù Shēn	6/20	Wù Yín	7/19	Dīng Wèi	8/17	Bǐng Zǐ
27	2/23	Xīn Sì	3/24	Gēng Xū	4/23	Gēng Chén	5/22	Jǐ Yǒu	6/21	Jǐ Mǎo	7/20	Wù Shēn	8/18	Dīng Chǒu
28	2/24	Rén Wǔ	3/25	Xīn Hài	4/24	Xīn Sì	5/23	Gēng Xū	6/22	Gēng Chén	7/21	Jǐ Yǒu	8/19	Wù Yín
29	2/25	Guǐ Wèi	3/26	Rén Zǐ	4/25	Rén Wǔ	5/24	Xīn Hài	6/23	Xīn Sì	7/22	Gēng Xū	8/20	Jǐ Mǎo
30			3/27	Guǐ Chǒu			5/25	Rén Zǐ					8/21	Gēng Chén
Jie	Li Chun		Jing Zhi		Qing Ming		Li Xia		Mang Zhong		Xiao Shu			
	2/3	11:49p	3/5	5:36p	4/4	10:20p	5/5	3:42p	6/5	7:57p	7/7	6:21a		
Qi	Yu Shui		Chun Fen		Gu Yu		Xiao Man		Xia Zhi		Da Shu			
	2/18	7:31p	3/20	6:25p	4/20	5:29a	5/21	4:42a	6/21	12:46p	7/22	11:51p		

針灸大成 · 卷之五

YEAR: 2017 Dīng Yǒu -- Last six months.												
7TH MONTH		8TH MONTH		9TH MONTH		10TH MONTH		11TH MONTH		12TH MONTH		
Wù Shēn		Jǐ Yǒu		Gēng Xū		Xīn Hài		Rén Zǐ		Guǐ Chǒu		
								2017 - 2018				
8/22	Xīn Sì	9/20	Gēng Xū	10/20	Gēng Chén	11/18	Jǐ Yǒu	12/18	Jǐ Mǎo	1/17	Jǐ Yǒu	1
8/23	Rén Wǔ	9/21	Xīn Hài	10/21	Xīn Sì	11/19	Gēng Xū	12/19	Gēng Chén	1/18	Gēng Xū	2
8/24	Guǐ Wèi	9/22	Rén Zǐ	10/22	Rén Wǔ	11/20	Xīn Hài	12/20	Xīn Sì	1/19	Xīn Hài	3
8/25	Jiǎ Shēn	9/23	Guǐ Chǒu	10/23	Guǐ Wèi	11/21	Rén Zǐ	12/21	Rén Wǔ	1/20	Rén Zǐ	4
8/26	Yǐ Yǒu	9/24	Jiǎ Yín	10/24	Jiǎ Shēn	11/22	Guǐ Chǒu	12/22	Guǐ Wèi	1/21	Guǐ Chǒu	5
8/27	Bǐng Xū	9/25	Yǐ Mǎo	10/25	Yǐ Yǒu	11/23	Jiǎ Yín	12/23	Jiǎ Shēn	1/22	Jiǎ Yín	6
8/28	Dīng Hài	9/26	Bǐng Chén	10/26	Bǐng Xū	11/24	Yǐ Mǎo	12/24	Yǐ Yǒu	1/23	Yǐ Mǎo	7
8/29	Wù Zǐ	9/27	Dīng Sì	10/27	Dīng Hài	11/25	Bǐng Chén	12/25	Bǐng Xū	1/24	Bǐng Chén	8
8/30	Jǐ Chǒu	9/28	Wù Wǔ	10/28	Wù Zǐ	11/26	Dīng Sì	12/26	Dīng Hài	1/25	Dīng Sì	9
8/31	Gēng Yín	9/29	Jǐ Wèi	10/29	Jǐ Chǒu	11/27	Wù Wǔ	12/27	Wù Zǐ	1/26	Wù Wǔ	10
9/1	Xīn Mǎo	9/30	Gēng Shēn	10/30	Gēng Yín	11/28	Jǐ Wèi	12/28	Jǐ Chǒu	1/27	Jǐ Wèi	11
9/2	Rén Chén	10/1	Xīn Yǒu	10/31	Xīn Mǎo	11/29	Gēng Shēn	12/29	Gēng Yín	1/28	Gēng Shēn	12
9/3	Guǐ Sì	10/2	Rén Xū	11/1	Rén Chén	11/30	Xīn Yǒu	12/30	Xīn Mǎo	1/29	Xīn Yǒu	13
9/4	Jiǎ Wǔ	10/3	Guǐ Hài	11/2	Guǐ Sì	12/1	Rén Xū	12/31	Rén Chén	1/30	Rén Xū	14
9/5	Yǐ Wèi	10/4	Jiǎ Zǐ	11/3	Jiǎ Wǔ	12/2	Guǐ Hài	1/1	Guǐ Sì	1/31	Guǐ Hài	15
9/6	Bǐng Shēn	10/5	Yǐ Chǒu	11/4	Yǐ Wèi	12/3	Jiǎ Zǐ	1/2	Jiǎ Wǔ	2/1	Jiǎ Zǐ	16
9/7	Dīng Yǒu	10/6	Bǐng Yín	11/5	Bǐng Shēn	12/4	Yǐ Chǒu	1/3	Yǐ Wèi	2/2	Yǐ Chǒu	17
9/8	Wù Xū	10/7	Dīng Mǎo	11/6	Dīng Yǒu	12/5	Bǐng Yín	1/4	Bǐng Shēn	2/3	Bǐng Yín	18
9/9	Jǐ Hài	**10/8**	Wù Chén	**11/7**	Wù Xū	12/6	Dīng Mǎo	**1/5**	Dīng Yǒu	**2/4**	Dīng Mǎo	19
9/10	Gēng Zǐ	10/9	Jǐ Sì	11/8	Jǐ Hài	**12/7**	Wù Chén	1/6	Wù Xū	2/5	Wù Chén	20
9/11	Xīn Chǒu	10/10	Gēng Wǔ	11/9	Gēng Zǐ	12/8	Jǐ Sì	1/7	Jǐ Hài	2/6	Jǐ Sì	21
9/12	Rén Yín	10/11	Xīn Wèi	11/10	Xīn Chǒu	12/9	Gēng Wǔ	1/8	Gēng Zǐ	2/7	Gēng Wǔ	22
9/13	Guǐ Mǎo	10/12	Rén Shēn	11/11	Rén Yín	12/10	Xīn Wèi	1/9	Xīn Chǒu	2/8	Xīn Wèi	23
9/14	Jiǎ Chén	10/13	Guǐ Yǒu	11/12	Guǐ Mǎo	12/11	Rén Shēn	1/10	Rén Yín	2/9	Rén Shēn	24
9/15	Yǐ Sì	10/14	Jiǎ Xū	11/13	Jiǎ Chén	12/12	Guǐ Yǒu	1/11	Guǐ Mǎo	2/10	Guǐ Yǒu	25
9/16	Bǐng Wǔ	10/15	Yǐ Hài	11/14	Yǐ Sì	12/13	Jiǎ Xū	1/12	Jiǎ Chén	2/11	Jiǎ Xū	26
9/17	Dīng Wèi	10/16	Bǐng Zǐ	11/15	Bǐng Wǔ	12/14	Yǐ Hài	1/13	Yǐ Sì	2/12	Yǐ Hài	27
9/18	Wù Shēn	10/17	Dīng Chǒu	11/16	Dīng Wèi	12/15	Bǐng Zǐ	1/14	Bǐng Wǔ	2/13	Bǐng Zǐ	28
9/19	Jǐ Yǒu	10/18	Wù Yín	11/17	Wù Shēn	12/16	Dīng Chǒu	1/15	Dīng Wèi	2/14	Dīng Chǒu	29
		10/19	Jǐ Mǎo			12/17	Wù Yín	1/16	Wù Shēn	2/15	Wù Yín	30
Li Qiu		Bai Lu		Han Lu		Li Dong		Da Xue		Xiao Han		Jie
8/7	4:27a	9/7	7:46p	10/8	11:47a	11/7	3:03p	12/7	7:40a	1/5	6:26p	
Chu Shu		Qiu Fen		Shuang Jiang		Xiao Xue		Dong Zhi		Da Han		Qi
8/23	7:18a	9/23	5:22a	10/23	2:58p	11/22	12:26p	12/22	1:24a	1/20	11:34a	

	1ST MONTH		2ND MONTH		3RD MONTH		4TH MONTH		5TH MONTH		6TH MONTH	
	Jiǎ Yín		Yǐ Mǎo		Bǐng Chén		Dīng Sì		Wù Wǔ		Jǐ Wèi	
1	2/16	Jǐ Mǎo	3/17	Wù Shēn	4/16	Wù Yín	5/15	Dīng Wèi	6/14	Dīng Chǒu	7/13	Bǐng Wǔ
2	2/17	Gēng Chén	3/18	Jǐ Yǒu	4/17	Jǐ Mǎo	5/16	Wù Shēn	6/15	Wù Yín	7/14	Dīng Wèi
3	2/18	Xīn Sì	3/19	Gēng Xū	4/18	Gēng Chén	5/17	Jǐ Yǒu	6/16	Jǐ Mǎo	7/15	Wù Shēn
4	2/19	Rén Wǔ	3/20	Xīn Hài	4/19	Xīn Sì	5/18	Gēng Xū	6/17	Gēng Chén	7/16	Jǐ Yǒu
5	2/20	Guǐ Wèi	3/21	Rén Zǐ	4/20	Rén Wǔ	5/19	Xīn Hài	6/18	Xīn Sì	7/17	Gēng Xū
6	2/21	Jiǎ Shēn	3/22	Guǐ Chǒu	4/21	Guǐ Wèi	5/20	Rén Zǐ	6/19	Rén Wǔ	7/18	Xīn Hài
7	2/22	Yǐ Yǒu	3/23	Jiǎ Yín	4/22	Jiǎ Shēn	5/21	Guǐ Chǒu	6/20	Guǐ Wèi	7/19	Rén Zǐ
8	2/23	Bǐng Xū	3/24	Yǐ Mǎo	4/23	Yǐ Yǒu	5/22	Jiǎ Yín	6/21	Jiǎ Shēn	7/20	Guǐ Chǒu
9	2/24	Dīng Hài	3/25	Bǐng Chén	4/24	Bǐng Xū	5/23	Yǐ Mǎo	6/22	Yǐ Yǒu	7/21	Jiǎ Yín
10	2/25	Wù Zǐ	3/26	Dīng Sì	4/25	Dīng Hài	5/24	Bǐng Chén	6/23	Bǐng Xū	7/22	Yǐ Mǎo
11	2/26	Jǐ Chǒu	3/27	Wù Wǔ	4/26	Wù Zǐ	5/25	Dīng Sì	6/24	Dīng Hài	7/23	Bǐng Chén
12	2/27	Gēng Yín	3/28	Jǐ Wèi	4/27	Jǐ Chǒu	5/26	Wù Wǔ	6/25	Wù Zǐ	7/24	Dīng Sì
13	2/28	Xīn Mǎo	3/29	Gēng Shēn	4/28	Gēng Yín	5/27	Jǐ Wèi	6/26	Jǐ Chǒu	7/25	Wù Wǔ
14	3/1	Rén Chén	3/30	Xīn Yǒu	4/29	Xīn Mǎo	5/28	Gēng Shēn	6/27	Gēng Yín	7/26	Jǐ Wèi
15	3/2	Guǐ Sì	3/31	Rén Xū	4/30	Rén Chén	5/29	Xīn Yǒu	6/28	Xīn Mǎo	7/27	Gēng Shēn
16	3/3	Jiǎ Wǔ	4/1	Guǐ Hài	5/1	Guǐ Sì	5/30	Rén Xū	6/29	Rén Chén	7/28	Xīn Yǒu
17	3/4	Yǐ Wèi	4/2	Jiǎ Zǐ	5/2	Jiǎ Wǔ	5/31	Guǐ Hài	6/30	Guǐ Sì	7/29	Rén Xū
18	3/5	Bǐng Shēn	4/3	Yǐ Chǒu	5/3	Yǐ Wèi	6/1	Jiǎ Zǐ	7/1	Jiǎ Wǔ	7/30	Guǐ Hài
19	3/6	Dīng Yǒu	4/4	Bǐng Yín	5/4	Bǐng Shēn	6/2	Yǐ Chǒu	7/2	Yǐ Wèi	7/31	Jiǎ Zǐ
20	3/7	Wù Xū	4/5	Dīng Mǎo	5/5	Dīng Yǒu	6/3	Bǐng Yín	7/3	Bǐng Shēn	8/1	Yǐ Chǒu
21	3/8	Jǐ Hài	4/6	Wù Chén	5/6	Wù Xū	6/4	Dīng Mǎo	7/4	Dīng Yǒu	8/2	Bǐng Yín
22	3/9	Gēng Zǐ	4/7	Jǐ Sì	5/7	Jǐ Hài	6/5	Wù Chén	7/5	Wù Xū	8/3	Dīng Mǎo
23	3/10	Xīn Chǒu	4/8	Gēng Wǔ	5/8	Gēng Zǐ	6/6	Jǐ Sì	7/6	Jǐ Hài	8/4	Wù Chén
24	3/11	Rén Yín	4/9	Xīn Wèi	5/9	Xīn Chǒu	6/7	Gēng Wǔ	7/7	Gēng Zǐ	8/5	Jǐ Sì
25	3/12	Guǐ Mǎo	4/10	Rén Shēn	5/10	Rén Yín	6/8	Xīn Wèi	7/8	Xīn Chǒu	8/6	Gēng Wǔ
26	3/13	Jiǎ Chén	4/11	Guǐ Yǒu	5/11	Guǐ Mǎo	6/9	Rén Shēn	7/9	Rén Yín	8/7	Xīn Wèi
27	3/14	Yǐ Sì	4/12	Jiǎ Xū	5/12	Jiǎ Chén	6/10	Guǐ Yǒu	7/10	Guǐ Mǎo	8/8	Rén Shēn
28	3/15	Bǐng Wǔ	4/13	Yǐ Hài	5/13	Yǐ Sì	6/11	Jiǎ Xū	7/11	Jiǎ Chén	8/9	Guǐ Yǒu
29	3/16	Dīng Wèi	4/14	Bǐng Zǐ	5/14	Bǐng Wǔ	6/12	Yǐ Hài	7/12	Yǐ Sì	8/10	Jiǎ Xū
30			4/15	Dīng Chǒu			6/13	Bǐng Zǐ				
Jie	Li Chun		Jing Zhi		Qing Ming		Li Xia		Mang Zhong		Xiao Shu	
	2/4	5:38a	3/5	11:25p	4/5	4:20a	5/5	9:31p	6/6	1:29a	7/7	12:09p
Qi	Yu Shui		Chun Fen		Gu Yu		Xiao Man		Xia Zhi		Da Shu	
	2/19	1:22a	3/21	12:13a	4/20	11:18a	5/21	10:30a	6/21	6:33p	7/23	5:40a

針灸大成 · 卷之五

YEAR: 2018 Wù Xū -- Last six months.												
7TH MONTH		8TH MONTH		9TH MONTH		10TH MONTH		11TH MONTH		12TH MONTH		
Gēng Shēn		Xīn Yǒu		Rén Xū		Guǐ Hài		Jiǎ Zǐ		Yǐ Chǒu		
								2018 - 2019				
8/11	Yǐ Hài	9/10	Yǐ Sì	10/9	Jiǎ Xū	11/8	Jiǎ Chén	12/7	Guǐ Yǒu	1/6	Guǐ Mǎo	1
8/12	Bǐng Zǐ	9/11	Bǐng Wǔ	10/10	Yǐ Hài	11/9	Yǐ Sì	12/8	Jiǎ Xū	1/7	Jiǎ Chén	2
8/13	Dīng Chǒu	9/12	Dīng Wèi	10/11	Bǐng Zǐ	11/10	Bǐng Wǔ	12/9	Yǐ Hài	1/8	Yǐ Sì	3
8/14	Wù Yín	9/13	Wù Shēn	10/12	Dīng Chǒu	11/11	Dīng Wèi	12/10	Bǐng Zǐ	1/9	Bǐng Wǔ	4
8/15	Jǐ Mǎo	9/14	Jǐ Yǒu	10/13	Wù Yín	11/12	Wù Shēn	12/11	Dīng Chǒu	1/10	Dīng Wèi	5
8/16	Gēng Chén	9/15	Gēng Xū	10/14	Jǐ Mǎo	11/13	Jǐ Yǒu	12/12	Wù Yín	1/11	Wù Shēn	6
8/17	Xīn Sì	9/16	Xīn Hài	10/15	Gēng Chén	11/14	Gēng Xū	12/13	Jǐ Mǎo	1/12	Jǐ Yǒu	7
8/18	Rén Wǔ	9/17	Rén Zǐ	10/16	Xīn Sì	11/15	Xīn Hài	12/14	Gēng Chén	1/13	Gēng Xū	8
8/19	Guǐ Wèi	9/18	Guǐ Chǒu	10/17	Rén Wǔ	11/16	Rén Zǐ	12/15	Xīn Sì	1/14	Xīn Hài	9
8/20	Jiǎ Shēn	9/19	Jiǎ Yín	10/18	Guǐ Wèi	11/17	Guǐ Chǒu	12/16	Rén Wǔ	1/15	Rén Zǐ	10
8/21	Yǐ Yǒu	9/20	Yǐ Mǎo	10/19	Jiǎ Shēn	11/18	Jiǎ Yín	12/17	Guǐ Wèi	1/16	Guǐ Chǒu	11
8/22	Bǐng Xū	9/21	Bǐng Chén	10/20	Yǐ Yǒu	11/19	Yǐ Mǎo	12/18	Jiǎ Shēn	1/17	Jiǎ Yín	12
8/23	Dīng Hài	9/22	Dīng Sì	10/21	Bǐng Xū	11/20	Bǐng Chén	12/19	Yǐ Yǒu	1/18	Yǐ Mǎo	13
8/24	Wù Zǐ	9/23	Wù Wǔ	10/22	Dīng Hài	11/21	Dīng Sì	12/20	Bǐng Xū	1/19	Bǐng Chén	14
8/25	Jǐ Chǒu	9/24	Jǐ Wèi	10/23	Wù Zǐ	11/22	Wù Wǔ	12/21	Dīng Hài	1/20	Dīng Sì	15
8/26	Gēng Yín	9/25	Gēng Shēn	10/24	Jǐ Chǒu	11/23	Jǐ Wèi	12/22	Wù Zǐ	1/21	Wù Wǔ	16
8/27	Xīn Mǎo	9/26	Xīn Yǒu	10/25	Gēng Yín	11/24	Gēng Shēn	12/23	Jǐ Chǒu	1/22	Jǐ Wèi	17
8/28	Rén Chén	9/27	Rén Xū	10/26	Xīn Mǎo	11/25	Xīn Yǒu	12/24	Gēng Yín	1/23	Gēng Shēn	18
8/29	Guǐ Sì	9/28	Guǐ Hài	10/27	Rén Chén	11/26	Rén Xū	12/25	Xīn Mǎo	1/24	Xīn Yǒu	19
8/30	Jiǎ Wǔ	9/29	Jiǎ Zǐ	10/28	Guǐ Sì	11/27	Guǐ Hài	12/26	Rén Chén	1/25	Rén Xū	20
8/31	Yǐ Wèi	9/30	Yǐ Chǒu	10/29	Jiǎ Wǔ	11/28	Jiǎ Zǐ	12/27	Guǐ Sì	1/26	Guǐ Hài	21
9/1	Bǐng Shēn	10/1	Bǐng Yín	10/30	Yǐ Wèi	11/29	Yǐ Chǒu	12/28	Jiǎ Wǔ	1/27	Jiǎ Zǐ	22
9/2	Dīng Yǒu	10/2	Dīng Mǎo	10/31	Bǐng Shēn	11/30	Bǐng Yín	12/29	Yǐ Wèi	1/28	Yǐ Chǒu	23
9/3	Wù Xū	10/3	Wù Chén	11/1	Dīng Yǒu	12/1	Dīng Mǎo	12/30	Bǐng Shēn	1/29	Bǐng Yín	24
9/4	Jǐ Hài	10/4	Jǐ Sì	11/2	Wù Xū	12/2	Wù Chén	12/31	Dīng Yǒu	1/30	Dīng Mǎo	25
9/5	Gēng Zǐ	10/5	Gēng Wǔ	11/3	Jǐ Hài	12/3	Jǐ Sì	1/1	Wù Xū	1/31	Wù Chén	26
9/6	Xīn Chǒu	10/6	Xīn Wèi	11/4	Gēng Zǐ	12/4	Gēng Wǔ	1/2	Jǐ Hài	2/1	Jǐ Sì	27
9/7	Rén Yín	10/7	Rén Shēn	11/5	Xīn Chǒu	12/5	Xīn Wèi	1/3	Gēng Zǐ	2/2	Gēng Wǔ	28
9/8	Guǐ Mǎo	10/8	Guǐ Yǒu	11/6	Rén Yín	12/6	Rén Shēn	1/4	Xīn Chǒu	2/3	Xīn Wèi	29
9/9	Jiǎ Chén			11/7	Guǐ Mǎo			1/5	Rén Yín	2/4	Rén Shēn	30
Li Qiu		Bai Lu		Han Lu		Li Dong		Da Xue		Xiao Han		Jie
8/7	10:15p	9/8	1:35a	10/8	5:36p	11/7	8:54p	12/7	1:30p	1/6	12:16a	
Chu Shu		Qiu Fen		Shuang Jiang		Xiao Xue		Dong Zhi		Da Han		Qi
8/23	1:07p	9/23	11:11a	10/23	8:47p	11/22	8:17p	12/22	7:14a	1/20	5:28p	

	YEAR: 2019 Jǐ Hài -- First six months.										
	1ST MONTH		2ND MONTH		3RD MONTH		4TH MONTH		5TH MONTH		6TH MONTH
	Bǐng Yín		Dīng Mǎo		Wù Chén		Jǐ Sì		Gēng Wǔ		Xīn Wèi
1	2/5	Guǐ Yǒu	**3/6**	Rén Yín	**4/5**	Rén Shēn	5/5	Rén Yín	6/3	Xīn Wèi	7/3	Xīn Chǒu
2	2/6	Jiǎ Xū	3/7	Guǐ Mǎo	4/6	Guǐ Yǒu	**5/6**	Guǐ Mǎo	6/4	Rén Shēn	7/4	Rén Yín
3	2/7	Yǐ Hài	3/8	Jiǎ Chén	4/7	Jiǎ Xū	5/7	Jiǎ Chén	6/5	Guǐ Yǒu	7/5	Guǐ Mǎo
4	2/8	Bǐng Zǐ	3/9	Yǐ Sì	4/8	Yǐ Hài	5/8	Yǐ Sì	6/6	Jiǎ Xū	7/6	Jiǎ Chén
5	2/9	Dīng Chǒu	3/10	Bǐng Wǔ	4/9	Bǐng Zǐ	5/9	Bǐng Wǔ	6/7	Yǐ Hài	7/7	Yǐ Sì
6	2/10	Wù Yín	3/11	Dīng Wèi	4/10	Dīng Chǒu	5/10	Dīng Wèi	6/8	Bǐng Zǐ	7/8	Bǐng Wǔ
7	2/11	Jǐ Mǎo	3/12	Wù Shēn	4/11	Wù Yín	5/11	Wù Shēn	6/9	Dīng Chǒu	7/9	Dīng Wèi
8	2/12	Gēng Chén	3/13	Jǐ Yǒu	4/12	Jǐ Mǎo	5/12	Jǐ Yǒu	6/10	Wù Yín	7/10	Wù Shēn
9	2/13	Xīn Sì	3/14	Gēng Xū	4/13	Gēng Chén	5/13	Gēng Xū	6/11	Jǐ Mǎo	7/11	Jǐ Yǒu
10	2/14	Rén Wǔ	3/15	Xīn Hài	4/14	Xīn Sì	5/14	Xīn Hài	6/12	Gēng Chén	7/12	Gēng Xū
11	2/15	Guǐ Wèi	3/16	Rén Zǐ	4/15	Rén Wǔ	5/15	Rén Zǐ	6/13	Xīn Sì	7/13	Xīn Hài
12	2/16	Jiǎ Shēn	3/17	Guǐ Chǒu	4/16	Guǐ Wèi	5/16	Guǐ Chǒu	6/14	Rén Wǔ	7/14	Rén Zǐ
13	2/17	Yǐ Yǒu	3/18	Jiǎ Yín	4/17	Jiǎ Shēn	5/17	Jiǎ Yín	6/15	Guǐ Wèi	7/15	Guǐ Chǒu
14	2/18	Bǐng Xū	3/19	Yǐ Mǎo	4/18	Yǐ Yǒu	5/18	Yǐ Mǎo	6/16	Jiǎ Shēn	7/16	Jiǎ Yín
15	2/19	Dīng Hài	3/20	Bǐng Chén	4/19	Bǐng Xū	5/19	Bǐng Chén	6/17	Yǐ Yǒu	7/17	Yǐ Mǎo
16	2/20	Wù Zǐ	3/21	Dīng Sì	4/20	Dīng Hài	5/20	Dīng Sì	6/18	Bǐng Xū	7/18	Bǐng Chén
17	2/21	Jǐ Chǒu	3/22	Wù Wǔ	4/21	Wù Zǐ	5/21	Wù Wǔ	6/19	Dīng Hài	7/19	Dīng Sì
18	2/22	Gēng Yín	3/23	Jǐ Wèi	4/22	Jǐ Chǒu	5/22	Jǐ Wèi	6/20	Wù Zǐ	7/20	Wù Wǔ
19	2/23	Xīn Mǎo	3/24	Gēng Shēn	4/23	Gēng Yín	5/23	Gēng Shēn	6/21	Jǐ Chǒu	7/21	Jǐ Wèi
20	2/24	Rén Chén	3/25	Xīn Yǒu	4/24	Xīn Mǎo	5/24	Xīn Yǒu	6/22	Gēng Yín	7/22	Gēng Shēn
21	2/25	Guǐ Sì	3/26	Rén Xū	4/25	Rén Chén	5/25	Rén Xū	6/23	Xīn Mǎo	7/23	Xīn Yǒu
22	2/26	Jiǎ Wǔ	3/27	Guǐ Hài	4/26	Guǐ Sì	5/26	Guǐ Hài	6/24	Rén Chén	7/24	Rén Xū
23	2/27	Yǐ Wèi	3/28	Jiǎ Zǐ	4/27	Jiǎ Wǔ	5/27	Jiǎ Zǐ	6/25	Guǐ Sì	7/25	Guǐ Hài
24	2/28	Bǐng Shēn	3/29	Yǐ Chǒu	4/28	Yǐ Wèi	5/28	Yǐ Chǒu	6/26	Jiǎ Wǔ	7/26	Jiǎ Zǐ
25	3/1	Dīng Yǒu	3/30	Bǐng Yín	4/29	Bǐng Shēn	5/29	Bǐng Yín	6/27	Yǐ Wèi	7/27	Yǐ Chǒu
26	3/2	Wù Xū	3/31	Dīng Mǎo	4/30	Dīng Yǒu	5/30	Dīng Mǎo	6/28	Bǐng Shēn	7/28	Bǐng Yín
27	3/3	Jǐ Hài	4/1	Wù Chén	5/1	Wù Xū	5/31	Wù Chén	6/29	Dīng Yǒu	7/29	Dīng Mǎo
28	3/4	Gēng Zǐ	4/2	Jǐ Sì	5/2	Jǐ Hài	6/1	Jǐ Sì	6/30	Wù Xū	7/30	Wù Chén
29	3/5	Xīn Chǒu	4/3	Gēng Wǔ	5/3	Gēng Zǐ	6/2	Gēng Wǔ	7/1	Jǐ Hài	7/31	Jǐ Sì
30			4/4	Xīn Wèi	5/4	Xīn Chǒu			7/2	Gēng Zǐ		
Jie	Li Chun		Jing Zhi		Qing Ming		Li Xia		Mang Zhong		Xiao Shu
	2/4	11:28a	3/6	5:14a	4/5	9:59a	5/6	3:20p	6/6	7:33a	7/7	5:57p
Qi	Yu Shui		Chun Fen		Gu Yu		Xiao Man		Xia Zhi		Da Shu
	2/19	7:12a	3/21	6:04a	4/20	5:07p	5/21	4:19p	6/22	12:22a	7/23	11:28a

YEAR: 2019 Jǐ Hài -- Last six months.												
7TH MONTH		8TH MONTH		9TH MONTH		10TH MONTH		11TH MONTH		12TH MONTH		
Rén Shēn		Guǐ Yǒu		Jiǎ Xū		Yǐ Hài		Bǐng Zǐ		Dīng Chǒu		
										2019 - 2020		
8/1	Gēng Wǔ	8/30	Jǐ Hài	9/29	Jǐ Sì	10/28	Wù Xū	11/26	Dīng Mǎo	12/26	Dīng Yǒu	1
8/2	Xīn Wèi	8/31	Gēng Zǐ	9/30	Gēng Wǔ	10/29	Jǐ Hài	11/27	Wù Chén	12/27	Wù Xū	2
8/3	Rén Shēn	9/1	Xīn Chǒu	10/1	Xīn Wèi	10/30	Gēng Zǐ	11/28	Jǐ Sì	12/28	Jǐ Hài	3
8/4	Guǐ Yǒu	9/2	Rén Yín	10/2	Rén Shēn	10/31	Xīn Chǒu	11/29	Gēng Wǔ	12/29	Gēng Zǐ	4
8/5	Jiǎ Xū	9/3	Guǐ Mǎo	10/3	Guǐ Yǒu	11/1	Rén Yín	11/30	Xīn Wèi	12/30	Xīn Chǒu	5
8/6	Yǐ Hài	9/4	Jiǎ Chén	10/4	Jiǎ Xū	11/2	Guǐ Mǎo	12/1	Rén Shēn	12/31	Rén Yín	6
8/7	Bǐng Zǐ	9/5	Yǐ Sì	10/5	Yǐ Hài	11/3	Jiǎ Chén	12/2	Guǐ Yǒu	1/1	Guǐ Mǎo	7
8/8	Dīng Chǒu	9/6	Bǐng Wǔ	10/6	Bǐng Zǐ	11/4	Yǐ Sì	12/3	Jiǎ Xū	1/2	Jiǎ Chén	8
8/9	Wù Yín	9/7	Dīng Wèi	10/7	Dīng Chǒu	11/5	Bǐng Wǔ	12/4	Yǐ Hài	1/3	Yǐ Sì	9
8/10	Jǐ Mǎo	9/8	Wù Shēn	10/8	Wù Yín	11/6	Dīng Wèi	12/5	Bǐng Zǐ	1/4	Bǐng Wǔ	10
8/11	Gēng Chén	9/9	Jǐ Yǒu	10/9	Jǐ Mǎo	11/7	Wù Shēn	12/6	Dīng Chǒu	1/5	Dīng Wèi	11
8/12	Xīn Sì	9/10	Gēng Xū	10/10	Gēng Chén	11/8	Jǐ Yǒu	12/7	Wù Yín	1/6	Wù Shēn	12
8/13	Rén Wǔ	9/11	Xīn Hài	10/11	Xīn Sì	11/9	Gēng Xū	12/8	Jǐ Mǎo	1/7	Jǐ Yǒu	13
8/14	Guǐ Wèi	9/12	Rén Zǐ	10/12	Rén Wǔ	11/10	Xīn Hài	12/9	Gēng Chén	1/8	Gēng Xū	14
8/15	Jiǎ Shēn	9/13	Guǐ Chǒu	10/13	Guǐ Wèi	11/11	Rén Zǐ	12/10	Xīn Sì	1/9	Xīn Hài	15
8/16	Yǐ Yǒu	9/14	Jiǎ Yín	10/14	Jiǎ Shēn	11/12	Guǐ Chǒu	12/11	Rén Wǔ	1/10	Rén Zǐ	16
8/17	Bǐng Xū	9/15	Yǐ Mǎo	10/15	Yǐ Yǒu	11/13	Jiǎ Yín	12/12	Guǐ Wèi	1/11	Guǐ Chǒu	17
8/18	Dīng Hài	9/16	Bǐng Chén	10/16	Bǐng Xū	11/14	Yǐ Mǎo	12/13	Jiǎ Shēn	1/12	Jiǎ Yín	18
8/19	Wù Zǐ	9/17	Dīng Sì	10/17	Dīng Hài	11/15	Bǐng Chén	12/14	Yǐ Yǒu	1/13	Yǐ Mǎo	19
8/20	Jǐ Chǒu	9/18	Wù Wǔ	10/18	Wù Zǐ	11/16	Dīng Sì	12/15	Bǐng Xū	1/14	Bǐng Chén	20
8/21	Gēng Yín	9/19	Jǐ Wèi	10/19	Jǐ Chǒu	11/17	Wù Wǔ	12/16	Dīng Hài	1/15	Dīng Sì	21
8/22	Xīn Mǎo	9/20	Gēng Shēn	10/20	Gēng Yín	11/18	Jǐ Wèi	12/17	Wù Zǐ	1/16	Wù Wǔ	22
8/23	Rén Chén	9/21	Xīn Yǒu	10/21	Xīn Mǎo	11/19	Gēng Shēn	12/18	Jǐ Chǒu	1/17	Jǐ Wèi	23
8/24	Guǐ Sì	9/22	Rén Xū	10/22	Rén Chén	11/20	Xīn Yǒu	12/19	Gēng Yín	1/18	Gēng Shēn	24
8/25	Jiǎ Wǔ	9/23	Guǐ Hài	10/23	Guǐ Sì	11/21	Rén Xū	12/20	Xīn Mǎo	1/19	Xīn Yǒu	25
8/26	Yǐ Wèi	9/24	Jiǎ Zǐ	10/24	Jiǎ Wǔ	11/22	Guǐ Hài	12/21	Rén Chén	1/20	Rén Xū	26
8/27	Bǐng Shēn	9/25	Yǐ Chǒu	10/25	Yǐ Wèi	11/23	Jiǎ Zǐ	12/22	Guǐ Sì	1/21	Guǐ Hài	27
8/28	Dīng Yǒu	9/26	Bǐng Yín	10/26	Bǐng Shēn	11/24	Yǐ Chǒu	12/23	Jiǎ Wǔ	1/22	Jiǎ Zǐ	28
8/29	Wù Xū	9/27	Dīng Mǎo	10/27	Dīng Yǒu	11/25	Bǐng Yín	12/24	Yǐ Wèi	1/23	Yǐ Chǒu	29
		9/28	Wù Chén					12/25	Bǐng Shēn	1/24	Bǐng Yín	30
Li Qiu		Bai Lu		Han Lu		Li Dong		Da Xue		Xiao Han		Jie
8/8	4:03a	9/8	7:24a	10/8	11:25p	11/8	2:42a	12/7	7:20p	1/6	6:06a	
Chu Shu		Qiu Fen		Shuang Jiang		Xiao Xue		Dong Zhi		Da Han		Qi
8/23	6:55p	9/23	5:00p	10/24	2:36a	11/23	12:06a	12/22	1:04p	1/20	11:10p	

	1ST MONTH		2ND MONTH		3RD MONTH		4TH MONTH		LEAP MONTH		5TH MONTH		6TH MONTH	
YEAR: 2020 Gēng Zǐ -- First six months.														
	Wù Yín		Jǐ Mǎo		Gēng Chén		Xīn Sì				Rén Wǔ		Guǐ Wèi	
1	1/25	Dīng Mǎo	2/23	Bǐng Shēn	3/24	Bǐng Yín	4/23	Bǐng Shēn	5/23	Bǐng Yín	6/21	Yǐ Wèi	7/21	Yǐ Chǒu
2	1/26	Wù Chén	2/24	Dīng Yǒu	3/25	Dīng Mǎo	4/24	Dīng Yǒu	5/24	Dīng Mǎo	6/22	Bǐng Shēn	7/22	Bǐng Yín
3	1/27	Jǐ Sì	2/25	Wù Xū	3/26	Wù Chén	4/25	Wù Xū	5/25	Wù Chén	6/23	Dīng Yǒu	7/23	Dīng Mǎo
4	1/28	Gēng Wǔ	2/26	Jǐ Hài	3/27	Jǐ Sì	4/26	Jǐ Hài	5/26	Jǐ Sì	6/24	Wù Xū	7/24	Wù Chén
5	1/29	Xīn Wèi	2/27	Gēng Zǐ	3/28	Gēng Wǔ	4/27	Gēng Zǐ	5/27	Gēng Wǔ	6/25	Jǐ Hài	7/25	Jǐ Sì
6	1/30	Rén Shēn	2/28	Xīn Chǒu	3/29	Xīn Wèi	4/28	Xīn Chǒu	5/28	Xīn Wèi	6/26	Gēng Zǐ	7/26	Gēng Wǔ
7	1/31	Guǐ Yǒu	2/29	Rén Yín	3/30	Rén Shēn	4/29	Rén Yín	5/29	Rén Shēn	6/27	Xīn Chǒu	7/27	Xīn Wèi
8	2/1	Jiǎ Xū	3/1	Guǐ Mǎo	3/31	Guǐ Yǒu	4/30	Guǐ Mǎo	5/30	Guǐ Yǒu	6/28	Rén Yín	7/28	Rén Shēn
9	2/2	Yǐ Hài	3/2	Jiǎ Chén	4/1	Jiǎ Xū	5/1	Jiǎ Chén	5/31	Jiǎ Xū	6/29	Guǐ Mǎo	7/29	Guǐ Yǒu
10	2/3	Bǐng Zǐ	3/3	Yǐ Sì	4/2	Yǐ Hài	5/2	Yǐ Sì	6/1	Yǐ Hài	6/30	Jiǎ Chén	7/30	Jiǎ Xū
11	2/4	Dīng Chǒu	3/4	Bǐng Wǔ	4/3	Bǐng Zǐ	5/3	Bǐng Wǔ	6/2	Bǐng Zǐ	7/1	Yǐ Sì	7/31	Yǐ Hài
12	2/5	Wù Yín	3/5	Dīng Wèi	4/4	Dīng Chǒu	5/4	Dīng Wèi	6/3	Dīng Chǒu	7/2	Bǐng Wǔ	8/1	Bǐng Zǐ
13	2/6	Jǐ Mǎo	3/6	Wù Shēn	4/5	Wù Yín	5/5	Wù Shēn	6/4	Wù Yín	7/3	Dīng Wèi	8/2	Dīng Chǒu
14	2/7	Gēng Chén	3/7	Jǐ Yǒu	4/6	Jǐ Mǎo	5/6	Jǐ Yǒu	6/5	Jǐ Mǎo	7/4	Wù Shēn	8/3	Wù Yín
15	2/8	Xīn Sì	3/8	Gēng Xū	4/7	Gēng Chén	5/7	Gēng Xū	6/6	Gēng Chén	7/5	Jǐ Yǒu	8/4	Jǐ Mǎo
16	2/9	Rén Wǔ	3/9	Xīn Hài	4/8	Xīn Sì	5/8	Xīn Hài	6/7	Xīn Sì	7/6	Gēng Xū	8/5	Gēng Chén
17	2/10	Guǐ Wèi	3/10	Rén Zǐ	4/9	Rén Wǔ	5/9	Rén Zǐ	6/8	Rén Wǔ	7/7	Xīn Hài	8/6	Xīn Sì
18	2/11	Jiǎ Shēn	3/11	Guǐ Chǒu	4/10	Guǐ Wèi	5/10	Guǐ Chǒu	6/9	Guǐ Wèi	7/8	Rén Zǐ	8/7	Rén Wǔ
19	2/12	Yǐ Yǒu	3/12	Jiǎ Yín	4/11	Jiǎ Shēn	5/11	Jiǎ Yín	6/10	Jiǎ Shēn	7/9	Guǐ Chǒu	8/8	Guǐ Wèi
20	2/13	Bǐng Xū	3/13	Yǐ Mǎo	4/12	Yǐ Yǒu	5/12	Yǐ Mǎo	6/11	Yǐ Yǒu	7/10	Jiǎ Yín	8/9	Jiǎ Shēn
21	2/14	Dīng Hài	3/14	Bǐng Chén	4/13	Bǐng Xū	5/13	Bǐng Chén	6/12	Bǐng Xū	7/11	Yǐ Mǎo	8/10	Yǐ Yǒu
22	2/15	Wù Zǐ	3/15	Dīng Sì	4/14	Dīng Hài	5/14	Dīng Sì	6/13	Dīng Hài	7/12	Bǐng Chén	8/11	Bǐng Xū
23	2/16	Jǐ Chǒu	3/16	Wù Wǔ	4/15	Wù Zǐ	5/15	Wù Wǔ	6/14	Wù Zǐ	7/13	Dīng Sì	8/12	Dīng Hài
24	2/17	Gēng Yín	3/17	Jǐ Wèi	4/16	Jǐ Chǒu	5/16	Jǐ Wèi	6/15	Jǐ Chǒu	7/14	Wù Wǔ	8/13	Wù Zǐ
25	2/18	Xīn Mǎo	3/18	Gēng Shēn	4/17	Gēng Yín	5/17	Gēng Shēn	6/16	Gēng Yín	7/15	Jǐ Wèi	8/14	Jǐ Chǒu
26	2/19	Rén Chén	3/19	Xīn Yǒu	4/18	Xīn Mǎo	5/18	Xīn Yǒu	6/17	Xīn Mǎo	7/16	Gēng Shēn	8/15	Gēng Yín
27	2/20	Guǐ Sì	3/20	Rén Xū	4/19	Rén Chén	5/19	Rén Xū	6/18	Rén Chén	7/17	Xīn Yǒu	8/16	Xīn Mǎo
28	2/21	Jiǎ Wǔ	3/21	Guǐ Hài	4/20	Guǐ Sì	5/20	Guǐ Hài	6/19	Guǐ Sì	7/18	Rén Xū	8/17	Rén Chén
29	2/22	Yǐ Wèi	3/22	Jiǎ Zǐ	4/21	Jiǎ Wǔ	5/21	Jiǎ Zǐ	6/20	Jiǎ Wǔ	7/19	Guǐ Hài	8/18	Guǐ Sì
30			3/23	Yǐ Chǒu	4/22	Yǐ Wèi	5/22	Yǐ Chǒu			7/20	Jiǎ Zǐ		
Jie	Li Chun		Jing Zhi		Qing Ming		Li Xia				Mang Zhong		Xiao Shu	
	2/4	5:18p	3/5	11:03a	4/4	3:48p	5/5	9:08a			6/5	1:22p	7/6	11:46p
Qi	Yu Shui		Chun Fen		Gu Yu		Xiao Man				Xia Zhi		Da Shu	
	2/19	1:02p	3/20	11:53a	4/19	10:55p	5/20	8:07p			6/21	6:10a	7/22	5:16p

針灸大成 · 卷之五

7TH MONTH		8TH MONTH		9TH MONTH		10TH MONTH		11TH MONTH		12TH MONTH		
Jiǎ Shēn		Yǐ Yǒu		Bǐng Xū		Dīng Hài		Wù Zǐ		Jǐ Chǒu		
						2020 - 2021						
8/19	Jiǎ Wǔ	9/17	Guǐ Hài	10/17	Guǐ Sì	11/15	Rén Xū	12/15	Rén Chén	1/13	Xīn Yǒu	1
8/20	Yǐ Wèi	9/18	Jiǎ Zǐ	10/18	Jiǎ Wǔ	11/16	Guǐ Hài	12/16	Guǐ Sì	1/14	Rén Xū	2
8/21	Bǐng Shēn	9/19	Yǐ Chǒu	10/19	Yǐ Wèi	11/17	Jiǎ Zǐ	12/17	Jiǎ Wǔ	1/15	Guǐ Hài	3
8/22	Dīng Yǒu	9/20	Bǐng Yín	10/20	Bǐng Shēn	11/18	Yǐ Chǒu	12/18	Yǐ Wèi	1/16	Jiǎ Zǐ	4
8/23	Wù Xū	9/21	Dīng Mǎo	10/21	Dīng Yǒu	11/19	Bǐng Yín	12/19	Bǐng Shēn	1/17	Yǐ Chǒu	5
8/24	Jǐ Hài	9/22	Wù Chén	10/22	Wù Xū	11/20	Dīng Mǎo	12/20	Dīng Yǒu	1/18	Bǐng Yín	6
8/25	Gēng Zǐ	9/23	Jǐ Sì	10/23	Jǐ Hài	11/21	Wù Chén	12/21	Wù Xū	1/19	Dīng Mǎo	7
8/26	Xīn Chǒu	9/24	Gēng Wǔ	10/24	Gēng Zǐ	11/22	Jǐ Sì	12/22	Jǐ Hài	1/20	Wù Chén	8
8/27	Rén Yín	9/25	Xīn Wèi	10/25	Xīn Chǒu	11/23	Gēng Wǔ	12/23	Gēng Zǐ	1/21	Jǐ Sì	9
8/28	Guǐ Mǎo	9/26	Rén Shēn	10/26	Rén Yín	11/24	Xīn Wèi	12/24	Xīn Chǒu	1/22	Gēng Wǔ	10
8/29	Jiǎ Chén	9/27	Guǐ Yǒu	10/27	Guǐ Mǎo	11/25	Rén Shēn	12/25	Rén Yín	1/23	Xīn Wèi	11
8/30	Yǐ Sì	9/28	Jiǎ Xū	10/28	Jiǎ Chén	11/26	Guǐ Yǒu	12/26	Guǐ Mǎo	1/24	Rén Shēn	12
8/31	Bǐng Wǔ	9/29	Yǐ Hài	10/29	Yǐ Sì	11/27	Jiǎ Xū	12/27	Jiǎ Chén	1/25	Guǐ Yǒu	13
9/1	Dīng Wèi	9/30	Bǐng Zǐ	10/30	Bǐng Wǔ	11/28	Yǐ Hài	12/28	Yǐ Sì	1/26	Jiǎ Xū	14
9/2	Wù Shēn	10/1	Dīng Chǒu	10/31	Dīng Wèi	11/29	Bǐng Zǐ	12/29	Bǐng Wǔ	1/27	Yǐ Hài	15
9/3	Jǐ Yǒu	10/2	Wù Yín	11/1	Wù Shēn	11/30	Dīng Chǒu	12/30	Dīng Wèi	1/28	Bǐng Zǐ	16
9/4	Gēng Xū	10/3	Jǐ Mǎo	11/2	Jǐ Yǒu	12/1	Wù Yín	12/31	Wù Shēn	1/29	Dīng Chǒu	17
9/5	Xīn Hài	10/4	Gēng Chén	11/3	Gēng Xū	12/2	Jǐ Mǎo	1/1	Jǐ Yǒu	1/30	Wù Yín	18
9/6	Rén Zǐ	10/5	Xīn Sì	11/4	Xīn Hài	12/3	Gēng Chén	1/2	Gēng Xū	1/31	Jǐ Mǎo	19
9/7	Guǐ Chǒu	10/6	Rén Wǔ	11/5	Rén Zǐ	12/4	Xīn Sì	1/3	Xīn Hài	2/1	Gēng Chén	20
9/8	Jiǎ Yín	10/7	Guǐ Wèi	11/6	Guǐ Chǒu	12/5	Rén Wǔ	1/4	Rén Zǐ	2/2	Xīn Sì	21
9/9	Yǐ Mǎo	**10/8**	Jiǎ Shēn	**11/7**	Jiǎ Yín	12/6	Guǐ Wèi	**1/5**	Guǐ Chǒu	**2/3**	Rén Wǔ	22
9/10	Bǐng Chén	10/9	Yǐ Yǒu	11/8	Yǐ Mǎo	**12/7**	Jiǎ Shēn	1/6	Jiǎ Yín	2/4	Guǐ Wèi	23
9/11	Dīng Sì	10/10	Bǐng Xū	11/9	Bǐng Chén	12/8	Yǐ Yǒu	1/7	Yǐ Mǎo	2/5	Jiǎ Shēn	24
9/12	Wù Wǔ	10/11	Dīng Hài	11/10	Dīng Sì	12/9	Bǐng Xū	1/8	Bǐng Chén	2/6	Yǐ Yǒu	25
9/13	Jǐ Wèi	10/12	Wù Zǐ	11/11	Wù Wǔ	12/10	Dīng Hài	1/9	Dīng Sì	2/7	Bǐng Xū	26
9/14	Gēng Shēn	10/13	Jǐ Chǒu	11/12	Jǐ Wèi	12/11	Wù Zǐ	1/10	Wù Wǔ	2/8	Dīng Hài	27
9/15	Xīn Yǒu	10/14	Gēng Yín	11/13	Gēng Shēn	12/12	Jǐ Chǒu	1/11	Jǐ Wèi	2/9	Wù Zǐ	28
9/16	Rén Xū	10/15	Xīn Mǎo	11/14	Xīn Yǒu	12/13	Gēng Yín	1/12	Gēng Shēn	2/10	Jǐ Chǒu	29
		10/16	Rén Chén			12/14	Xīn Mǎo			2/11	Gēng Yín	30
Li Qiu		Bai Lu		Han Lu		Li Dong		Da Xue		Xiao Han		Jie
8/7	9:51a	9/7	1:12p	10/8	5:15a	11/7	8:31a	12/7	1:09a	1/5	11:55a	
Chu Shu		Qiu Fen		Shuang Jiang		Xiao Xue		Dong Zhi		Da Han		Qi
8/23	12:43a	9/22	8:49p	10/23	8:26a	11/22	5:56a	12/21	6:54p	1/20	5:04a	

YEAR: 2020 Gēng Zǐ -- Last six months.

YEAR: 2021 Xīn Chǒu -- First six months.												
	1ST MONTH		2ND MONTH		3RD MONTH		4TH MONTH		5TH MONTH		6TH MONTH	
	Gēng Yín		Xīn Mǎo		Rén Chén		Guǐ Sì		Jiǎ Wǔ		Yǐ Wèi	
1	2/12	Xīn Mǎo	3/13	Gēng Shēn	4/12	Gēng Yín	5/12	Gēng Shēn	6/10	Jǐ Chǒu	7/10	Jǐ Wèi
2	2/13	Rén Chén	3/14	Xīn Yǒu	4/13	Xīn Mǎo	5/13	Xīn Yǒu	6/11	Gēng Yín	7/11	Gēng Shēn
3	2/14	Guǐ Sì	3/15	Rén Xū	4/14	Rén Chén	5/14	Rén Xū	6/12	Xīn Mǎo	7/12	Xīn Yǒu
4	2/15	Jiǎ Wǔ	3/16	Guǐ Hài	4/15	Guǐ Sì	5/15	Guǐ Hài	6/13	Rén Chén	7/13	Rén Xū
5	2/16	Yǐ Wèi	3/17	Jiǎ Zǐ	4/16	Jiǎ Wǔ	5/16	Jiǎ Zǐ	6/14	Guǐ Sì	7/14	Guǐ Hài
6	2/17	Bǐng Shēn	3/18	Yǐ Chǒu	4/17	Yǐ Wèi	5/17	Yǐ Chǒu	6/15	Jiǎ Wǔ	7/15	Jiǎ Zǐ
7	2/18	Dīng Yǒu	3/19	Bǐng Yín	4/18	Bǐng Shēn	5/18	Bǐng Yín	6/16	Yǐ Wèi	7/16	Yǐ Chǒu
8	2/19	Wù Xū	3/20	Dīng Mǎo	4/19	Dīng Yǒu	5/19	Dīng Mǎo	6/17	Bǐng Shēn	7/17	Bǐng Yín
9	2/20	Jǐ Hài	3/21	Wù Chén	4/20	Wù Xū	5/20	Wù Chén	6/18	Dīng Yǒu	7/18	Dīng Mǎo
10	2/21	Gēng Zǐ	3/22	Jǐ Sì	4/21	Jǐ Hài	5/21	Jǐ Sì	6/19	Wù Xū	7/19	Wù Chén
11	2/22	Xīn Chǒu	3/23	Gēng Wǔ	4/22	Gēng Zǐ	5/22	Gēng Wǔ	6/20	Jǐ Hài	7/20	Jǐ Sì
12	2/23	Rén Yín	3/24	Xīn Wèi	4/23	Xīn Chǒu	5/23	Xīn Wèi	6/21	Gēng Zǐ	7/21	Gēng Wǔ
13	2/24	Guǐ Mǎo	3/25	Rén Shēn	4/24	Rén Yín	5/24	Rén Shēn	6/22	Xīn Chǒu	7/22	Xīn Wèi
14	2/25	Jiǎ Chén	3/26	Guǐ Yǒu	4/25	Guǐ Mǎo	5/25	Guǐ Yǒu	6/23	Rén Yín	7/23	Rén Shēn
15	2/26	Yǐ Sì	3/27	Jiǎ Xū	4/26	Jiǎ Chén	5/26	Jiǎ Xū	6/24	Guǐ Mǎo	7/24	Guǐ Yǒu
16	2/27	Bǐng Wǔ	3/28	Yǐ Hài	4/27	Yǐ Sì	5/27	Yǐ Hài	6/25	Jiǎ Chén	7/25	Jiǎ Xū
17	2/28	Dīng Wèi	3/29	Bǐng Zǐ	4/28	Bǐng Wǔ	5/28	Bǐng Zǐ	6/26	Yǐ Sì	7/26	Yǐ Hài
18	3/1	Wù Shēn	3/30	Dīng Chǒu	4/29	Dīng Wèi	5/29	Dīng Chǒu	6/27	Bǐng Wǔ	7/27	Bǐng Zǐ
19	3/2	Jǐ Yǒu	3/31	Wù Yín	4/30	Wù Shēn	5/30	Wù Yín	6/28	Dīng Wèi	7/28	Dīng Chǒu
20	3/3	Gēng Xū	4/1	Jǐ Mǎo	5/1	Jǐ Yǒu	5/31	Jǐ Mǎo	6/29	Wù Shēn	7/29	Wù Yín
21	3/4	Xīn Hài	4/2	Gēng Chén	5/2	Gēng Xū	6/1	Gēng Chén	6/30	Jǐ Yǒu	7/30	Jǐ Mǎo
22	3/5	Rén Zǐ	4/3	Xīn Sì	5/3	Xīn Hài	6/2	Xīn Sì	7/1	Gēng Xū	7/31	Gēng Chén
23	3/6	Guǐ Chǒu	4/4	Rén Wǔ	5/4	Rén Zǐ	6/3	Rén Wǔ	7/2	Xīn Hài	8/1	Xīn Sì
24	3/7	Jiǎ Yín	4/5	Guǐ Wèi	5/5	Guǐ Chǒu	6/4	Guǐ Wèi	7/3	Rén Zǐ	8/2	Rén Wǔ
25	3/8	Yǐ Mǎo	4/6	Jiǎ Shēn	5/6	Jiǎ Yín	6/5	Jiǎ Shēn	7/4	Guǐ Chǒu	8/3	Guǐ Wèi
26	3/9	Bǐng Chén	4/7	Yǐ Yǒu	5/7	Yǐ Mǎo	6/6	Yǐ Yǒu	7/5	Jiǎ Yín	8/4	Jiǎ Shēn
27	3/10	Dīng Sì	4/8	Bǐng Xū	5/8	Bǐng Chén	6/7	Bǐng Xū	7/6	Yǐ Mǎo	8/5	Yǐ Yǒu
28	3/11	Wù Wǔ	4/9	Dīng Hài	5/9	Dīng Sì	6/8	Dīng Hài	7/7	Bǐng Chén	8/6	Bǐng Xū
29	3/12	Jǐ Wèi	4/10	Wù Zǐ	5/10	Wù Wǔ	6/9	Wù Zǐ	7/8	Dīng Sì	8/7	Dīng Hài
30			4/11	Jǐ Chǒu	5/11	Jǐ Wèi			7/9	Wù Wǔ		
Jie	Li Chun		Jing Zhi		Qing Ming		Li Xia		Mang Zhong		Xiao Shu	
	2/3	11:08p	3/5	4:54p	4/4	9:37p	5/5	2:57p	6/5	7:09p	7/7	5:33a
Qi	Yu Shui		Chun Fen		Gu Yu		Xiao Man		Xia Zhi		Da Shu	
	2/18	6:51p	3/20	5:42p	4/20	4:44a	5/21	3:56a	6/21	11:58a	7/22	11:05p

針灸大成 · 卷之五

YEAR: 2021 Xīn Chǒu -- Last six months.												
7TH MONTH		8TH MONTH		9TH MONTH		10TH MONTH		11TH MONTH		12TH MONTH		
Bǐng Shēn		Dīng Yǒu		Wù Xū		Jǐ Hài		Gēng Zǐ		Xīn Chǒu		
								2021 - 2022				
8/8	Wù Zǐ	9/7	Wù Wǔ	10/6	Dīng Hài	11/5	Dīng Sì	12/4	Bǐng Xū	1/3	Bǐng Chén	1
8/9	Jǐ Chǒu	9/8	Jǐ Wèi	10/7	Wù Zǐ	11/6	Wù Wǔ	12/5	Dīng Hài	1/4	Dīng Sì	2
8/10	Gēng Yín	9/9	Gēng Shēn	10/8	Jǐ Chǒu	11/7	Jǐ Wèi	12/6	Wù Zǐ	1/5	Wù Wǔ	3
8/11	Xīn Mǎo	9/10	Xīn Yǒu	10/9	Gēng Yín	11/8	Gēng Shēn	12/7	Jǐ Chǒu	1/6	Jǐ Wèi	4
8/12	Rén Chén	9/11	Rén Xū	10/10	Xīn Mǎo	11/9	Xīn Yǒu	12/8	Gēng Yín	1/7	Gēng Shēn	5
8/13	Guǐ Sì	9/12	Guǐ Hài	10/11	Rén Chén	11/10	Rén Xū	12/9	Xīn Mǎo	1/8	Xīn Yǒu	6
8/14	Jiǎ Wǔ	9/13	Jiǎ Zǐ	10/12	Guǐ Sì	11/11	Guǐ Hài	12/10	Rén Chén	1/9	Rén Xū	7
8/15	Yǐ Wèi	9/14	Yǐ Chǒu	10/13	Jiǎ Wǔ	11/12	Jiǎ Zǐ	12/11	Guǐ Sì	1/10	Guǐ Hài	8
8/16	Bǐng Shēn	9/15	Bǐng Yín	10/14	Yǐ Wèi	11/13	Yǐ Chǒu	12/12	Jiǎ Wǔ	1/11	Jiǎ Zǐ	9
8/17	Dīng Yǒu	9/16	Dīng Mǎo	10/15	Bǐng Shēn	11/14	Bǐng Yín	12/13	Yǐ Wèi	1/12	Yǐ Chǒu	10
8/18	Wù Xū	9/17	Wù Chén	10/16	Dīng Yǒu	11/15	Dīng Mǎo	12/14	Bǐng Shēn	1/13	Bǐng Yín	11
8/19	Jǐ Hài	9/18	Jǐ Sì	10/17	Wù Xū	11/16	Wù Chén	12/15	Dīng Yǒu	1/14	Dīng Mǎo	12
8/20	Gēng Zǐ	9/19	Gēng Wǔ	10/18	Jǐ Hài	11/17	Jǐ Sì	12/16	Wù Xū	1/15	Wù Chén	13
8/21	Xīn Chǒu	9/20	Xīn Wèi	10/19	Gēng Zǐ	11/18	Gēng Wǔ	12/17	Jǐ Hài	1/16	Jǐ Sì	14
8/22	Rén Yín	9/21	Rén Shēn	10/20	Xīn Chǒu	11/19	Xīn Wèi	12/18	Gēng Zǐ	1/17	Gēng Wǔ	15
8/23	Guǐ Mǎo	9/22	Guǐ Yǒu	10/21	Rén Yín	11/20	Rén Shēn	12/19	Xīn Chǒu	1/18	Xīn Wèi	16
8/24	Jiǎ Chén	9/23	Jiǎ Xū	10/22	Guǐ Mǎo	11/21	Guǐ Yǒu	12/20	Rén Yín	1/19	Rén Shēn	17
8/25	Yǐ Sì	9/24	Yǐ Hài	10/23	Jiǎ Chén	11/22	Jiǎ Xū	12/21	Guǐ Mǎo	1/20	Guǐ Yǒu	18
8/26	Bǐng Wǔ	9/25	Bǐng Zǐ	10/24	Yǐ Sì	11/23	Yǐ Hài	12/22	Jiǎ Chén	1/21	Jiǎ Xū	19
8/27	Dīng Wèi	9/26	Dīng Chǒu	10/25	Bǐng Wǔ	11/24	Bǐng Zǐ	12/23	Yǐ Sì	1/22	Yǐ Hài	20
8/28	Wù Shēn	9/27	Wù Yín	10/26	Dīng Wèi	11/25	Dīng Chǒu	12/24	Bǐng Wǔ	1/23	Bǐng Zǐ	21
8/29	Jǐ Yǒu	9/28	Jǐ Mǎo	10/27	Wù Shēn	11/26	Wù Yín	12/25	Dīng Wèi	1/24	Dīng Chǒu	22
8/30	Gēng Xū	9/29	Gēng Chén	10/28	Jǐ Yǒu	11/27	Jǐ Mǎo	12/26	Wù Shēn	1/25	Wù Yín	23
8/31	Xīn Hài	9/30	Xīn Sì	10/29	Gēng Xū	11/28	Gēng Chén	12/27	Jǐ Yǒu	1/26	Jǐ Mǎo	24
9/1	Rén Zǐ	10/1	Rén Wǔ	10/30	Xīn Hài	11/29	Xīn Sì	12/28	Gēng Xū	1/27	Gēng Chén	25
9/2	Guǐ Chǒu	10/2	Guǐ Wèi	10/31	Rén Zǐ	11/30	Rén Wǔ	12/29	Xīn Hài	1/28	Xīn Sì	26
9/3	Jiǎ Yín	10/3	Jiǎ Shēn	11/1	Guǐ Chǒu	12/1	Guǐ Wèi	12/30	Rén Zǐ	1/29	Rén Wǔ	27
9/4	Yǐ Mǎo	10/4	Yǐ Yǒu	11/2	Jiǎ Yín	12/2	Jiǎ Shēn	12/31	Guǐ Chǒu	1/30	Guǐ Wèi	28
9/5	Bǐng Chén	10/5	Bǐng Xū	11/3	Yǐ Mǎo	12/3	Yǐ Yǒu	1/1	Jiǎ Yín	1/31	Jiǎ Shēn	29
9/6	Dīng Sì			11/4	Bǐng Chén			1/2	Yǐ Mǎo			30
Li Qiu		Bai Lu		Han Lu		Li Dong		Da Xue		Xiao Han		Jie
8/7	3:40p	9/7	7:01p	10/8	11:04a	11/7	2:21p	12/7	7:00a	1/5	5:46p	
Chu Shu		Qiu Fen		Shuang Jiang		Xiao Xue		Dong Zhi		Da Han		Qi
8/23	6:32a	9/23	4:37a	10/23	2:15p	11/22	11:46a	12/22	12:44a	1/20	10:54a	

		YEAR: 2022 Rén Yín -- First six months.									
	1ST MONTH		2ND MONTH		3RD MONTH		4TH MONTH		5TH MONTH		6TH MONTH
	Rén Yín		Guǐ Mǎo		Jiǎ Chén		Yǐ Sì		Bǐng Wǔ		Dīng Wèi
1	2/1	Yǐ Yǒu	3/3	Yǐ Mǎo	4/1	Jiǎ Shēn	5/1	Jiǎ Yín	5/30	Guǐ Wèi	6/29	Guǐ Chǒu
2	2/2	Bǐng Xū	3/4	Bǐng Chén	4/2	Yǐ Yǒu	5/2	Yǐ Mǎo	5/31	Jiǎ Shēn	6/30	Jiǎ Yín
3	2/3	Dīng Hài	3/5	Dīng Sì	4/3	Bǐng Xū	5/3	Bǐng Chén	6/1	Yǐ Yǒu	7/1	Yǐ Mǎo
4	2/4	Wù Zǐ	3/6	Wù Wǔ	4/4	Dīng Hài	5/4	Dīng Sì	6/2	Bǐng Xū	7/2	Bǐng Chén
5	2/5	Jǐ Chǒu	3/7	Jǐ Wèi	4/5	Wù Zǐ	5/5	Wù Wǔ	6/3	Dīng Hài	7/3	Dīng Sì
6	2/6	Gēng Yín	3/8	Gēng Shēn	4/6	Jǐ Chǒu	5/6	Jǐ Wèi	6/4	Wù Zǐ	7/4	Wù Wǔ
7	2/7	Xīn Mǎo	3/9	Xīn Yǒu	4/7	Gēng Yín	5/7	Gēng Shēn	6/5	Jǐ Chǒu	7/5	Jǐ Wèi
8	2/8	Rén Chén	3/10	Rén Xū	4/8	Xīn Mǎo	5/8	Xīn Yǒu	6/6	Gēng Yín	7/6	Gēng Shēn
9	2/9	Guǐ Sì	3/11	Guǐ Hài	4/9	Rén Chén	5/9	Rén Xū	6/7	Xīn Mǎo	7/7	Xīn Yǒu
10	2/10	Jiǎ Wǔ	3/12	Jiǎ Zǐ	4/10	Guǐ Sì	5/10	Guǐ Hài	6/8	Rén Chén	7/8	Rén Xū
11	2/11	Yǐ Wèi	3/13	Yǐ Chǒu	4/11	Jiǎ Wǔ	5/11	Jiǎ Zǐ	6/9	Guǐ Sì	7/9	Guǐ Hài
12	2/12	Bǐng Shēn	3/14	Bǐng Yín	4/12	Yǐ Wèi	5/12	Yǐ Chǒu	6/10	Jiǎ Wǔ	7/10	Jiǎ Zǐ
13	2/13	Dīng Yǒu	3/15	Dīng Mǎo	4/13	Bǐng Shēn	5/13	Bǐng Yín	6/11	Yǐ Wèi	7/11	Yǐ Chǒu
14	2/14	Wù Xū	3/16	Wù Chén	4/14	Dīng Yǒu	5/14	Dīng Mǎo	6/12	Bǐng Shēn	7/12	Bǐng Yín
15	2/15	Jǐ Hài	3/17	Jǐ Sì	4/15	Wù Xū	5/15	Wù Chén	6/13	Dīng Yǒu	7/13	Dīng Mǎo
16	2/16	Gēng Zǐ	3/18	Gēng Wǔ	4/16	Jǐ Hài	5/16	Jǐ Sì	6/14	Wù Xū	7/14	Wù Chén
17	2/17	Xīn Chǒu	3/19	Xīn Wèi	4/17	Gēng Zǐ	5/17	Gēng Wǔ	6/15	Jǐ Hài	7/15	Jǐ Sì
18	2/18	Rén Yín	3/20	Rén Shēn	4/18	Xīn Chǒu	5/18	Xīn Wèi	6/16	Gēng Zǐ	7/16	Gēng Wǔ
19	2/19	Guǐ Mǎo	3/21	Guǐ Yǒu	4/19	Rén Yín	5/19	Rén Shēn	6/17	Xīn Chǒu	7/17	Xīn Wèi
20	2/20	Jiǎ Chén	3/22	Jiǎ Xū	4/20	Guǐ Mǎo	5/20	Guǐ Yǒu	6/18	Rén Yín	7/18	Rén Shēn
21	2/21	Yǐ Sì	3/23	Yǐ Hài	4/21	Jiǎ Chén	5/21	Jiǎ Xū	6/19	Guǐ Mǎo	7/19	Guǐ Yǒu
22	2/22	Bǐng Wǔ	3/24	Bǐng Zǐ	4/22	Yǐ Sì	5/22	Yǐ Hài	6/20	Jiǎ Chén	7/20	Jiǎ Xū
23	2/23	Dīng Wèi	3/25	Dīng Chǒu	4/23	Bǐng Wǔ	5/23	Bǐng Zǐ	6/21	Yǐ Sì	7/21	Yǐ Hài
24	2/24	Wù Shēn	3/26	Wù Yín	4/24	Dīng Wèi	5/24	Dīng Chǒu	6/22	Bǐng Wǔ	7/22	Bǐng Zǐ
25	2/25	Jǐ Yǒu	3/27	Jǐ Mǎo	4/25	Wù Shēn	5/25	Wù Yín	6/23	Dīng Wèi	7/23	Dīng Chǒu
26	2/26	Gēng Xū	3/28	Gēng Chén	4/26	Jǐ Yǒu	5/26	Jǐ Mǎo	6/24	Wù Shēn	7/24	Wù Yín
27	2/27	Xīn Hài	3/29	Xīn Sì	4/27	Gēng Xū	5/27	Gēng Chén	6/25	Jǐ Yǒu	7/25	Jǐ Mǎo
28	2/28	Rén Zǐ	3/30	Rén Wǔ	4/28	Xīn Hài	5/28	Xīn Sì	6/26	Gēng Xū	7/26	Gēng Chén
29	3/1	Guǐ Chǒu	3/31	Guǐ Wèi	4/29	Rén Zǐ	5/29	Rén Wǔ	6/27	Xīn Hài	7/27	Xīn Sì
30	3/2	Jiǎ Yín			4/30	Guǐ Chǒu			6/28	Rén Zǐ	7/28	Rén Wǔ
Jie	Li Chun		Jing Zhi		Qing Ming		Li Xia		Mang Zhong		Xiao Shu	
	2/4	4:58a	3/5	10:42p	4/5	3:22a	5/5	8:45p	6/6	12:58a	7/7	11:22a
Qi	Yu Shui		Chun Fen		Gu Yu		Xiao Man		Xia Zhi		Da Shu	
	2/19	12:42a	3/20	11:32p	4/20	1/0	5/21	9:44a	6/21	5:46p	7/23	4:52a

YEAR: 2022 Rén Yín -- Last six months.												
7TH MONTH		8TH MONTH		9TH MONTH		10TH MONTH		11TH MONTH		12TH MONTH		
Wù Shēn		Jǐ Yǒu		Gēng Xū		Xīn Hài		Rén Zǐ		Guǐ Chǒu		
										2022 - 2023		
7/29	Guǐ Wèi	8/27	Rén Zǐ	9/26	Rén Wǔ	10/25	Xīn Hài	11/24	Xīn Sì	12/23	Gēng Xū	1
7/30	Jiǎ Shēn	8/28	Guǐ Chǒu	9/27	Guǐ Wèi	10/26	Rén Zǐ	11/25	Rén Wǔ	12/24	Xīn Hài	2
7/31	Yǐ Yǒu	8/29	Jiǎ Yín	9/28	Jiǎ Shēn	10/27	Guǐ Chǒu	11/26	Guǐ Wèi	12/25	Rén Zǐ	3
8/1	Bǐng Xū	8/30	Yǐ Mǎo	9/29	Yǐ Yǒu	10/28	Jiǎ Yín	11/27	Jiǎ Shēn	12/26	Guǐ Chǒu	4
8/2	Dīng Hài	8/31	Bǐng Chén	9/30	Bǐng Xū	10/29	Yǐ Mǎo	11/28	Yǐ Yǒu	12/27	Jiǎ Yín	5
8/3	Wù Zǐ	9/1	Dīng Sì	10/1	Dīng Hài	10/30	Bǐng Chén	11/29	Bǐng Xū	12/28	Yǐ Mǎo	6
8/4	Jǐ Chǒu	9/2	Wù Wǔ	10/2	Wù Zǐ	10/31	Dīng Sì	11/30	Dīng Hài	12/29	Bǐng Chén	7
8/5	Gēng Yín	9/3	Jǐ Wèi	10/3	Jǐ Chǒu	11/1	Wù Wǔ	12/1	Wù Zǐ	12/30	Dīng Sì	8
8/6	Xīn Mǎo	9/4	Gēng Shēn	10/4	Gēng Yín	11/2	Jǐ Wèi	12/2	Jǐ Chǒu	12/31	Wù Wǔ	9
8/7	Rén Chén	9/5	Xīn Yǒu	10/5	Xīn Mǎo	11/3	Gēng Shēn	12/3	Gēng Yín	1/1	Jǐ Wèi	10
8/8	Guǐ Sì	9/6	Rén Xū	10/6	Rén Chén	11/4	Xīn Yǒu	12/4	Xīn Mǎo	1/2	Gēng Shēn	11
8/9	Jiǎ Wǔ	9/7	Guǐ Hài	10/7	Guǐ Sì	11/5	Rén Xū	12/5	Rén Chén	1/3	Xīn Yǒu	12
8/10	Yǐ Wèi	9/8	Jiǎ Zǐ	10/8	Jiǎ Wǔ	11/6	Guǐ Hài	12/6	Guǐ Sì	1/4	Rén Xū	13
8/11	Bǐng Shēn	9/9	Yǐ Chǒu	10/9	Yǐ Wèi	11/7	Jiǎ Zǐ	12/7	Jiǎ Wǔ	1/5	Guǐ Hài	14
8/12	Dīng Yǒu	9/10	Bǐng Yín	10/10	Bǐng Shēn	11/8	Yǐ Chǒu	12/8	Yǐ Wèi	1/6	Jiǎ Zǐ	15
8/13	Wù Xū	9/11	Dīng Mǎo	10/11	Dīng Yǒu	11/9	Bǐng Yín	12/9	Bǐng Shēn	1/7	Yǐ Chǒu	16
8/14	Jǐ Hài	9/12	Wù Chén	10/12	Wù Xū	11/10	Dīng Mǎo	12/10	Dīng Yǒu	1/8	Bǐng Yín	17
8/15	Gēng Zǐ	9/13	Jǐ Sì	10/13	Jǐ Hài	11/11	Wù Chén	12/11	Wù Xū	1/9	Dīng Mǎo	18
8/16	Xīn Chǒu	9/14	Gēng Wǔ	10/14	Gēng Zǐ	11/12	Jǐ Sì	12/12	Jǐ Hài	1/10	Wù Chén	19
8/17	Rén Yín	9/15	Xīn Wèi	10/15	Xīn Chǒu	11/13	Gēng Wǔ	12/13	Gēng Zǐ	1/11	Jǐ Sì	20
8/18	Guǐ Mǎo	9/16	Rén Shēn	10/16	Rén Yín	11/14	Xīn Wèi	12/14	Xīn Chǒu	1/12	Gēng Wǔ	21
8/19	Jiǎ Chén	9/17	Guǐ Yǒu	10/17	Guǐ Mǎo	11/15	Rén Shēn	12/15	Rén Yín	1/13	Xīn Wèi	22
8/20	Yǐ Sì	9/18	Jiǎ Xū	10/18	Jiǎ Chén	11/16	Guǐ Yǒu	12/16	Guǐ Mǎo	1/14	Rén Shēn	23
8/21	Bǐng Wǔ	9/19	Yǐ Hài	10/19	Yǐ Sì	11/17	Jiǎ Xū	12/17	Jiǎ Chén	1/15	Guǐ Yǒu	24
8/22	Dīng Wèi	9/20	Bǐng Zǐ	10/20	Bǐng Wǔ	11/18	Yǐ Hài	12/18	Yǐ Sì	1/16	Jiǎ Xū	25
8/23	Wù Shēn	9/21	Dīng Chǒu	10/21	Dīng Wèi	11/19	Bǐng Zǐ	12/19	Bǐng Wǔ	1/17	Yǐ Hài	26
8/24	Jǐ Yǒu	9/22	Wù Yín	10/22	Wù Shēn	11/20	Dīng Chǒu	12/20	Dīng Wèi	1/18	Bǐng Zǐ	27
8/25	Gēng Xū	9/23	Jǐ Mǎo	10/23	Jǐ Yǒu	11/21	Wù Yín	12/21	Wù Shēn	1/19	Dīng Chǒu	28
8/26	Xīn Hài	9/24	Gēng Chén	10/24	Gēng Xū	11/22	Jǐ Mǎo	12/22	Jǐ Yǒu	1/20	Wù Yín	29
		9/25	Xīn Sì			11/23	Gēng Chén			1/21	Jǐ Mǎo	30
Li Qiu		Bai Lu		Han Lu		Li Dong		Da Xue		Xiao Han		Jie
8/7	7:28p	9/8	12:50a	10/8	4:53p	11/7	8:11p	12/7	12:49p	1/5	11:35p	
Chu Shu		Qiu Fen		Shuang Jiang		Xiao Xue		Dong Zhi		Da Han		Qi
8/23	12:20p	9/23	10:27a	10/23	8:04p	11/22	5:35p	12/22	6:33a	1/20	4:43p	

針灸大成・卷之五

	|	YEAR: 2023 Guǐ Mǎo -- First six months.												
	1ST MONTH		2ND MONTH		LEAP YEAR		3RD MONTH		4TH MONTH		5TH MONTH		6TH MONTH	
	Jiǎ Yín		Yǐ Mǎo				Bǐng Chén		Dīng Sì		Wù Wǔ		Jǐ Wèi	
1	1/22	Gēng Chén	2/20	Jǐ Yǒu	3/22	Jǐ Mǎo	4/20	Wù Shēn	5/20	Wù Yín	6/18	Dīng Wèi	7/18	Dīng Chǒu
2	1/23	Xīn Sì	2/21	Gēng Xū	3/23	Gēng Chén	4/21	Jǐ Yǒu	5/21	Jǐ Mǎo	6/19	Wù Shēn	7/19	Wù Yín
3	1/24	Rén Wǔ	2/22	Xīn Hài	3/24	Xīn Sì	4/22	Gēng Xū	5/22	Gēng Chén	6/20	Jǐ Yǒu	7/20	Jǐ Mǎo
4	1/25	Guǐ Wèi	2/23	Rén Zǐ	3/25	Rén Wǔ	4/23	Xīn Hài	5/23	Xīn Sì	6/21	Gēng Xū	7/21	Gēng Chén
5	1/26	Jiǎ Shēn	2/24	Guǐ Chǒu	3/26	Guǐ Wèi	4/24	Rén Zǐ	5/24	Rén Wǔ	6/22	Xīn Hài	7/22	Xīn Sì
6	1/27	Yǐ Yǒu	2/25	Jiǎ Yín	3/27	Jiǎ Shēn	4/25	Guǐ Chǒu	5/25	Guǐ Wèi	6/23	Rén Zǐ	7/23	Rén Wǔ
7	1/28	Bǐng Xū	2/26	Yǐ Mǎo	3/28	Yǐ Yǒu	4/26	Jiǎ Yín	5/26	Jiǎ Shēn	6/24	Guǐ Chǒu	7/24	Guǐ Wèi
8	1/29	Dīng Hài	2/27	Bǐng Chén	3/29	Bǐng Xū	4/27	Yǐ Mǎo	5/27	Yǐ Yǒu	6/25	Jiǎ Yín	7/25	Jiǎ Shēn
9	1/30	Wù Zǐ	2/28	Dīng Sì	3/30	Dīng Hài	4/28	Bǐng Chén	5/28	Bǐng Xū	6/26	Yǐ Mǎo	7/26	Yǐ Yǒu
10	1/31	Jǐ Chǒu	3/1	Wù Wǔ	3/31	Wù Zǐ	4/29	Dīng Sì	5/29	Dīng Hài	6/27	Bǐng Chén	7/27	Bǐng Xū
11	2/1	Gēng Yín	3/2	Jǐ Wèi	4/1	Jǐ Chǒu	4/30	Wù Wǔ	5/30	Wù Zǐ	6/28	Dīng Sì	7/28	Dīng Hài
12	2/2	Xīn Mǎo	3/3	Gēng Shēn	4/2	Gēng Yín	5/1	Jǐ Wèi	5/31	Jǐ Chǒu	6/29	Wù Wǔ	7/29	Wù Zǐ
13	2/3	Rén Chén	3/4	Xīn Yǒu	4/3	Xīn Mǎo	5/2	Gēng Shēn	6/1	Gēng Yín	6/30	Jǐ Wèi	7/30	Jǐ Chǒu
14	2/4	Guǐ Sì	3/5	Rén Xū	4/4	Rén Chén	5/3	Xīn Yǒu	6/2	Xīn Mǎo	7/1	Gēng Shēn	7/31	Gēng Yín
15	2/5	Jiǎ Wǔ	3/6	Guǐ Hài	4/5	Guǐ Sì	5/4	Rén Xū	6/3	Rén Chén	7/2	Xīn Yǒu	8/1	Xīn Mǎo
16	2/6	Yǐ Wèi	3/7	Jiǎ Zǐ	4/6	Jiǎ Wǔ	5/5	Guǐ Hài	6/4	Guǐ Sì	7/3	Rén Xū	8/2	Rén Chén
17	2/7	Bǐng Shēn	3/8	Yǐ Chǒu	4/7	Yǐ Wèi	5/6	Jiǎ Zǐ	6/5	Jiǎ Wǔ	7/4	Guǐ Hài	8/3	Guǐ Sì
18	2/8	Dīng Yǒu	3/9	Bǐng Yín	4/8	Bǐng Shēn	5/7	Yǐ Chǒu	6/6	Yǐ Wèi	7/5	Jiǎ Zǐ	8/4	Jiǎ Wǔ
19	2/9	Wù Xū	3/10	Dīng Mǎo	4/9	Dīng Yǒu	5/8	Bǐng Yín	6/7	Bǐng Shēn	7/6	Yǐ Chǒu	8/5	Yǐ Wèi
20	2/10	Jǐ Hài	3/11	Wù Chén	4/10	Wù Xū	5/9	Dīng Mǎo	6/8	Dīng Yǒu	7/7	Bǐng Yín	8/6	Bǐng Shēn
21	2/11	Gēng Zǐ	3/12	Jǐ Sì	4/11	Jǐ Hài	5/10	Wù Chén	6/9	Wù Xū	7/8	Dīng Mǎo	8/7	Dīng Yǒu
22	2/12	Xīn Chǒu	3/13	Gēng Wǔ	4/12	Gēng Zǐ	5/11	Jǐ Sì	6/10	Jǐ Hài	7/9	Wù Chén	8/8	Wù Xū
23	2/13	Rén Yín	3/14	Xīn Wèi	4/13	Xīn Chǒu	5/12	Gēng Wǔ	6/11	Gēng Zǐ	7/10	Jǐ Sì	8/9	Jǐ Hài
24	2/14	Guǐ Mǎo	3/15	Rén Shēn	4/14	Rén Yín	5/13	Xīn Wèi	6/12	Xīn Chǒu	7/11	Gēng Wǔ	8/10	Gēng Zǐ
25	2/15	Jiǎ Chén	3/16	Guǐ Yǒu	4/15	Guǐ Mǎo	5/14	Rén Shēn	6/13	Rén Yín	7/12	Xīn Wèi	8/11	Xīn Chǒu
26	2/16	Yǐ Sì	3/17	Jiǎ Xū	4/16	Jiǎ Chén	5/15	Guǐ Yǒu	6/14	Guǐ Mǎo	7/13	Rén Shēn	8/12	Rén Yín
27	2/17	Bǐng Wǔ	3/18	Yǐ Hài	4/17	Yǐ Sì	5/16	Jiǎ Xū	6/15	Jiǎ Chén	7/14	Guǐ Yǒu	8/13	Guǐ Mǎo
28	2/18	Dīng Wèi	3/19	Bǐng Zǐ	4/18	Bǐng Wǔ	5/17	Yǐ Hài	6/16	Yǐ Sì	7/15	Jiǎ Xū	8/14	Jiǎ Chén
29	2/19	Wù Shēn	3/20	Dīng Chǒu	4/19	Dīng Wèi	5/18	Bǐng Zǐ	6/17	Bǐng Wǔ	7/16	Yǐ Hài	8/15	Yǐ Sì
30			3/21	Wù Yín			5/19	Dīng Chǒu			7/17	Bǐng Zǐ		
Jie	Li Chun		Jing Zhi				Qing Ming		Li Xia		Mang Zhong		Xiao Shu	
	2/4	10:47a	3/6	4:31a			4/5	9:14a	5/6	2:33a	6/6	6:46a	7/7	6:10p
Qi	Yu Shui		Chun Fen				Gu Yu		Xiao Man		Xia Zhi		Da Shu	
	2/19	6:30a	3/21	5:20a			4/20	4:21p	5/21	3:32p	6/21	11:35p	7/23	10:10a

針灸大成 · 卷之五

YEAR: 2023 Guǐ Mǎo -- Last six months.												
7TH MONTH		8TH MONTH		9TH MONTH		10TH MONTH		11TH MONTH		12TH MONTH		
Gēng Shēn		Xīn Yǒu		Rén Xū		Guǐ Hài		Jiǎ Zǐ		Yǐ Chǒu		
								2023 - 2024				
8/16	Bǐng Wǔ	9/15	Bǐng Zǐ	10/15	Bǐng Wǔ	11/13	Yǐ Hài	12/13	Yǐ Sì	1/11	Jiǎ Xū	1
8/17	Dīng Wèi	9/16	Dīng Chǒu	10/16	Dīng Wèi	11/14	Bǐng Zǐ	12/14	Bǐng Wǔ	1/12	Yǐ Hài	2
8/18	Wù Shēn	9/17	Wù Yín	10/17	Wù Shēn	11/15	Dīng Chǒu	12/15	Dīng Wèi	1/13	Bǐng Zǐ	3
8/19	Jǐ Yǒu	9/18	Jǐ Mǎo	10/18	Jǐ Yǒu	11/16	Wù Yín	12/16	Wù Shēn	1/14	Dīng Chǒu	4
8/20	Gēng Xū	9/19	Gēng Chén	10/19	Gēng Xū	11/17	Jǐ Mǎo	12/17	Jǐ Yǒu	1/15	Wù Yín	5
8/21	Xīn Hài	9/20	Xīn Sì	10/20	Xīn Hài	11/18	Gēng Chén	12/18	Gēng Xū	1/16	Jǐ Mǎo	6
8/22	Rén Zǐ	9/21	Rén Wǔ	10/21	Rén Zǐ	11/19	Xīn Sì	12/19	Rén Zǐ	1/17	Gēng Chén	7
8/23	Guǐ Chǒu	9/22	Guǐ Wèi	10/22	Guǐ Chǒu	11/20	Rén Wǔ	12/20	Rén Zǐ	1/18	Xīn Sì	8
8/24	Jiǎ Yín	9/23	Jiǎ Shēn	10/23	Jiǎ Yín	11/21	Guǐ Wèi	12/21	Guǐ Chǒu	1/19	Rén Wǔ	9
8/25	Yǐ Mǎo	9/24	Yǐ Yǒu	10/24	Yǐ Mǎo	11/22	Jiǎ Shēn	12/22	Jiǎ Yín	1/20	Guǐ Wèi	10
8/26	Bǐng Chén	9/25	Bǐng Xū	10/25	Bǐng Chén	11/23	Yǐ Yǒu	12/23	Yǐ Mǎo	1/21	Jiǎ Shēn	11
8/27	Dīng Sì	9/26	Dīng Hài	10/26	Dīng Sì	11/24	Bǐng Xū	12/24	Bǐng Chén	1/22	Yǐ Yǒu	12
8/28	Wù Wǔ	9/27	Wù Zǐ	10/27	Wù Wǔ	11/25	Dīng Hài	12/25	Dīng Sì	1/23	Bǐng Xū	13
8/29	Jǐ Wèi	9/28	Jǐ Chǒu	10/28	Jǐ Wèi	11/26	Wù Zǐ	12/26	Wù Wǔ	1/24	Dīng Hài	14
8/30	Gēng Shēn	9/29	Gēng Yín	10/29	Gēng Shēn	11/27	Jǐ Chǒu	12/27	Jǐ Wèi	1/25	Wù Zǐ	15
8/31	Xīn Yǒu	9/30	Xīn Mǎo	10/30	Xīn Yǒu	11/28	Gēng Yín	12/28	Gēng Shēn	1/26	Jǐ Chǒu	16
9/1	Rén Xū	10/1	Rén Chén	10/31	Rén Xū	11/29	Xīn Mǎo	12/29	Xīn Yǒu	1/27	Gēng Yín	17
9/2	Guǐ Hài	10/2	Guǐ Sì	11/1	Guǐ Hài	11/30	Rén Chén	12/30	Rén Xū	1/28	Xīn Mǎo	18
9/3	Jiǎ Zǐ	10/3	Jiǎ Wǔ	11/2	Jiǎ Zǐ	12/1	Guǐ Sì	12/31	Guǐ Hài	1/29	Rén Chén	19
9/4	Yǐ Chǒu	10/4	Yǐ Wèi	11/3	Yǐ Chǒu	12/2	Jiǎ Wǔ	1/1	Jiǎ Zǐ	1/30	Guǐ Sì	20
9/5	Bǐng Yín	10/5	Bǐng Shēn	11/4	Bǐng Yín	12/3	Yǐ Wèi	1/2	Yǐ Chǒu	1/31	Jiǎ Wǔ	21
9/6	Dīng Mǎo	10/6	Dīng Yǒu	11/5	Dīng Mǎo	12/4	Bǐng Shēn	1/3	Bǐng Yín	2/1	Yǐ Wèi	22
9/7	Wù Chén	10/7	Wù Xū	11/6	Wù Chén	12/5	Dīng Yǒu	1/4	Dīng Mǎo	2/2	Bǐng Shēn	23
9/8	Jǐ Sì	10/8	Jǐ Hài	11/7	Jǐ Sì	12/6	Wù Xū	1/5	Wù Chén	2/3	Dīng Yǒu	24
9/9	Gēng Wǔ	10/9	Gēng Zǐ	11/8	Gēng Wǔ	12/7	Jǐ Hài	1/6	Jǐ Sì	2/4	Wù Xū	25
9/10	Xīn Wèi	10/10	Xīn Chǒu	11/9	Xīn Wèi	12/8	Gēng Zǐ	1/7	Gēng Wǔ	2/5	Jǐ Hài	26
9/11	Rén Shēn	10/11	Rén Yín	11/10	Rén Shēn	12/9	Xīn Chǒu	1/8	Xīn Wèi	2/6	Gēng Zǐ	27
9/12	Guǐ Yǒu	10/12	Guǐ Mǎo	11/11	Guǐ Yǒu	12/10	Rén Yín	1/9	Rén Shēn	2/7	Xīn Chǒu	28
9/13	Jiǎ Xū	10/13	Jiǎ Chén	11/12	Jiǎ Xū	12/11	Guǐ Mǎo	1/10	Guǐ Yǒu	2/8	Rén Yín	29
9/14	Yǐ Hài	10/14	Yǐ Sì			12/12	Jiǎ Chén			2/9	Guǐ Mǎo	30
Li Qiu		Bai Lu		Han Lu		Li Dong		Da Xue		Xiao Han		Jie
8/8	3:16a	9/8	6:38a	10/8	10:41p	11/8	2:00a	12/7	6:38p	1/6	5:25a	
Chu Shu		Qiu Fen		Shuang Jiang		Xiao Xue		Dong Zhi		Da Han		Qi
8/23	2:23a	9/23	4:15p	10/24	1:53a	11/22	11:24p	12/22	12:23p	1/20	10:33p	

YEAR: 2024 Jiǎ Chén -- First six months.												
	1ST MONTH		2ND MONTH		3RD MONTH		4TH MONTH		5TH MONTH		6TH MONTH	
	Bǐng Yín		Dīng Mǎo		Wù Chén		Jǐ Sì		Gēng Wǔ		Xīn Wèi	
1	2/10	Jiǎ Chén	3/10	Guǐ Yǒu	4/9	Guǐ Mǎo	5/8	Rén Shēn	6/6	Xīn Chǒu	7/6	Xīn Wèi
2	2/11	Yǐ Sì	3/11	Jiǎ Xū	4/10	Jiǎ Chén	5/9	Guǐ Yǒu	6/7	Rén Yín	7/7	Rén Shēn
3	2/12	Bǐng Wǔ	3/12	Yǐ Hài	4/11	Yǐ Sì	5/10	Jiǎ Xū	6/8	Guǐ Mǎo	7/8	Guǐ Yǒu
4	2/13	Dīng Wèi	3/13	Bǐng Zǐ	4/12	Bǐng Wǔ	5/11	Yǐ Hài	6/9	Jiǎ Chén	7/9	Jiǎ Xū
5	2/14	Wù Shēn	3/14	Dīng Chǒu	4/13	Dīng Wèi	5/12	Bǐng Zǐ	6/10	Yǐ Sì	7/10	Yǐ Hài
6	2/15	Jǐ Yǒu	3/15	Wù Yín	4/14	Wù Shēn	5/13	Dīng Chǒu	6/11	Bǐng Wǔ	7/11	Bǐng Zǐ
7	2/16	Gēng Xū	3/16	Jǐ Mǎo	4/15	Jǐ Yǒu	5/14	Wù Yín	6/12	Dīng Wèi	7/12	Dīng Chǒu
8	2/17	Xīn Hài	3/17	Gēng Chén	4/16	Gēng Xū	5/15	Jǐ Mǎo	6/13	Wù Shēn	7/13	Wù Yín
9	2/18	Rén Zǐ	3/18	Xīn Sì	4/17	Xīn Hài	5/16	Gēng Chén	6/14	Jǐ Yǒu	7/14	Jǐ Mǎo
10	2/19	Guǐ Chǒu	3/19	Rén Wǔ	4/18	Rén Zǐ	5/17	Xīn Sì	6/15	Gēng Xū	7/15	Gēng Chén
11	2/20	Jiǎ Yín	3/20	Guǐ Wèi	4/19	Guǐ Chǒu	5/18	Rén Wǔ	6/16	Xīn Hài	7/16	Xīn Sì
12	2/21	Yǐ Mǎo	3/21	Jiǎ Shēn	4/20	Jiǎ Yín	5/19	Guǐ Wèi	6/17	Rén Zǐ	7/17	Rén Wǔ
13	2/22	Bǐng Chén	3/22	Yǐ Yǒu	4/21	Yǐ Mǎo	5/20	Jiǎ Shēn	6/18	Guǐ Chǒu	7/18	Guǐ Wèi
14	2/23	Dīng Sì	3/23	Bǐng Xū	4/22	Bǐng Chén	5/21	Yǐ Yǒu	6/19	Jiǎ Yín	7/19	Jiǎ Shēn
15	2/24	Wù Wǔ	3/24	Dīng Hài	4/23	Dīng Sì	5/22	Bǐng Xū	6/20	Yǐ Mǎo	7/20	Yǐ Yǒu
16	2/25	Jǐ Wèi	3/25	Wù Zǐ	4/24	Wù Wǔ	5/23	Dīng Hài	6/21	Bǐng Chén	7/21	Bǐng Xū
17	2/26	Gēng Shēn	3/26	Jǐ Chǒu	4/25	Jǐ Wèi	5/24	Wù Zǐ	6/22	Dīng Sì	7/22	Dīng Hài
18	2/27	Xīn Yǒu	3/27	Gēng Yín	4/26	Gēng Shēn	5/25	Jǐ Chǒu	6/23	Wù Wǔ	7/23	Wù Zǐ
19	2/28	Rén Xū	3/28	Xīn Mǎo	4/27	Xīn Yǒu	5/26	Gēng Yín	6/24	Jǐ Wèi	7/24	Jǐ Chǒu
20	2/29	Guǐ Hài	3/29	Rén Chén	4/28	Rén Xū	5/27	Xīn Mǎo	6/25	Gēng Shēn	7/25	Gēng Yín
21	3/1	Jiǎ Zǐ	3/30	Guǐ Sì	4/29	Guǐ Hài	5/28	Rén Chén	6/26	Xīn Yǒu	7/26	Xīn Mǎo
22	3/2	Yǐ Chǒu	3/31	Jiǎ Wǔ	4/30	Jiǎ Zǐ	5/29	Guǐ Sì	6/27	Rén Xū	7/27	Rén Chén
23	3/3	Bǐng Yín	4/1	Yǐ Wèi	5/1	Yǐ Chǒu	5/30	Jiǎ Wǔ	6/28	Guǐ Hài	7/28	Guǐ Sì
24	3/4	Dīng Mǎo	4/2	Bǐng Shēn	5/2	Bǐng Yín	5/31	Yǐ Wèi	6/29	Jiǎ Zǐ	7/29	Jiǎ Wǔ
25	3/5	Wù Chén	4/3	Dīng Yǒu	5/3	Dīng Mǎo	6/1	Bǐng Shēn	6/30	Yǐ Chǒu	7/30	Yǐ Wèi
26	3/6	Jǐ Sì	4/4	Wù Xū	5/4	Wù Chén	6/2	Dīng Yǒu	7/1	Bǐng Yín	7/31	Bǐng Shēn
27	3/7	Gēng Wǔ	4/5	Jǐ Hài	5/5	Jǐ Sì	6/3	Wù Xū	7/2	Dīng Mǎo	8/1	Dīng Yǒu
28	3/8	Xīn Wèi	4/6	Gēng Zǐ	5/6	Gēng Wǔ	6/4	Jǐ Hài	7/3	Wù Chén	8/2	Wù Xū
29	3/9	Rén Shēn	4/7	Xīn Chǒu	5/7	Xīn Wèi	6/5	Gēng Zǐ	7/4	Jǐ Sì	8/3	Jǐ Hài
30			4/8	Rén Yín					7/5	Gēng Wǔ		
Jie	Li Chun		Jing Zhi		Qing Ming		Li Xia		Mang Zhong		Xiao Shu	
	2/4	4:37p	3/5	10:21a	4/4	3:03p	5/5	8:22a	6/5	12:34p	7/6	10:58p
Qi	Yu Shui		Chun Fen		Gu Yu		Xiao Man		Xia Zhi		Da Shu	
	2/19	12:20p	3/20	11:10a	4/19	10:10p	5/20	9:20p	6/21	5:22a	7/22	4:29p

針灸大成 · 卷之五

YEAR: 2024 Jiǎ Chén -- Last six months.												
7TH MONTH		8TH MONTH		9TH MONTH		10TH MONTH		11TH MONTH		12TH MONTH		
Rén Shēn		Guǐ Yǒu		Jiǎ Xū		Yǐ Hài		Bǐng Zǐ		Dīng Chǒu		
										2024 - 2025		
8/4	Gēng Zǐ	9/3	Gēng Wǔ	10/3	Gēng Zǐ	11/1	Jǐ Sì	12/1	Jǐ Hài	12/31	Jǐ Sì	1
8/5	Xīn Chǒu	9/4	Xīn Wèi	10/4	Xīn Chǒu	11/2	Gēng Wǔ	12/2	Gēng Zǐ	1/1	Gēng Wǔ	2
8/6	Rén Yín	9/5	Rén Shēn	10/5	Rén Yín	11/3	Xīn Wèi	12/3	Xīn Chǒu	1/2	Xīn Wèi	3
8/7	Guǐ Mǎo	9/6	Guǐ Yǒu	10/6	Guǐ Mǎo	11/4	Rén Shēn	12/4	Rén Yín	1/3	Rén Shēn	4
8/8	Jiǎ Chén	9/7	Jiǎ Xū	10/7	Jiǎ Chén	11/5	Guǐ Yǒu	12/5	Guǐ Mǎo	1/4	Guǐ Yǒu	5
8/9	Yǐ Sì	9/8	Yǐ Hài	10/8	Yǐ Sì	11/6	Jiǎ Xū	12/6	Jiǎ Chén	1/5	Jiǎ Xū	6
8/10	Bǐng Wǔ	9/9	Bǐng Zǐ	10/9	Bǐng Wǔ	11/7	Yǐ Hài	12/7	Yǐ Sì	1/6	Yǐ Hài	7
8/11	Dīng Wèi	9/10	Dīng Chǒu	10/10	Dīng Wèi	11/8	Bǐng Zǐ	12/8	Bǐng Wǔ	1/7	Bǐng Zǐ	8
8/12	Wù Shēn	9/11	Wù Yín	10/11	Wù Shēn	11/9	Dīng Chǒu	12/9	Dīng Wèi	1/8	Dīng Chǒu	9
8/13	Jǐ Yǒu	9/12	Jǐ Mǎo	10/12	Jǐ Yǒu	11/10	Wù Yín	12/10	Wù Shēn	1/9	Wù Yín	10
8/14	Gēng Xū	9/13	Gēng Chén	10/13	Gēng Xū	11/11	Jǐ Mǎo	12/11	Jǐ Yǒu	1/10	Jǐ Mǎo	11
8/15	Xīn Hài	9/14	Xīn Sì	10/14	Xīn Hài	11/12	Gēng Chén	12/12	Gēng Xū	1/11	Gēng Chén	12
8/16	Rén Zǐ	9/15	Rén Wǔ	10/15	Rén Zǐ	11/13	Xīn Sì	12/13	Xīn Hài	1/12	Xīn Sì	13
8/17	Guǐ Chǒu	9/16	Guǐ Wèi	10/16	Guǐ Chǒu	11/14	Rén Wǔ	12/14	Rén Zǐ	1/13	Rén Wǔ	14
8/18	Jiǎ Yín	9/17	Jiǎ Shēn	10/17	Jiǎ Yín	11/15	Guǐ Wèi	12/15	Guǐ Chǒu	1/14	Guǐ Wèi	15
8/19	Yǐ Mǎo	9/18	Yǐ Yǒu	10/18	Yǐ Mǎo	11/16	Jiǎ Shēn	12/16	Jiǎ Yín	1/15	Jiǎ Shēn	16
8/20	Bǐng Chén	9/19	Bǐng Xū	10/19	Bǐng Chén	11/17	Yǐ Yǒu	12/17	Yǐ Mǎo	1/16	Yǐ Yǒu	17
8/21	Dīng Sì	9/20	Dīng Hài	10/20	Dīng Sì	11/18	Bǐng Xū	12/18	Bǐng Chén	1/17	Bǐng Xū	18
8/22	Wù Wǔ	9/21	Wù Zǐ	10/21	Wù Wǔ	11/19	Dīng Hài	12/19	Dīng Sì	1/18	Dīng Hài	19
8/23	Jǐ Wèi	9/22	Jǐ Chǒu	10/22	Jǐ Wèi	11/20	Wù Zǐ	12/20	Wù Wǔ	1/19	Wù Zǐ	20
8/24	Gēng Shēn	9/23	Gēng Yín	10/23	Gēng Shēn	11/21	Jǐ Chǒu	12/21	Jǐ Wèi	1/20	Jǐ Chǒu	21
8/25	Xīn Yǒu	9/24	Xīn Mǎo	10/24	Xīn Yǒu	11/22	Gēng Yín	12/22	Gēng Shēn	1/21	Gēng Yín	22
8/26	Rén Xū	9/25	Rén Chén	10/25	Rén Xū	11/23	Xīn Mǎo	12/23	Xīn Yǒu	1/22	Xīn Mǎo	23
8/27	Guǐ Hài	9/26	Guǐ Sì	10/26	Guǐ Hài	11/24	Rén Chén	12/24	Rén Xū	1/23	Rén Chén	24
8/28	Jiǎ Zǐ	9/27	Jiǎ Wǔ	10/27	Jiǎ Zǐ	11/25	Guǐ Sì	12/25	Guǐ Hài	1/24	Guǐ Sì	25
8/29	Yǐ Chǒu	9/28	Yǐ Wèi	10/28	Yǐ Chǒu	11/26	Jiǎ Wǔ	12/26	Jiǎ Zǐ	1/25	Jiǎ Wǔ	26
8/30	Bǐng Yín	9/29	Bǐng Shēn	10/29	Bǐng Yín	11/27	Yǐ Wèi	12/27	Yǐ Chǒu	1/26	Yǐ Wèi	27
8/31	Dīng Mǎo	9/30	Dīng Yǒu	10/30	Dīng Mǎo	11/28	Bǐng Shēn	12/28	Bǐng Yín	1/27	Bǐng Shēn	28
9/1	Wù Chén	10/1	Wù Xū	10/31	Wù Chén	11/29	Dīng Yǒu	12/29	Dīng Mǎo	1/28	Dīng Yǒu	29
9/2	Jǐ Sì	10/2	Jǐ Hài			11/30	Wù Xū	12/30	Wù Chén			30
Li Qiu		Bai Lu		Han Lu		Li Dong		Da Xue		Xiao Han		Jie
8/7	9:05a	9/7	12:27p	10/8	4:31a	11/7	7:49a	12/7	12:29a	1/5	11:15a	
Chu Shu		Qiu Fen		Shuang Jiang		Xiao Xue		Dong Zhi		Da Han		Qi
8/22	11:57p	9/22	10:04p	10/23	7:43a	11/22	5:14a	12/21	8:13p	1/20	4:23a	

YEAR: 2025 Yǐ Sì -- First six months.													
	1ST MONTH		2ND MONTH		3RD MONTH		4TH MONTH		5TH MONTH		6TH MONTH		LEAP MONTH
	Wù Yín		Jǐ Mǎo		Gēng Chén		Xīn Sì		Rén Wǔ		Guǐ Wèi		
1	1/29	Wù Xū	2/28	Wù Chén	3/29	Dīng Yǒu	4/28	Dīng Mǎo	5/27	Bǐng Shēn	6/25	Yǐ Chǒu	7/25	Yǐ Wèi
2	1/30	Jǐ Hài	3/1	Jǐ Sì	3/30	Wù Xū	4/29	Wù Chén	5/28	Dīng Yǒu	6/26	Bǐng Yín	7/26	Bǐng Shēn
3	1/31	Gēng Zǐ	3/2	Gēng Wǔ	3/31	Jǐ Hài	4/30	Jǐ Sì	5/29	Wù Xū	6/27	Dīng Mǎo	7/27	Dīng Yǒu
4	2/1	Xīn Chǒu	3/3	Xīn Wèi	4/1	Gēng Zǐ	5/1	Gēng Wǔ	5/30	Jǐ Hài	6/28	Wù Chén	7/28	Wù Xū
5	2/2	Rén Yín	3/4	Rén Shēn	4/2	Xīn Chǒu	5/2	Xīn Wèi	5/31	Gēng Zǐ	6/29	Jǐ Sì	7/29	Jǐ Hài
6	2/3	Guǐ Mǎo	3/5	Guǐ Yǒu	4/3	Rén Yín	5/3	Rén Shēn	6/1	Xīn Chǒu	6/30	Gēng Wǔ	7/30	Gēng Zǐ
7	2/4	Jiǎ Chén	3/6	Jiǎ Xū	4/4	Guǐ Mǎo	5/4	Guǐ Yǒu	6/2	Rén Yín	7/1	Xīn Wèi	7/31	Xīn Chǒu
8	2/5	Yǐ Sì	3/7	Yǐ Hài	4/5	Jiǎ Chén	5/5	Jiǎ Xū	6/3	Guǐ Mǎo	7/2	Rén Shēn	8/1	Rén Yín
9	2/6	Bǐng Wǔ	3/8	Bǐng Zǐ	4/6	Yǐ Sì	5/6	Yǐ Hài	6/4	Jiǎ Chén	7/3	Guǐ Yǒu	8/2	Guǐ Mǎo
10	2/7	Dīng Wèi	3/9	Dīng Chǒu	4/7	Bǐng Wǔ	5/7	Bǐng Zǐ	6/5	Yǐ Sì	7/4	Jiǎ Xū	8/3	Jiǎ Chén
11	2/8	Wù Shēn	3/10	Wù Yín	4/8	Dīng Wèi	5/8	Dīng Chǒu	6/6	Bǐng Wǔ	7/5	Yǐ Hài	8/4	Yǐ Sì
12	2/9	Jǐ Yǒu	3/11	Jǐ Mǎo	4/9	Wù Shēn	5/9	Wù Yín	6/7	Dīng Wèi	7/6	Bǐng Zǐ	8/5	Bǐng Wǔ
13	2/10	Gēng Xū	3/12	Gēng Chén	4/10	Jǐ Yǒu	5/10	Jǐ Mǎo	6/8	Wù Shēn	7/7	Dīng Chǒu	8/6	Dīng Wèi
14	2/11	Xīn Hài	3/13	Xīn Sì	4/11	Gēng Xū	5/11	Gēng Chén	6/9	Jǐ Yǒu	7/8	Wù Yín	8/7	Wù Shēn
15	2/12	Rén Zǐ	3/14	Rén Wǔ	4/12	Xīn Hài	5/12	Xīn Sì	6/10	Gēng Xū	7/9	Jǐ Mǎo	8/8	Jǐ Yǒu
16	2/13	Guǐ Chǒu	3/15	Guǐ Wèi	4/13	Rén Zǐ	5/13	Rén Wǔ	6/11	Xīn Hài	7/10	Gēng Chén	8/9	Gēng Xū
17	2/14	Jiǎ Yín	3/16	Jiǎ Shēn	4/14	Guǐ Chǒu	5/14	Guǐ Wèi	6/12	Rén Zǐ	7/11	Xīn Sì	8/10	Xīn Hài
18	2/15	Yǐ Mǎo	3/17	Yǐ Yǒu	4/15	Jiǎ Yín	5/15	Jiǎ Shēn	6/13	Guǐ Chǒu	7/12	Rén Wǔ	8/11	Rén Zǐ
19	2/16	Bǐng Chén	3/18	Bǐng Xū	4/16	Yǐ Mǎo	5/16	Yǐ Yǒu	6/14	Jiǎ Yín	7/13	Guǐ Wèi	8/12	Guǐ Chǒu
20	2/17	Dīng Sì	3/19	Dīng Hài	4/17	Bǐng Chén	5/17	Bǐng Xū	6/15	Yǐ Mǎo	7/14	Jiǎ Shēn	8/13	Jiǎ Yín
21	2/18	Wù Wǔ	3/20	Wù Zǐ	4/18	Dīng Sì	5/18	Dīng Hài	6/16	Bǐng Chén	7/15	Yǐ Yǒu	8/14	Yǐ Mǎo
22	2/19	Jǐ Wèi	3/21	Jǐ Chǒu	4/19	Wù Wǔ	5/19	Wù Zǐ	6/17	Dīng Sì	7/16	Bǐng Xū	8/15	Bǐng Chén
23	2/20	Gēng Shēn	3/22	Gēng Yín	4/20	Jǐ Wèi	5/20	Jǐ Chǒu	6/18	Wù Wǔ	7/17	Dīng Hài	8/16	Dīng Sì
24	2/21	Xīn Yǒu	3/23	Xīn Mǎo	4/21	Gēng Shēn	5/21	Gēng Yín	6/19	Jǐ Wèi	7/18	Wù Zǐ	8/17	Wù Wǔ
25	2/22	Rén Xū	3/24	Rén Chén	4/22	Xīn Yǒu	5/22	Xīn Mǎo	6/20	Gēng Shēn	7/19	Jǐ Chǒu	8/18	Jǐ Wèi
26	2/23	Guǐ Hài	3/25	Guǐ Sì	4/23	Rén Xū	5/23	Rén Chén	6/21	Xīn Yǒu	7/20	Gēng Yín	8/19	Gēng Shēn
27	2/24	Jiǎ Zǐ	3/26	Jiǎ Wǔ	4/24	Guǐ Hài	5/24	Guǐ Sì	6/22	Rén Xū	7/21	Xīn Mǎo	8/20	Xīn Yǒu
28	2/25	Yǐ Chǒu	3/27	Yǐ Wèi	4/25	Jiǎ Zǐ	5/25	Jiǎ Wǔ	6/23	Guǐ Hài	7/22	Rén Chén	8/21	Rén Xū
29	2/26	Bǐng Yín	3/28	Bǐng Shēn	4/26	Yǐ Chǒu	5/26	Yǐ Wèi	6/24	Jiǎ Zǐ	7/23	Guǐ Sì	8/22	Guǐ Hài
30	2/27	Dīng Mǎo			4/27	Bǐng Yín					7/24	Jiǎ Wǔ		
Jie	Li Chun		Jing Zhi		Qing Ming		Li Xia		Mang Zhong		Xiao Shu		
	2/3	10:27p	3/5	4:11p	4/4	8:52p	5/5	2:11p	6/5	6:22p	7/7	4:46a		
Qi	Yu Shui		Chun Fen		Gu Yu		Xiao Man		Xia Zhi		Da Shu		
	2/18	6:10p	3/20	4:59p	4/20	3:57a	5/21	3:09a	6/21	11:11a	7/22	10:17p		

針灸大成 · 卷之五

YEAR: 2025 Yǐ Sì -- Last six months.												
7TH MONTH		8TH MONTH		9TH MONTH		10TH MONTH		11TH MONTH		12TH MONTH		
Jiǎ Shēn		Yǐ Yǒu		Bǐng Xū		Dīng Hài		Wù Zǐ		Jǐ Chǒu		
								2025 - 2026				
8/23	Jiǎ Zǐ	9/22	Jiǎ Wǔ	10/21	Guǐ Hài	11/20	Guǐ Sì	12/20	Guǐ Hài	1/19	Guǐ Sì	1
8/24	Yǐ Chǒu	9/23	Yǐ Wèi	10/22	Jiǎ Zǐ	11/21	Jiǎ Wǔ	12/21	Jiǎ Zǐ	1/20	Jiǎ Wǔ	2
8/25	Bǐng Yín	9/24	Bǐng Shēn	10/23	Yǐ Chǒu	11/22	Yǐ Wèi	12/22	Yǐ Chǒu	1/21	Yǐ Wèi	3
8/26	Dīng Mǎo	9/25	Dīng Yǒu	10/24	Bǐng Yín	11/23	Bǐng Shēn	12/23	Bǐng Yín	1/22	Bǐng Shēn	4
8/27	Wù Chén	9/26	Wù Xū	10/25	Dīng Mǎo	11/24	Dīng Yǒu	12/24	Dīng Mǎo	1/23	Dīng Yǒu	5
8/28	Jǐ Sì	9/27	Jǐ Hài	10/26	Wù Chén	11/25	Wù Xū	12/25	Wù Chén	1/24	Wù Xū	6
8/29	Gēng Wǔ	9/28	Gēng Zǐ	10/27	Jǐ Sì	11/26	Jǐ Hài	12/26	Jǐ Sì	1/25	Jǐ Hài	7
8/30	Xīn Wèi	9/29	Xīn Chǒu	10/28	Gēng Wǔ	11/27	Gēng Zǐ	12/27	Gēng Wǔ	1/26	Gēng Zǐ	8
8/31	Rén Shēn	9/30	Rén Yín	10/29	Xīn Wèi	11/28	Xīn Chǒu	12/28	Xīn Wèi	1/27	Xīn Chǒu	9
9/1	Guǐ Yǒu	10/1	Guǐ Mǎo	10/30	Rén Shēn	11/29	Rén Yín	12/29	Rén Shēn	1/28	Rén Yín	10
9/2	Jiǎ Xū	10/2	Jiǎ Chén	10/31	Guǐ Yǒu	11/30	Guǐ Mǎo	12/30	Guǐ Yǒu	1/29	Guǐ Mǎo	11
9/3	Yǐ Hài	10/3	Yǐ Sì	11/1	Jiǎ Xū	12/1	Jiǎ Chén	12/31	Jiǎ Xū	1/30	Jiǎ Chén	12
9/4	Bǐng Zǐ	10/4	Bǐng Wǔ	11/2	Yǐ Hài	12/2	Yǐ Sì	1/1	Yǐ Hài	1/31	Yǐ Sì	13
9/5	Dīng Chǒu	10/5	Dīng Wèi	11/3	Bǐng Zǐ	12/3	Bǐng Wǔ	1/2	Bǐng Zǐ	2/1	Bǐng Wǔ	14
9/6	Wù Yín	10/6	Wù Shēn	11/4	Dīng Chǒu	12/4	Dīng Wèi	1/3	Dīng Chǒu	2/2	Dīng Wèi	15
9/7	Jǐ Mǎo	10/7	Jǐ Yǒu	11/5	Wù Yín	12/5	Wù Shēn	1/4	Wù Yín	2/3	Wù Shēn	16
9/8	Gēng Chén	10/8	Gēng Xū	11/6	Jǐ Mǎo	12/6	Jǐ Yǒu	1/5	Jǐ Mǎo	2/4	Jǐ Yǒu	17
9/9	Xīn Sì	10/9	Xīn Hài	11/7	Gēng Chén	12/7	Gēng Xū	1/6	Gēng Chén	2/5	Gēng Xū	18
9/10	Rén Wǔ	10/10	Rén Zǐ	11/8	Xīn Sì	12/8	Xīn Hài	1/7	Xīn Sì	2/6	Xīn Hài	19
9/11	Guǐ Wèi	10/11	Guǐ Chǒu	11/9	Rén Wǔ	12/9	Rén Zǐ	1/8	Rén Wǔ	2/7	Rén Zǐ	20
9/12	Jiǎ Shēn	10/12	Jiǎ Yín	11/10	Guǐ Wèi	12/10	Guǐ Chǒu	1/9	Guǐ Wèi	2/8	Guǐ Chǒu	21
9/13	Yǐ Yǒu	10/13	Yǐ Mǎo	11/11	Jiǎ Shēn	12/11	Jiǎ Yín	1/10	Jiǎ Shēn	2/9	Jiǎ Yín	22
9/14	Bǐng Xū	10/14	Bǐng Chén	11/12	Yǐ Yǒu	12/12	Yǐ Mǎo	1/11	Yǐ Yǒu	2/10	Yǐ Mǎo	23
9/15	Dīng Hài	10/15	Dīng Sì	11/13	Bǐng Xū	12/13	Bǐng Chén	1/12	Bǐng Xū	2/11	Bǐng Chén	24
9/16	Wù Zǐ	10/16	Wù Wǔ	11/14	Dīng Hài	12/14	Dīng Sì	1/13	Dīng Hài	2/12	Dīng Sì	25
9/17	Jǐ Chǒu	10/17	Jǐ Wèi	11/15	Wù Zǐ	12/15	Wù Wǔ	1/14	Wù Zǐ	2/13	Wù Wǔ	26
9/18	Gēng Yín	10/18	Gēng Shēn	11/16	Jǐ Chǒu	12/16	Jǐ Wèi	1/15	Jǐ Chǒu	2/14	Jǐ Wèi	27
9/19	Xīn Mǎo	10/19	Xīn Yǒu	11/17	Gēng Yín	12/17	Gēng Shēn	1/16	Gēng Yín	2/15	Gēng Shēn	28
9/20	Rén Chén	10/20	Rén Xū	11/18	Xīn Mǎo	12/18	Xīn Yǒu	1/17	Xīn Mǎo	2/16	Xīn Yǒu	29
9/21	Guǐ Sì			11/19	Rén Chén	12/19	Rén Xū	1/18	Rén Chén			30
Li Qiu		Bai Lu		Han Lu		Li Dong		Da Xue		Xiao Han		Jie
8/7	2:53p	9/7	6:15p	10/8	10:19a	11/7	1:40p	12/7	6:18a	1/5	5:05p	
Chu Shu		Qiu Fen		Shuang Jiang		Xiao Xue		Dong Zhi		Da Han		Qi
8/23	5:45a	9/23	3:53a	10/23	1:32p	11/22	11:04a	12/22	12:03a	1/20	10:13a	

Bibliography

Anonymous. 1997. 《 難經 》 *Classic of Difficulties*. Chongqing: Southwest Teacher Training University Publishing House.

Cheng, B.S. 程寶書. 1995. 《 新編針灸大辭典 》 *Newly re-edited great dictionary of acupuncture-moxibustion*. Beijing: Cathay Publishing House.

Deng, T.T., 1999. *Practical diagnosis in traditional Chinese medicine*. Edinburgh: Churchill Livingstone.

Ellis, A., Wiseman, N., and Boss, K. 1989. *Grasping the wind*. Brookline: Paradigm Press.

Gao, W. 高武. 1999. 《 針灸聚英 》 *Gatherings from eminent acupuncturists*. Beijing: Chinese Medicine Ancient Book Publishing House.

Guo, A.C. 郭靄春. 1999. 《 黃帝內經素問校注語譯 》 *Yellow Emperor's inner classic, elementary questions, revised, annotated, and interpreted*. Tianjin: Tianjin Science and Technology Publishing House.

Guo, A.C. 郭靄春. 1999. 《 黃帝內經靈樞校注語譯 》 *Yellow Emperor's inner classic, magic pivot, revised, annotated, and interpreted*. Tianjin: Tianjin Science and Technology Publishing House.

Huang, L.X. 黃龍祥, ed. 1996. 《 針灸名著集成 》 *Grand compendium of famous works on acupuncture and moxibustion*. Beijing: Cathay Publishing House.

Huangfu, M. 皇甫謐. 1993; *The systematic classic of acupuncture and moxibustion*. Trans. Yang, S.Z. and Chace, C. Boulder, CO: Blue Poppy Press.

———1997. 《 針灸甲乙經 》 The systematic classic of acupuncture and moxibustion. Liaoning: Liaoning Science and Technology Publishing House.

Li, C. 李梴. 1999. 《 醫學入門 》 *Entering the gate of medicine*. Tianjin: Tianjin Science and Technology Publishing House.

Li, J. W. 李經緯. 1995. 《 中醫大辭典 》 *Great dictionary of Chinese medicine*. Beijing: People's Health Publishing House.

Li, S.B. 李順保. 2001. 《 中醫中藥醫古文難字字典 》 *Dictionary of difficult characters from ancient Chinese medicine and Chinese herbal texts*. Beijing: Xueyuan Publishing.

Liu B.Q. 劉炳權 et al. 1995. 《 八卦與時間醫學 》 *Medicine of the eight gua and time*. Guangdong: Guangdong Science and Technology Publishing House.

Mathews, R.H. 1943. *Mathews' Chinese-English dictionary*. Cambridge: Harvard University Press.

O'Connor, J. and Bensky, D. 1981. *Acupuncture: A comprehensive text*. Seattle: Eastland Press.

Sun, J. S. 孫吉山. 1995. 《 時辰開穴全書 》 *Complete book of time and open points*. Shanghai: Shanghai Far East Publishing House.

Sun, S.M. 孫思邈. 1994. 《 千金方 》 *Prescriptions worth a thousand pieces of gold*. Beijing: Cathay Publishing House.

Unschuld, P.U. 1985. 1986. *Nan-ching: The classic of difficult issues.* Berkeley: University of California Press.

———. 2003. *Huang di nei jing su wen: Nature, knowledge, imagery in an ancient Chinese medical text.* Berkeley: University of California Press.

Wang, B. 王冰, ed. 1994. 《黃帝內經素問》 *The Yellow Emperor's inner canon: elementary questions.* Beijing: People's Health Publishing House.

———. 2006. 《王冰醫學全書》 *Wang Bing's complete medical writings.* Beijing: China Press of Traditional Chinese Medicine.

Wiseman, N. 1995. *English-Chinese Chinese-English dictionary of Chinese medicine.* Changsha: Hunan Science and Technology Publishing House.

Wiseman, N. and Ye, F. 1998. *A practical dictionary of Chinese medicine.* Brookline MA: Paradigm Publications.

Wu, J.N., trans., 1993. *Ling shu or the spiritual pivot.* Washington D.C. The Taoist Center.

Wu, L.S. and Wu, A.Q., 1997. *Yellow Emperor's canon of internal medicine.* Beijing: China Science and Technology Press.

Yang, J.Z. 楊繼洲. 1908. 《繪圖針灸大成》 *Illustrated great compendium of acupuncture and moxibustion.* Shanghai: Shanghai Zhang Fu Ji Shi Yin.

———. 1998. 《針灸大成》 *Great compendium of acupuncture and moxibustion.* Beijing: Chinese Medicine Ancient Book Publishing House.

———. 2006. 《針灸大成》 *Great compendium of acupuncture and moxibustion.* Beijing: People's Health Publishing House.

Zhang, F.J. 張芳杰. 1992. *Far East Chinese-English dictionary.* Taibei: The Far East Book Company, LTD.

針灸大成・卷之五

Book Index

Points Index

Alternate point names are in ( )'s

針灸大成・卷之五

245

Indications Index

針灸大成・卷之五

針灸大成・卷之五

針灸大成・卷之五

針灸大成・卷之五

253

The Chinese Medicine Database

www.cm-db.com

The Chinese Medicine Database has been organized around one central principle -- translation of Classical Chinese texts, and dissemination of that information.

There are thousands of Chinese medicine texts that have never been translated. We have compiled a small list on our website of the ones that we have found, but we believe that there are tens of thousands of documents that span from the Hàn dynasty to pre-Republican times. Most of these documents will never be read by people in the West, simply because of lack of translation.

We have created a vehicle, that allows interested practitioners, students, institutions, and scholars to help support and fund the translation of these documents, and then mine and synthesize the data that is gained from these texts.

The Database contains:

Monographs on:
673 Single Herbs
1485 Formulas
Mayway's Patents
ITM's Formulations
Golden Flowers Formulations
Health Concerns Formulations
Blue Poppy's Patents
Classical Pearls Formulations by Heiner Fruehauf
OBGYN Modifications to Formulas
Single Points: the 361 Regular Points

Beer Hall Lecture Series
Watch videos from our monthly Beer Hall lecture series with guest speakers such as: Arnaud Versluys, Subhuti Dharmananda, Jason Robertson, Craig Mitchell, Michael Max, Lorraine Wilcox, and Ed Neal.

Play STORT
Play our free online game STORT where you can learn Chinese while having a bit of fun (www.cm-db.com/stort).

15,000 Western Diagnoses with ICD-9 Codes

A Chinese-English dictionary:
Containing over 100,000 terms, including the Eastland and the WHO term sets.

A Western Book search containing:
Fenner's Complete Formulary
    by B. Fenner
The 1918 Dispensatory of the United States of America
    Edited by Joseph P. Remington, Horatio C. Woods and others

The Eclectic Materia Medica, Pharmacology and Therapeutics
    by Harvey Wickes Felter, M.D.

A Personal Dashboard, which allows users to:
Blog
Take notes on any monograph.
Search for other users by city, state, country and name.
Make friends all around the world.
Share and compare notes with friends.
Personalize your dashboard by adding photos, and information about your practice.

Translations:

Shāng Hán Lái Sū Jí	傷寒來蘇集	Renewal of Treatise on Cold Damage
Qí Jīng Bā Mài Kǎo	奇經八脈考	Explanation of the Eight Vessels of the Marvellous Meridians
Shāng Hán Míng Lǐ Lùn	傷寒明理論	Treatise on Enlightening the Principles of Cold Damage
Wú Jū Tōng Yī Àn	吳鞠通医案	Case Studies of Wú Jūtōng
The Nàn Jīng	難經	The Classic of Difficulties
The Zàng Fǔ Biāo Běn Hán Rè Xū Shí Yòng Yào Shì	臟腑標本寒熱 虛實用藥式	Viscera and Bowels, Tip and Root, Cold and Heat, Vacuity and Repletion Model for Using Medicinals
Bèi Jí Qiān Jīn Yào Fāng	備急千金要方	Essential Prescriptions Worth a Thousand Gold Pieces For Emergencies. vol. 2-4
Wēn Rè Lún	温熱論	Treatise on Warm Heat Disease
Shāng Hán Shé Jiàn	傷寒舌鑒	Tongue Mirror of Cold Damage
Xǔ Shì Yī Àn	許氏醫案	Case Histories of Master Xǔ
Fǔ Xíng Jué Zāng Fǔ Yòng Yào Fǎ Yào	輔行決臟腑用 藥法要	Secret Instructions for Assisting the Body: Essential Methods for the Application of Drugs to the Viscera & Bowels
Biāo Yōu Fù	標幽賦	Indicating the Obscure
Liú Juān Zǐ Guǐ Yí Fāng	劉涓子鬼遺方	Liu Juanzi's Formulas Inherited from Ghosts
Shèn Jí Chú Yán	慎疾芻言	Precautions in Illness: My Humble Thoughts
Yào Zhèng Jì Yí	藥症忌宜	Medicinals & Patterns Contraindications & Appropriate [Choices]
Fù Kē Wèn Dá	婦科問答	Questions and Answers in Gynecology

Benefits:
Subscribers to the Database receive a 10% discount on our published books when they are in pre-release.

We translate texts as often, and in quantities that reflect our user base. The larger amount of subscribers that we have, the more translation that we can accomplish.

Published Books:

2008 Bèi Jí Qiān Jīn Yào Fāng 備急千金要方: Essential Prescriptions Worth a Thousand Gold Pieces For Emergencies. vol. 2-4 by Sūn Sīmiǎo 孫思邈
    Translated by Sabine Wilms.
    ISBN 978-0-9799552-0-4

2010 Zhēn Jiǔ Dà Chéng 針灸大成: The Great Compendium of Acupuncture & Moxabustion vol. I by
       Yáng Jìzhōu 楊繼洲
       Translated by Sabine Wilms.
       ISBN 978-0-9799552-2-8

2010 Jīn Guì Fāng Gē Kuò 金匱方歌括: Formulas from the Golden Cabinet with Songs vol. I - III by
       Chén Xiūyuán 陳修園
       Translated by Sabine Wilms.
       ISBN 978-0-9799552-5-9

2011 Zhēn Jiǔ Dà Chéng 針灸大成: The Great Compendium of Acupuncture & Moxabustion vol. IX by
       Yáng Jìzhōu 楊繼洲
       Translated by Lorraine Wilcox.
       ISBN 978-0-9799552-6-6

Forthcoming in 2011

2011 Zhēn Jiǔ Dà Chéng 針灸大成: The Great Compendium of Acupuncture & Moxabustion vol. VIII by
       Yáng Jìzhōu 楊繼洲
       Translated by Yue Lu.
       ISBN 978-0-9799552-7-3

2011 Zhēn Jiǔ Dà Chéng 針灸大成: The Great Compendium of Acupuncture & Moxabustion vol. II by
       Yáng Jìzhōu 楊繼洲
       Translated by Steve Jackowicz L.Ac.
       ISBN 978-0-9799552-8-0

2011 Bèi Jí Qiān Jīn Yào Fāng 備急千金要方: Essential Prescriptions Worth a Thousand Gold Pieces For
       Emergencies. vol. 5 by Sūn Sīmiǎo 孫思邈
       Translated by Sabine Wilms.

2011 Jīn Guì Fāng Gē Kuò 金匱方歌括: Formulas from the Golden Cabinet with Songs vol. IV - VI by
       Chén Xiūyuán 陳修園
       Translated by Sabine Wilms.

www.ingramcontent.com/pod-product-compliance
Lightning Source LLC
Chambersburg PA
CBHW061359210326
41598CB00035B/6036